Qin Bo-Wei's
56 Treatment Methods:
Writing Precise Prescriptions

QIN BO-WEI'S
56 TREATMENT METHODS

Writing Precise Prescriptions

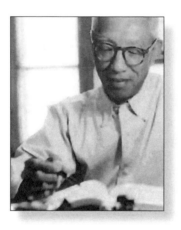

CLINICAL COMMENTARY BY
Wu Bo-Ping

TRANSLATED AND EDITED BY
Jason Blalack

EASTLAND PRESS ▶ SEATTLE

Published by Eastland Press, Inc.
P.O. Box 99749
Seattle, WA 98139, USA
www.eastlandpress.com

Library of Congress Control Number: 2011933929
ISBN: 978-0-939616-74-9

2 4 6 8 10 9 7 5 3 1

Indexes prepared by Sybil Ihrig
Cover photo of Qin Bo-Wei (c. 1960), hand-colored by Clare O'Connor
Cover design by Gary Niemeier and Patricia O'Connor
Book design by Gary Niemeier

Table of Contents

Foreword

WHEN I FIRST BEGAN practicing Chinese medicine in 1984, I had a lot of time on my hands. I'd show up at the clinic every day and have ample time to study while waiting for the phone to ring. It was during this time that I first became acquainted with the writings of Qin Bo-Wei. A few years previously, my friend Bob Flaws had picked up an anthology of Qin's writings on the recommendation of a particularly enthusiastic bookstore clerk in Beijing. Bob was a little vague on who Qin Bo-Wei really was but he assured me that everyone he had talked to in China agreed that Qin was an important figure in Chinese medicine. Bob was kind enough to loan me the book and I quickly became fascinated with Qin's approach to medicine. It took a number of years and a great deal of pleading before Bob finally got his book back.

As a fledgling clinician, I loved how Qin Bo-Wei clarified so many of the points that my education had thus far left unresolved. His essay on Liver disharmonies not only shaped my approach to Liver problems, but showed me how to think about all *zang fu* patterns. Another essay on herbal prescribing taught me to think more clearly about combining herbs. Yet another introduced me to the wonders of the case history literature. Although Qin's writings were liberally seeded with clinical pearls, the most significant thing that I learned from him was an overall mode of thinking. He exemplified a synthesis of rigor and flexibility that remains an inspiration to this day. I eventually translated a number of my favorite Qin Bo-Wei essays and cases. This collection became *A Qin Bowei Anthology*, the first real introduction to Qin Bo-Wei in a Western language.

Today, one can find many of Qin's works on the internet but access to Qin's writings in the late 1980s was quite limited, even in China. With only a single volume of Qin's work to draw from, I had to content myself with translating those essays that had been the most influential for me. Yet there was clearly so much more of Qin's thought to present, particularly the core tenets of his approach. But without access to more of his writings, and someone who was intimately familiar with them to elucidate them for me, I was clearly out of my depth. Other interests took me in different directions, but in my own way, I continued to try to think like Qin.

Almost twenty years later, upon returning from a trip to China to study with his teacher Wu Bo-Ping, my friend Jason Blalack mentioned that he had begun translating one of Qin's seminal texts, and that professor Wu was providing commentary. I remember grinning with a sense of things having somehow come full circle. Another generation was revealing a deeper layer of Qin's thought.

This book is a major step in the dissemination of Qin Bo-Wei's ideas. Perhaps more importantly, it represents a highly refined vision of how Chinese medicine can be understood in the West. Here we are presented with much more than a list of signs and symptoms linked to a pattern, which in turn is linked to a fixed formula. Instead, this book illustrates the nuances inherent in every step of the diagnostic and treatment process.

Many of the principles of practice that were most important to Dr. Qin were ignored in the schools that he was so instrumental in establishing. Yet these ideas survive in both his writings and in his own students. Qin Bo-Wei doesn't tell us what to do so much as he teaches us how to think. Ironically, that mode of thinking is almost antithetical to how many Westerners perceive TCM. In this, Qin Bo-Wei exemplifies Chinese medical thinking outside of the ossifying tendencies of institutionalization. He was also part of a very specific lineage of Chinese medical teaching.

The notion of oral traditions in Chinese medicine has recently been the topic of a great deal of discussion. Proponents of oral traditions often claim that they teach a more fluid and authentic way of thinking about Chinese medicine than the rigid methodologies characteristic of TCM. It is worth noting that Qin Bo-Wei was himself deeply embedded in a well-established tradition of oral transmission. His understanding of the medicine was fundamentally shaped by his teacher, Ding Gan-Ren, and that ever -evolving mode of thinking was passed on to Qin's students, most notably Wu Bo-Ping. Yet, at every step of the way, those oral teachings were necessarily grounded in a degree of familiarity with the Chinese medical literature that most Western practitioners can only vaguely comprehend. The memorization of dozens of medical texts was taken for granted. The fruit of this synthesis of literature and language has been an approach to practice that yields a profound capacity for fluidity and creativity and yet is balanced with a demand for rigor and critical thinking.

In this volume, Qin's straightforward prose is illuminated by Wu Bo-Ping's incisive commentary and his own clinical insights. No one is more qualified for this task than Doctor Wu, a modern master who has spent a lifetime making Qin's ideas his own. Yet this book is best understood as a three-way conversation between Qin Bo-Wei, Wu Bo-Ping, and Jason Blalack. Jason's contribution to this lineage extends well beyond his capacity to accurately record the words and writings of his mentors. The depth of Jason's own understanding of this material is evident in the way that it is organized and presented. He has asked the questions of the material that practitioners trained in the West must ask if we are to make use of it in our own cultural context. In this he represents a crucial bridge between indigenous Chinese medicine and its clinical practice in the West.

This volume, which presents some of Qin Bo-Wei's core ideas, has revitalized my own attempts to think like Qin and has shaped my practice in some remarkable ways. I'm a little less likely to indulge in sloppy thinking. My prescriptions are smaller and more tightly organized. My clinical outcomes are a bit better. And my love and respect for the medicine is that much deeper.

—— CHARLES CHACE
Capitol Peak, Colorado
September, 2010

Preface

BEFORE THE PRESENTATION OF Qin Bo-Wei's original text, I would like to make some important points.

New Guidelines for Treatment (治疗新律 *zhì liáo xīn lǜ*) is my teacher Qin Bo-Wei's summary of the fundamental rules of treatment based on the 113 methods that he was taught by his own teacher, the well-respected and influential early 20th century physician, Ding Gan-Ren (丁甘仁). It also incorporates ideas from the *Inner Classic's* section on the 19 pathomechanisms as well as the thought of Cheng Zhong-Ling (程钟龄)[1] and Mo Mei-Shi's (莫枚士)[2] on treatment principles and etiology. From these sources, Qin derived 13 categories and 56 fundamental treatment strategies, based on the core concepts of Chinese medicine, that form the interrelationship between pattern differentiation and treatment.

Practitioners and students of Chinese medicine have found this work to be of great value owing to its clear arrangement, easy-to-follow outline, and orientation toward clinical practice. Because few copies of *New Guidelines for Treatment* were printed when it was first published in 1953, there was a frenzy to make private copies. As these went through many different hands, errors were inevitably introduced.

In 1959, in an effort to make the correct version available to the public, Dr. Qin published a three-part series in the *Periodical of the Beijing College of Chinese Medicine* (October 1959, January 1960, and March 1960). The series was entitled, "An Outline for Pattern Identification in Chinese Medicine as the Basis for Determining Treatment." At that time, distribution of the periodical was essentially restricted to people within the college. But because there was a large public demand for the material, it was republished in 1961 in the *Journal of Chinese Medicine* (volumes 1–3).

Due to the passage of time over the next 20 years, and the upheavals of the Cultural Revolution, Dr. Qin's original text became very difficult to find. In 1988, my friends Wu Da-Zhen (吴大真), Wang Feng-Qi (王凤歧) and I collected Dr. Qin's original works, added our own comments where appropriate, and published them in a two-part series entitled "Chinese Medicine Treatment Guidelines" in the *Journal of Chinese Traditional Medicine and Pharmacy*. In 2007, Wu Da-Zhen and Wang Feng-Qi changed the title of this work

---

1. Cheng Zhong-Ling (1662-1735), also known as Cheng Guo-Peng, was an influential Qing dynasty physician who remains well known today. His books are easy to understand, clear, and very practical. One of his most famous works is *Awakening of the Mind in Medical Studies (Yī xué xīn wù)* (1732).

2. Mo Mei-Shi (1862-1933) was a late Qing dynasty and Republican era doctor who was famous for his commentary on the Chinese medicine classics and his writings on Chinese medical terminology. He wrote *Classic Formulas Explained (Jīng fāng lì shì)*, *Critical Annotations of Divine Husbandman's Classic of the Materia Medica (Shén Nóng běn cǎo jīng jiào zhù)*, and *A Study of the Language of the Classics (Yán jīng yán)*.

to "Treatment Guidelines" and included it in the book, *A Comprehensive Volume of Qin Bo-Wei's Famous Medical Works.*

The title of this book has been changed many times, and the material has gone through many revisions and expansions. Consequently, deviations from the original text were unavoidable. In an effort to retain the original essence of Dr. Qin's publication, the version that has been used for the present volume is taken directly from Qin's original work, published in 1953. This is the earliest known version. And to prevent further changes, his original words are presented here in shaded text.

Striving to make *New Guidelines for Treatment* even more suitable for the beginner's clinical use, Dr. Qin met with me outside of class over a two-month period in 1962, right before I graduated, and explained the text's meaning to me. He specifically explained how he had come to select the basic seven medicinals for each method along with the modifications. This information is of great benefit in understanding and applying the information in *New Guidelines for Treatment.*

—— Dr. Wu Bo-Ping
Translated by Jason Blalack

Acknowledgments

THIS BOOK WOULD NOT have been possible without the support of my loving family: Kate, Evan, Milton, Marcia, Shannon, and Bing. My wife Kate was not only exceptionally patient listening to almost daily rants as I tried to work out difficult issues in the book, but her reading and feedback from beginning to end was invaluable.

I would also like to acknowledge the people who directly contributed to making this project possible as well as improving it far beyond what I could have done alone: Jennifer Alberti, Sarito Carroll, Charles Chace (Chu Xing-Yan), Andy Ellis, Greg Livingston, Tina Morani, Volker Scheid, Tim Sharpe, Morgan Stanfield, Darren Stone (Wang Hui-Yu), Warren Sheir, and Kacey Wardle.

Finally, extra special thanks to Eastland Press's exceptional staff for their incredible attention to detail and their ability to turn my rough manuscript into a hopefully worthwhile text for the Chinese medicine community. Dan Bensky, the medical editor, with his unparalleled knowledge and expertise, was instrumental in helping me portray Dr. Qin's original thoughts correctly and forcing me to clarify and correct many unclear statements. Although he made more corrections than I would like to admit, any errors at this point are my own. The general editor, John O'Connor, and book designer, Gary Niemeier, did an exceptional job turning my string of words into this book. They had an unusually hard job trying to find a layout that stayed true to the original text, while at the same time making it accessible to the Western reader.

Introduction

IN THE SPRING OF 2007 I asked my teacher, Dr. Wu Bo-Ping (吴伯平), what he thought was the most important text to translate into English. After a few moments of thought, he reached behind some books on his shelf and pulled out a tattered paperback wrapped in a frayed cloth. It was the original version of Qin Bo-Wei's *New Guidelines for Treatment* (治疗新律 *zhì liáo xīn lǜ*, c. 1953), a book that for all intents and purposes had been lost during the Cultural Revolution.

Dr. Wu, who had been one of Dr. Qin's most prominent students, believed that this book was one of his masterpieces. As I read through the manuscript it became apparent that nothing like it existed in the English language and I began to appreciate why Dr. Wu was so enthusiastic about resurrecting it.

The book is a clinical guide, organized by 56 core treatment methods,[1] which brings together and synthesizes the most important ideas from the history of Chinese medicine. For each treatment method, Qin presents key diagnostic criteria and an exemplary seven-ingredient formula. Dr. Wu said that if you can understand these methods, you can treat the vast majority of conditions that we see in the contemporary clinic. It really is an extraordinary treasure house of knowledge.

Dr. Qin was a very clear thinker who paid exceptional attention to detail. The core formulas that he developed are extremely precise. Not only did he take great care in picking the ingredients based on how they interacted with each other, he also paid special attention to how they were prepared (*páo zhì*). One of his purposes in writing this book was to demonstrate that attention to such detail significantly improves clinical results.

Chinese medicine texts tend to be very terse, often requiring further explanation. This book was no exception. Dr. Qin spent a great deal of time explaining the intricacies of this book to Dr. Wu, adding commentary to flesh out the deeper meaning within the original text. Dr. Wu, in turn, taught this text to me over the past few years, adding further commentary based on nearly a half century of clinical experience utilizing Qin's ideas. Dr. Wu was very patient in answering a seemingly endless stream of questions that arose from my efforts to present this material in a clear, accurate, and easy-to-use manner.

Dr. Wu's extensive commentary transformed Qin's presentation of core principles into a detailed description of how to skillfully practice herbal medicine. As such, this is more than a mere translation of an important historical text; it is a hands-on manual filled with

---

1. *Translation note:* While proper terminology is an important issue in Chinese medicine, for the purposes of this book we use the term "principle" somewhat interchangeably with "method". Thus the 56 core methods are often understood as treatment principles, and consequently both terms are used.

clinical pearls that over time foster progressively deeper levels of understanding. Thus, the potential for this book goes far beyond its role as a handy reference for effective formulas and modifications.

Ultimately, this book teaches a method of thinking that enables one to accurately diagnose and write precise prescriptions for the individual rather than for the disease, which is one of the great strengths of Chinese medicine. It trains the practitioner to think clearly, logically, and flexibly. Thus, not only does it serve as an invaluable tool for experienced herbalists, it is an excellent bridge for those who wish to make the jump from prescribing prepared formulas, or who find themselves reflexively prescribing X formula for Y disease (or Z pattern), to becoming more skilled Chinese herbalists who write custom formulas. Finally, because in the end this book is teaching a method of thinking, it can serve as the foundation for a lifelong approach to herbal medicine based on precision.

There are a few aspects of this book that really make it unique, and deserve further discussion.

1. Treatment methods as a foundation for prescribing

The organization of this book differs from most, if not all, Western style clinical manuals. Instead of being organized by disease or chief complaint, such as headache or menstrual pain, it is arranged by pathology/pathogen and treatment methods. Each chapter corresponds to a pathogen (e.g., phlegm) or pathology (e.g., deficiency) and contains sections comprised of treatment methods for eliminating that problem.

Qin extracted these treatment methods from classical formulas and ideas. They are templates, which allow the physician a way to emulate the thinking behind a prescription without being tied down to the exact ingredients or original indications. They provide an important link between the diagnosis and the individual herbs that make up the formula. Thus they give one the capability to think flexibly and modify classic ideas (formulas) for the modern patient. Utilizing treatment methods in this way provides a unique opportunity to engage the medicine on a deeper level and emulate the thinking of many great Chinese physicians.

In the end, understanding how to use treatment methods opens up treatment possibilities that are often ignored in typical Chinese medical textbooks. They provide the foundation to address presentations that are unusual, lie in between two patterns, or encompass multiple patterns. This approach crystallizes the essence of Chinese herbal medicine.

2. Concise, gentle, and precise formulas based on a clear diagnosis

Qin Bo-Wei was part of the *Menghe* current (1626 and onward) and was heavily influenced by many of its famous physicians, like his teacher Ding Gan-Ren (丁甘仁), as well as clinicians such as Ye Tian-Shi (叶天士). These physicians favored prescriptions with a small number of ingredients, smaller dosages, and generally mild medicinals. Consequently, the formulas Qin constructed in this book are gentle, clear, and concise and are especially appropriate for modern patients. Each of Qin's seven ingredient formulas is based on one or more pre-modern formulas, some of which were quite large. Dr. Qin extracted the essential medicinals, creating formulas that elegantly accomplish a given treatment method. These well-considered formulas can be used either in their entirety or as building blocks.

The commentary allows the reader to understand how the formulas were constructed and to further grasp how the medicinals interact. This methodology keeps us focused on evaluating every medicinal and selecting only those that are essential for a particular problem.

The successful use of these methods rests on an accurate diagnosis. Dr. Qin provides key diagnostic criteria for each pathology. For example, he presents fine distinctions between locations of pathology, such as dampness in the upper burner, middle burner, lower burner, channels and collaterals, muscles, joints of the limbs, passages and pathways, skin, qi and blood, Lungs, Spleen, Liver, Kidneys, yang organs, and yin organs. Dr. Wu adds further commentary, rounding out the clinical picture, and presents treatment strategies based on his own clinical practice.

When one can diagnose with precision, precise prescriptions will follow.
Only when one has clarity and focus can the essential problem
be understood, and treated accordingly.

---

3. Herbal differentiation and herbal processing (炮制 *páo zhì*)

Learning how to prescribe with precision requires the ability to make distinctions among medicinals. This enables one to pick one medicinal instead of two or three, thus keeping one's prescriptions small. This book contains extensive discussions on differentiating among similar herbs, especially in relation to herbal processing methods that alter their properties. One will notice that Drs. Qin and Wu are very particular about the type of processing they use in each situation. For example, they might use steamed Rhei Radix et Rhizoma *(shú dà huáng)* instead of Rhei Radix et Rhizoma *(dà huáng)* or dry-fried Atractylodis macrocephalae Rhizoma *(chǎo bái zhú)* instead of unprepared Atractylodis macrocephalae Rhizoma *(bái zhú)*, which can have a profound clinical impact.

It should be noted that many medicinals that we commonly get from our distributors in the United States have already been processed but are not labeled as such. Some may be obvious, for example, *he shou wu* will most likely be Polygoni multiflori Radix preparata *(zhì hé shǒu wū)* and not the unprepared product. When one orders *bai bian dou*, it is often already dry-fried, making it dry-fried Lablab Semen album *(chǎo biǎn dòu)*. However, some preparations are less obvious and can lead to confusion. For example, *xiang fu* will almost always be processed Cyperi Rhizoma *(zhì xiāng fù)*, but processing methods may vary between distributors: it may be roasted, dry-fried with sand, or boiled together with yellow rice wine and rice vinegar, then dried in the sun.

Since clinical results may be affected by the type of processing the medicinal has undergone, it is important to ask your distributor exactly how the medicinals have been processed; the labeling is not always transparent. Appendix II of this book lists the most common processing methods in the United States for some key herbs found in this text.

4. A synthesis, not a compilation

One of the most important and unique characteristics of this material is that it represents a synthesis of the core ideas found throughout Chinese medical history. This vast body of material is filtered through Dr. Qin's personal experience and interpretation to produce a remarkably coherent system for the practice of Chinese medicine.

The formulas presented here took Qin over 20 years to develop. Although all of the formulas have their roots in a broad base of classical and pre-modern knowledge, they have been modified to incorporate further developments in theory as well as Dr. Qin's own clinical experience. For example, for the method *harmonize the nutritive and protective,* instead of just presenting Cinnamon Twig Decoction *(guì zhī tāng)* in its original form, he gives an updated version incorporating ideas that came after its original inception, thus making it more flexible and useful in the clinic.

One of the most intriguing aspects of this book is that the alterations and developments were all filtered through the mind of one person. This is in contrast to collections of formulas from multiple authors. Although such encyclopedic compilations can be useful, the wide variations in opinion and theoretical ideas throughout history make it difficult to develop a cohesive method of thinking.

For example, practitioners accessing typical Chinese medical textbooks may find five different formulas for an external contraction of wind-cold. The differences among these formulas may not be readily apparent to even seasoned readers. Doctors from different time periods invariably reflect different ideas concerning both pathology and the functions of individual medicinals. Their rationales for designing their respective formulas will quite naturally differ from one another in significant ways. Consequently, practitioners may find themselves unable to effectively differentiate among them, much less modify them, in clinical practice.

Dr. Qin sorted through the many schools of thought in Chinese medicine and developed a unified system that resolves many of its discrepancies. His formulas are thus rooted in tradition yet filtered through the prisms of his own lineage and experience and his wide reading of classical texts. For example, a formula might incorporate a warm disease concept into a cold damage formula. The original formulas are sourced in our text, enabling one to trace back the thought process, should one desire.

In my experience, following a single author's train of thought is invaluable. For example, following how Dr. Qin repeatedly uses a single herb or combination of herbs, how he formulates prescriptions (the number of medicinals and dosages), how he uses a particular method of processing to fine tune his formulas, and how he diagnoses—all open a window into his thinking process. This allows us to gain much more than merely finding a "suitable" formula.

Furthermore, observing this continuity—sticking to one train of thought—not only brings us back to the lineage-style roots of Chinese medicine, but is priceless in our ever-expanding world of information overload. Having hundreds if not thousands of disconnected, essentially random formulas at our fingertips sometimes only obscures our path. The system presented in this book roots practitioners in a remarkably flexible methodology that helps us realize the full potential of Chinese medicine.

Who Was Qin Bo-Wei (秦伯未)?

Qin Bo-Wei (1901-1970) is regarded as one of the most important physicians, educators, writers, and synthesizers of Chinese medicine of the 20th century. He began studying medicine with his father at a very early age. His grandfather, father, uncle, and wife were accomplished Chinese physicians.

Qin was born in Shanghai and attended Ding Gan-Ren's Shanghai Technical College of Chinese Medicine from 1919-1923. Graduating at the top of his class, Qin quickly became regarded as one of the "Ding Three," his most accomplished students. In addition, he was also a student of the renowned expert in classical formulas (*jīng fāng*), Cao Ying-Fu (曹颖甫). Qin became known as an expert in gynecology and the *Inner Classic (Neijing)*. Because of his devotion to this classic work and his ability to recite the text, he was nicknamed "Qin Neijing."

After graduation he founded the New Chinese Medicine Society and was chief editor of its journal, *The World of Chinese Medicine.* Throughout his life he founded, administered, and taught at numerous Chinese medical institutions including the Shanghai College of Traditional Chinese Medicine and the China Medicine College. It is estimated that he taught over 5,000 students and that his original material was so popular that his students later compiled it into numerous textbooks. He held many positions in hospitals, colleges and universities, publishing houses, and even government. In the 1950s, he was invited to serve as the TCM advisor to the Ministry of Health in Beijing. Dr. Qin was particularly renowned for his clinical skills and his ability to treat very complicated cases such as leukemia, hemophilia, and myasthenia gravis. He treated many high-level officials, even in foreign countries such as the Soviet Union and Mongolia.

Qin wrote over 50 books and innumerable articles. His first book, *Essential Case Records by Famous Qing Dynasty Physicians,* was written in 1928 and is still highly regarded. He was especially known for his ability to take complex ideas and contradictions in classical texts and present them in a clear, concise, and systematic format. One of his fundamental endeavors was collecting the doctrines of different physicians and creating principles that could be applied practically in the clinic. In this, he was a great integrator of ideas.

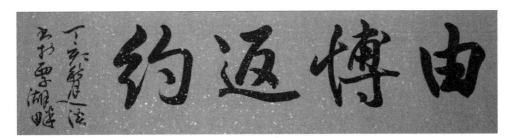

This is a classic Chinese idiom (four-character phrase) of which Qin Bo-Wei was especially fond: *yóu bó fǎn yuē.* Dr. Qin gave this phrase to my teacher, Wu Bo-Ping, as a sort of mantra, and Dr. Wu in turn gave it to me. A literal translation is, "From the plentiful, return to the simple." This can be further elaborated and understood as, "[The scholar] starts with extensive amounts of knowledge, but ultimately strives for a profound, yet concise, understanding." It now hangs above my desk in my home office.

Qin had no attachment to any single methodology or school of thought but merely sought out the most effective and practical methods. Although he had a very strong foundation in the Chinese medical classics, and thought that Chinese medicine should be firmly based in ancient wisdom, he warned against paying excessive attention to the exact wording of those texts.

Qin believed that Chinese medicine had its own distinctly scientific spirit. Although he was an advocate of the integration of Chinese and Western medicine, he believed that the Chinese medical model should be the primary context for such a synthesis. Consequently, when the Ministry of Health, under directives from Mao Ze-Dong (毛泽东), wanted to integrate Chinese medicine into a modern medical system guided by Western medicine, Qin and four other prominent physicians spoke out and directly confronted the government on this issue. They argued for an emphasis on the study of the Chinese medicine classical texts and the use of more traditional methods of learning. These efforts ultimately failed and consequently the TCM we now study lacks much of the foundation that Qin thought was so important. Such views cost Qin dearly during the Cultural Revolution. Prevented from practicing medicine, he was ridiculed and forced to clean toilets. This emotional blow likely contributed to his early death in 1970.

Qin's dedication and work in systematizing and synthesizing the most important ideas throughout the history of Chinese medicine nevertheless forms a cornerstone of what we recognize as traditional Chinese medicine (TCM) today. However, many of Qin's most important ideas did not make it into TCM textbooks. For example, his magnum opus, *Medical Lecture Notes of [Qin] Qian-Zhai (Qiān-Zhāi yī xué jiǎng gǎo)*, was destroyed in the Cultural Revolution and was only reconstituted later. In addition, when TCM was developing, much of Qin's work on differentiation and treatment was replaced by more simplified and politically aligned alternatives that we now see dominating our modern textbooks.

The text that we present here was actually a core part of Qin's vision for an integrated Chinese medicine. It directly competed with the system that later became TCM. There were a number of political reasons that Qin's approach was not chosen, and a full analysis of the history is beyond the scope of this introduction. However, one important point was that Qin's system did not allow for easy integration of Western diseases and thus was not easily exportable.

Although Qin lived and breathed Chinese medicine, he was adamant about the importance of a broad-based education and life experience in developing a high level clinical practice. Just like his teacher Ding Gan-Ren, he required his students to memorize many philosophical texts, especially Confucius and Mencius. Qin was also an accomplished calligrapher, artist, and poet. He actually published quite a bit of poetry throughout his life, one example of which is below on p. *xxi*. For Qin, a rounded life was essential to becoming a good doctor. Examples of his calligraphy, poetry, and painting can be found on p. *xxiv*.

死去原知万事空，生前殁后此心同，待到国医振兴日，家祭勿忘告乃翁。

When death comes I fundamentally know that all things are empty.
Yet in life and in death, this hope doesn't change.
When the day comes that the medicine of our country has fully flourished.
Don't forget to tell your old man when next you visit his grave.[2]

When reading such poetry it was expected that one understood the context and historical overtones in order to fully appreciate it. Although a full exploration of this poem is beyond the scope of this introduction, it is worth noting that it is based in part on the famous poem "To My Son" by the renowned Song dynasty poet, Lu You (陆游). This demonstrates Qin's link to an ongoing literary tradition. Qin also purposely noted his commitment to his country, keeping with the spirit of the times, while at the same time proclaiming his love for the medicine. Thus, Dr. Wu and I chose this poem because it shows Dr. Qin's love of poetry, medicine, and country.

I would like to end this very short biography with one of Qin's favorite sayings: "Stay lively until you're old, study until you're old, and never stop learning" (活到老，学到老，学不了 *huó dào lǎo, xué dào lǎo, xué bù liǎo*).

A Word about Wu Bo-Ping (吴伯平)

Wu Bo-Ping was born on June 20, 1935 in Shanghai. In addition to his long-term apprenticeship with Qin Bo-Wei, he studied with many other famous 20th-century physicians such as Zhao Bing-Nan (赵炳南), Ren Yin-Qiu (任应秋), and Zhu Yan (朱颜). He was also trained academically, graduating in 1962 in the first class of the newly-established Beijing College of Chinese Medicine.

Over his nearly 50 years of extensive clinical experience, he traveled the world teaching Chinese medicine and held key positions at schools such as the Zhejiang College of Chinese Medicine (Hangzhou), Academy of Chinese Medicine (Beijing), Seattle Institute of Oriental Medicine, Institute of Chinese Medicine (London), and European Institute of Oriental Medicine (Munich). In addition, he has been involved in many research projects and has edited such prestigious journals as the *Zhejiang Chinese Medicine Journal*. He currently resides in Hangzhou, where, until recently, he maintained a busy private practice.

Although he is known worldwide as a teacher, I believe Professor Wu's true talent lies in the clinic. His clinical approach followed in the footsteps of such great physicians as Qin Bo-Wei, Ding Gan-Ren, and Ye Tian-Shi. That is, he favored a therapeutic strategy that employs light and mild medicinals with smaller doses. He specialized in the treatment of complex diseases such as autoimmune disorders and dermatology. Not only is Dr. Wu known for his outstanding clinical results, but also his deep understanding of classical Chinese medicine and how to utilize this in the clinic.

Much like his mentor Qin Bo-Wei, Dr. Wu has an incredible knack for explaining complex

---

2. Translated by Charles Chace.

ideas in a straightforward manner. This, along with his close personal relationship with Dr. Qin, makes Wu an ideal person to provide clinical commentary on Qin's original text. All of the commentary contained in this book is Wu Bo-Ping's, except for small segments taken from Qin's other writings. Moreover, we have gone to considerable lengths to illustrate both Drs. Qin and Wu's clinical thought processes, instead of merely listing herbs and formulas for a particular pattern. Dr. Wu's commentary therefore provides an invaluable part of this book, explaining Dr. Qin's thinking and bringing it to life.

Structure of this Book

This book is composed of two interwoven parts. First is Dr. Qin's original text, which is always presented within a shaded background. Everything else—that is, the non-shaded text— is commentary, either of Dr. Wu's or drawn from information in Dr. Qin's other books.[3]

At the beginning of each of the thirteen chapters are important ideas describing the fundamental pathogen/pathology (e.g., phlegm, dampness, qi, etc.) that is the subject of that chapter, such as its etiology, pathodynamics, key symptoms, and diagnostic criteria. The remainder of the chapter is organized according to the treatment methods that one needs to correct that pathology.

For each treatment method, Qin's original text can be divided into three main parts. First is the title of the treatment method, for example, "warm and transform phlegm and thin mucus" (温化痰饮 *wēn huà tán yǐn*). This is the key point and should be kept in mind while reading the rest of the section. Next is what we call "presentation." This consists of the cause (pattern) and usually the most common manifestation, for example, "Spleen and Kidney cold-phlegm ascending counterflow; urgent breathing with phlegm and thin mucus." Finally, Qin presents his own herbal formula for the treatment method.

Qin's original text is quite concise in comparison to the commentary that follows it. As is often the case, Chinese medicine texts can be very terse, and leave the reader with more questions than answers. Qin's text is no exception. I think this is a purposeful feature that can be very beneficial in developing one's ability to solve problems and develop a method of thinking. However, many Westerners find it a little frustrating and require a more detailed explanation. Thus the ensuing commentary provides a fuller exposition of the clinical presentation (additional signs and symptoms), etiology, pathodynamics, treatment principles, how the herbs relate to them, and modifications of the formula. Interspersed within the text are Dr. Wu's own clinical pearls and tips that he has found to be important in applying this material over his many decades of clinical experience. There is further elaboration in a question and answer section, and in the addenda.

Each section also contains an analysis of the medicinals in the recommended formula. This differs from a standard materia medica entry in that it focuses on the relevant information related to the formula in which it is contained. Thus it may be useful to look at other sections of the book that use the same herb to further round out one's understanding of Drs. Qin and Wu's use of a given herb.

For more tips on how to use this book, the reader is referred to Appendix I (p. 279).

---

3. Dr. Wu's material came from lectures as well as personal conversations and emails spanning several years.

Notes on Translation

In general, the Chinese medicine terms are translated in accordance with the Eastland Press gloss, which can be found under the Resources tab of their website:

http://www.eastlandpress.com/resources/

Dr. Qin's original Chinese text is also posted there.

In those instances where the translated term is not clear, further explanation may be found in the Glossary (see p. 285) and at times in a footnote or endnote.

—— JASON BLALACK

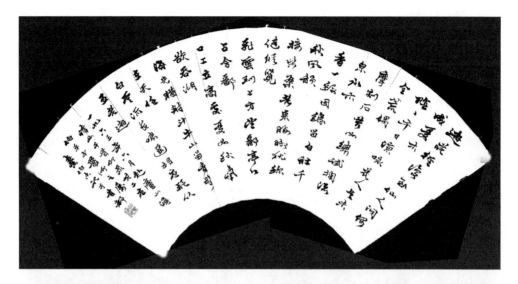

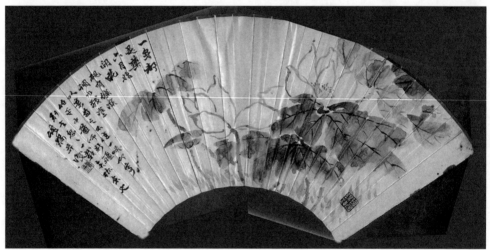

These two fans are examples of Qin Bo-Wei's calligraphy, poetry, and painting.

Treatment Guidelines for

Phlegm 痰 *(tán)*

SOURCE

- Phlegm is the result of a pathological transformation of fluids.

CAUSE

- There are many causes, ranging from overabundance of wind, cold, dampness, and heat to constraint due to the seven emotions or irregularities in diet.

MECHANISM

- Phlegm results from an abnormal flow of qi causing the fluids to become turbid. The turbid fluids transform into a large quantity of pathological liquid substance that is thin and sticky.   *

Essentially, the mechanism for phlegm production stems from a blockage of qi that causes fluids to stagnate and congeal, resulting in a pathological transformation of the physiological fluids. Therefore, anything that can cause the qi (and fluids) to stagnate is a potential cause of phlegm production; this would include the six excesses, internal damage due to the seven emotions, or harm from food and drink. For example, an irregular diet leads to food stagnation, which causes the qi (and thus the fluids) to stagnate, resulting in phlegm. In another example, the qi of the Lungs may be inhibited by an external pathogenic influence like wind-cold, resulting in phlegm.

---

* The shaded text throughout this book is taken directly from Qin Bo-Wei's *New Guidelines for Treatment*. All of the non-shaded text is elaboration and commentary by Wu Bo-Ping or drawn from information in Dr. Qin's other books. See Introduction, p. *xxii*, for further explanation.

DISEASE LOCATION

- Phlegm can come up and out via vomiting or expectoration.

The location is either in the Stomach (vomiting) or Lungs (expectoration).

- Phlegm can congeal and stagnate in the chest and diaphragm.
- Phlegm can lodge in the Intestines and Stomach.

Manifestations are symptoms like abdominal gurgling, diarrhea, nausea/vomiting, or stomachache.

- Phlegm can settle in the channels and network vessels of the limbs.

This refers to the sinews, muscles, and joints and can manifest in conditions such as carpal tunnel syndrome, painful obstruction syndrome, lipomas, or lymph nodules.

- Phlegm can follow qi that is ascending or descending, going up and down throughout the body. There is nowhere that phlegm cannot reach.

DISEASE MANIFESTATIONS

- Phlegm can manifest as coughing, wheezing, vomiting, nausea, focal distention and occlusion,[1] congestion in the chest, dizziness, indefinable epigastric discomfort, panicky throbbing,[2] palpitations, withdrawal-mania, fever and chills, or pain and swelling.

Phlegm can be substantial/visible, as with a cough, or insubstantial/invisible, as when phlegm and thin mucus lead to asthma.

Other phlegm-related disease manifestations include epileptic seizures, mental disorders, swelling and edema, and infertility. Essentially, any disease can have a component of phlegm.

This is especially true of difficult-to-cure conditions, in which case one should also consider blood stasis, as blood stasis and phlegm often combine to form phlegm-stasis. Thus it is said that "phlegm and stasis have the same source." For example, conditions commonly understood as blood stasis, such as endometriosis, are often mixed with phlegm. In these situations, medicinals like Arisaema cum Bile *(dǎn nán xīng)*, Gleditsiae Spina *(zào jiǎo cì)*, and Pinelliae Rhizoma preparatum *(zhì bàn xià)*, which eliminate phlegm, should be considered.

PRESENTING SYMPTOMS

- The area of the chest and diaphragm may have a moist appearance along with gurgling sounds.

---

1. This condition is quite severe in that nothing can pass down the throat/esophagus. This may be caused by an esophageal spasm or something like stomach cancer. *Translators note:* The original term (膈 *gé*) comes from *Basic Question (Sù wèn)* where it means blockage with no passage. It is a disease name that is defined as "food and drink are unable to descend and there is constipation."

2. This is severe heart palpitations that are not related to emotional stimulus.

- The small area at the center of the upper back may have an ice-cold sensation.

In addition, there may be tightness and spasm that feels as if the back has been exposed to a draft. Such sensations can precede asthma attacks. Often this is cold-dampness or phlegm and thin mucus. Many people with chronic bronchitis have an extreme sensitivity in this area of the back that is heightened when the weather changes to cold and damp. This pattern is often mixed with deficiency.

- There may be a feeling of insects crawling all over the body.
- Between the chest and the area of the throat, the two qi are twisted up.

The "two qi" refers to the normal qi and pathogenic qi contending and being twisted up in the throat. It may manifest in such conditions as difficulty swallowing, chest pain, plum pit qi, etc.

- There may also be nodules on the body that are neither red nor swollen.

Theses are palpable tumors, phlegm nodules, or lipomas. They can occur on the limbs or trunk, but similar masses are also commonly seen in the uterus (leiomyomas) and ovaries (polycystic ovaries). Key herbs are for treating these include Gleditsiae Spina *(zào jiǎo cì)*, Arisaema cum Bile *(dǎn nán xīng)*, Bambusae Caulis in taeniam *(zhú rú)*, Citri reticulatae Pericarpium *(chén pí)*, and Pinelliae Rhizoma preparatum *(zhì bàn xià)*.

- Lumps on the neck that are similar to scrofula, but not scrofula.
- Blockage in the throat like a plum pit.
- Expectoration of glue-like substances.
- The limbs can be stiff and swollen, with possible numbness and tingling.

This may also include some types of 'restless leg syndrome' where the presentation is usually not painful or burning, but feels like there is something inside the leg and there is a desire to beat or hit the leg.

- Ensconced lumps and accumulations may form in the flanks.
- There may be intermittent stabbing pain in the joints.

This is phlegm leading to qi and blood stagnation and causing pain. This demonstrates that sharp pain does not have to be due to blood stasis as in these cases one must treat the phlegm and not blood stasis to eliminate the problem. The difference is that blood stasis usually causes fixed, chronic, sharp pain that is worse at night.

- The lower back and legs may ache and be weak.
- There may be spitting up of cold saliva, green liquids, or black juices.

This refers to some substance that may contain mucus, food, bile, pus, and may be mixed with blood. It is a strange colored liquid that is usually dark green and not bright.

3

> • There may be nightmares of battles (with smoke, fire, swords, etc.).

In Ch. 43 of *Divine Pivot*, "Dreams Caused by Excess and Evils," it is said that hot-phlegm will cause fire-type dreams and cold-phlegm will cause dreams of wetlands and snakes. This is important because dreams can show pathology before symptoms manifest. One should still confirm suspected pathologies with other signs and symptoms.

> • There may be diarrhea; a mucus or pus-like substance may be mixed with the urine or stool.

Abnormal vaginal discharge can also represent phlegm.

CONCURRENT SYMPTOMS

Other symptoms related to occlusion and blockage; rapidly developing throat painful obstruction, toothache, tinnitus, consumption, paralysis, amenorrhea, vaginal discharge, childhood fright wind, tetany, and, if the condition is severe, the patient constantly hallucinates and sees ghosts, or has a condition that resembles being under the influence of an evil spirit but in fact is not.[i]

Rapidly developing throat painful obstruction is a disorder that can accompany serious epidemic throat diseases such as scarlet fever, in which the throat is swollen and blocked and the patient has a high fever. This is usually an emergency situation that develops quickly.

TREATMENT METHOD

To address phlegm: Clear, dry, scatter, open, soften, reduce, induce vomiting, and purge

To address the yin organs: Protect the Lungs and enrich the fluids, nurture the Spleen and transform oral mucus, tonify the Kidneys to return nourishment to the other organs

SUMMARY

Clear, descend, moisten, and reduce

1. Diffuse and Transform Phlegm (宣散化痰 *xuān sàn huà tán*)

[PRESENTATION] External contraction of wind-cold; cough with thick or thin phlegm

Perillae Folium (*zǐ sū yè*)/
   Perillae Caulis (*zǐ sū gěng*) . . . . 4.5g (each)
Dry-fried Arctii Fructus (*chǎo niú bàng zǐ*) 4.5g
Citri reticulatae Pericarpium (*chén pí*) 4.5g
Peucedani Radix (*qián hú*) 4.5g
Armeniacae Semen (*xìng rén*) 9g
Platycodi Radix (*jié gěng*) 2.4g
Zingiberis Rhizoma recens (*shēng jiāng*) . . . . 2 slices

1. Diffuse and Transform Phlegm

COMMENTARY

ADDITIONAL SIGNS AND SYMPTOMS

- Phlegm is thin, white, and profuse. It may also be slightly thick.
- Aversion to wind and drafts
- Chills
- Fever
- Itchy or sore throat (tight, not burning, not dry)
- Stabbing headache that is worse with cold
- The pulse is floating and tight
- The tongue has no change (normal) or may have a thin, white, moist coating

DISCUSSION

This presentation may begin with just a headache and sore throat. After a couple of days, the pathogen moves into the chest, causing discomfort and a cough with white phlegm.

LOCATION: Pathogen resides in the exterior and the disease is located in the Lungs.

TREATMENT PRINCIPLE: Eliminate the external pathogen (wind-cold) with acrid, warm medicinals by diffusing the Lungs and resolving the exterior in order to stop the cough, and simultaneously transform the phlegm.

MEDICINAL ANALYSIS

SUMMARY

- Perillae Folium *(zǐ sū yè)*, Peucedani Radix *(qián hú)*, Arctii Fructus *(niú bàng zǐ)*, Platycodi Radix *(jié gěng)*, and Zingiberis Rhizoma recens *(shēng jiāng)* all open and diffuse.

- Citri reticulatae Pericarpium *(chén pí)* and Perillae Caulis *(zǐ sū gěng)* primarily regulate the qi.

- Armeniacae Semen *(xìng rén)* and Peucedani Radix *(qián hú)* are the only medicinals here that cause the Lung qi to descend.

INDIVIDUAL CHARACTERISTICS

- Perillae Folium *(zǐ sū yè)* and Peucedani Radix *(qián hú)* are both acrid, scatter wind-cold, and diffuse the Lungs.

- Perillae Folium *(zǐ sū yè)* dredges, scatters, and resolves the exterior and also transforms phlegm in the upper burner. In addition, it enters the Spleen and can aromatically transform turbidity to treat phlegm. It is therefore suitable for exterior contraction of wind-cold with relatively severe phlegm-dampness.

- Peucedani Radix *(qián hú)* directs qi downward, transforms phlegm, and stops coughing. It is especially appropriate if there is intense coughing. It is a key ingredient of this formula.

5

- Perillae Caulis *(zǐ sū gěng)* circulates the qi in the chest, which aids in the elimination of phlegm and dampness.

- Armeniacae Semen *(xìng rén)* is acrid and warm, diffuses the Lungs, causes the Lung qi to descend, normalizes the qi, transforms phlegm, and stops coughing. It should be crushed.

- Platycodi Radix *(jié gěng)* has an opening, disseminating, and rising nature and dispels phlegm. A small dose is preferred since its ascending nature can cause nausea or headache.

- Dry-fried Arctii Fructus *(chǎo niú bàng zǐ)* is acrid, diffuses the Lungs, expels and transforms phlegm, and vents and disperses wind. Although Arctii Fructus *(niú bàng zǐ)* is cool to neutral and can be used for warm or cool conditions, stir frying it changes its thermal nature to warm, as well as moderates its slippery nature. This preparation is important to its use in treating this pattern.

- Citri reticulatae Pericarpium *(chén pí)* is warm, acrid, enters the Lungs, regulates qi, and transforms phlegm, making it useful for cough with profuse phlegm.

- Zingiberis Rhizoma recens *(shēng jiāng)* is acrid, dispersing, warm, and is able to release the exterior and expel wind-cold pathogens on the exterior. It is also able to transform phlegm and stop coughing. It is especially useful when there is strong wind-cold, nausea, and white, profuse, foamy phlegm. One should not substitute Zingiberis Rhizoma *(gān jiāng)* here because, while it warms the Lungs, it primarily acts on the interior and specifically on the Spleen. Zingiberis Rhizoma preparata *(páo jiāng)* is also not a suitable substitute, for it is bitter instead of acrid.

Dr. Qin's formula is based on Apricot Kernel and Perilla Leaf Powder *(xìng sū sǎn)*.

Apricot Kernel and Perilla Leaf Powder *(xìng sū sǎn)*

SOURCE: *Systematic Differentiation of Warm Pathogen* (1798)

Perillae Folium *(zǐ sū yè)* 6g
Peucedani Radix *(qián hú)* 6g
Armeniacae Semen *(xìng rén)* 6g
Platycodi Radix *(jié gěng)* 6g
Aurantii Fructus *(zhǐ ké)* 6g
Citri reticulatae Pericarpium *(chén pí)* 6g
Poria *(fú líng)* 6g
Pinelliae Rhizoma preparatum *(zhì bàn xià)* 6g
Zingiberis Rhizoma recens *(shēng jiāng)* 6g
Jujubae Fructus *(dà zǎo)* 2p
Glycyrrhizae Radix *(gān cǎo)* 3g

MODIFICATIONS OF DR. QIN'S FORMULA

Headache (general):

Menthae haplocalycis Herba *(bò hé)* 2-3g
Viticis Fructus *(màn jīng zǐ)* 4.5g

Headache (frontal) and nasal blockage:

Angelicae dahuricae Radix *(bái zhǐ)* 3g

Headache (vertex/back of head):

Ligustici Rhizoma *(gǎo běn)* 4.5g

Cough with nausea:

Dry-fried Aurantii Fructus *(chǎo zhǐ ké)*[ii] 4.5g

Itching in the throat:

Cicadae Periostracum *(chán tuì)* 1.5g

Sterculiae lychnophorae Semen *(pàng dà hǎi)* . . . . 2 pieces

Fullness and stifling sensation in the chest:

Aurantii Fructus *(zhǐ ké)* 4-6g

Profuse turbid phlegm:

Pinelliae Rhizoma preparatum *(zhì bàn xià)*[3] 4-6g

Poria *(fú líng)* 6-9g

QUESTIONS

1. *If the cough is strong, can one add medicinals to stop the coughing such as Eriobotryae Folium (pí pá yè) or Farfarae Flos (kuǎn dōng huā)?*

Adding these medicinals is a mistake with this presentation. These medicinals suppress the cough and do not treat the underlying pathodynamic. Quite simply, by diffusing the pathogen the cough will resolve on its own. Furthermore, utilizing these medicinals can cause the external pathogen to become constrained in the interior, making it difficult to eliminate the phlegm.

2. *If medicinals to stop the coughing are contraindicated for this method, then why does Dr. Qin use Peucedani Radix (qián hú)?*

Peucedani Radix *(qián hú)* is unique in that not only can it direct the qi downward to stop coughs, it also has the ability to expel exterior pathogenic factors. This makes it an effective medicinal for early-stage coughs.

3. *Many consider the thermal nature of Peucedani Radix (qián hú) to be cool, so why does Dr. Qin use it for a condition that is essentially cold?*

The thermal nature of this medicinal, which we consider to be neutral, is unimportant in this case, since it is chosen here for its expelling ability. Dr. Qin stated that, in the context of Apricot Kernel and Perilla Leaf Powder *(xìng sū sǎn)*, Peucedani Radix *(qián hú)* "expels wind cold."

4. *Pinelliae Rhizoma preparatum (zhì bàn xià) is a constituent of the original Apricot Kernel and Perilla Leaf Powder (xìng sū sǎn), so why is it omitted here?*

---

3. Ginger-fried Pinelliae Rhizoma preparatum *(jiāng bàn xià)* is best here.

Although Pinelliae Rhizoma preparatum *(zhì bàn xià)* can transform phlegm and treat cough, it primarily acts on the Spleen and Stomach, and does little to expel the external pathogen. It is therefore not needed for the resolution of the pathogen, which is the root cause of the phlegm and the cough in this case. Focusing on medicinals that work on the Lungs and the exterior is essential for dispelling the pathogen. In addition, there are enough other herbs in the formula to transform the phlegm.

5. *Since there is phlegm and possibly a moist tongue coating, could one add medicinals such as Eupatorii Herba (pèi lán) and Pogostemonis/Agastaches Herba (huò xiāng)?*

   Although both of these can be used for external conditions, they are not appropriate for wind-cold. They are best reserved for presentations that have a component of dampness, not phlegm. (For further elaboration, see Modifications on p. 6 and the method "dry dampness and transform phlegm" on p. 16.)

6. *With profuse amounts of phlegm, should one pay special attention to the Spleen?*

   When there are profuse amounts of phlegm, one might think that there is some Spleen involvement. This is not the case here, and medicinals for dampness, like Pogostemonis/Agastaches Herba *(huò xiāng)* and Eupatorii Herba *(pèi lán)*, or medicinals that tonify the Spleen, should not be included in the formula. One must focus the treatment on the cause of the phlegm, which is wind-cold. However, as mentioned in the modifications above, Pinelliae Rhizoma preparatum *(zhì bàn xià)*, with its acrid nature, can help eliminate the phlegm when it is profuse and serious, especially in combination with Perillae Folium *(zǐ sū yè)*.

7. *Besides stopping the cough, is there any other reason to use herbs that cause the Lung qi to descend?*

   The Lung qi should normally descend. When a pathogen inhibits its normal flow, there is Lung constraint, and normal disseminating and descending does not occur. This leads to numerous symptoms, including stifling sensation in the chest, cough, wheezing, shortness of breath, frequent urination, or edema, as well as dysfunction of other organs' qi dynamic.

8. *Besides causing the Lung qi to descend, is there any other way to stop the cough?*

   Yes. In this formula, for example, one does not just cause the Lung qi to descend to stop the coughing. One only slightly causes it to descend, while mostly diffusing, to re-establish the Lungs' normal movement. Notice the pairing of Platycodi Radix *(jié gěng)* and Armeniacae Semen *(xìng rén)*. Each herb provides complementary and opposing functions: one ascends and one descends. This creates a powerful herbal pairing that mimics, and hence restores, the normal qi function of the Lungs. Furthermore, all the medicinals in this formula that have a descending function on the Lungs also have a complimentary diffusing function.

2. Clear Heat and Transform Phlegm (清热化痰 *qīng rè huà tán*)

[PRESENTATION] Phlegm-heat lodged in the Lungs; thirst and cough

Mori Folium *(sāng yè)*[4]	4.5g
Eriobotryae Folium *(pí pá yè)*	9g
White Chrysanthemi Flos *(bái jú huā)*	4.5g
Trichosanthis Pericarpium *(guā lóu pí)*	9g
Cynanchi stauntonii Rhizoma *(bái qián)*	4.5g
Fritillariae cirrhosae Bulbus *(chuān bèi mǔ)* /	
Fritillariae thunbergii Bulbus *(zhè bèi mǔ)*	6g (each)
Eleocharitis Rhizoma *(bí qi)*	2p

COMMENTARY

ADDITIONAL SIGNS AND SYMPTOMS

- Phlegm is sticky with difficult expectoration (also possibly dry)
- Mild fever
- Only a slight aversion to wind and drafts (no chills)
- Slight sweating
- Dry mouth, dry throat, or burning, sore throat (not tight)
- Dull headache that is aggravated by heat or anything that increases heat or phlegm in the body (e.g. eating sweet and sticky foods)
- The pulse is floating, edgy,[5] forceful, and rapid
- The tongue has a dry, yellow coating

DISCUSSION

PATTERN AND LOCATION: The pathogen resides in the Lungs. This is a pathogen of the interior, not an exterior presentation (see discussion below).

ETIOLOGY: This pattern can arise from either one of the following causes:

1. External attack: This usually comes from wind-warmth, where a wind-heat pathogen enters the Lungs, or a wind-cold pathogen enters the Lungs and transforms into internal heat. In both situations, the external aspect is resolved.

2. Internal generation of heat: This may arise because of a constitutional tendency toward heat that is exacerbated by something like drinking alcohol or eating hot-natured foods. In this scenario, there are usually chronic signs and symptoms of internal heat.

This is not a very severe presentation.

---

4. Originally, Dr. Qin used 4.5g of the leaves collected after the first frost, which are called 'frost mulberry leaves' (霜桑葉 *shuāng sāng yè*). However, most Mori Folium *(sāng yè)* available in the West are a combination of regular leaves and the older leaves. Traditionally, 'frost mulberry leaves' are thought to be less expulsive, slightly cooler, and more moistening than the mixed product.

5. Consult the glossary for a full explanation.

TREATMENT PRINCIPLE: Generally, in cases of early stages of wind-warmth leading to phlegm-heat in the Lungs, the appropriate strategy is to clear and diffuse. In chronic, severe Lung heat patterns, one can use the method of clearing and draining the Lungs. This treatment pattern lies someone in between the two, by clearing, cooling, and transforming the phlegm. In addition, the secondary strategy of moistening, to protect the fluids as well as directly alleviate the cough, is used.

MEDICINAL ANALYSIS

SUMMARY

COOLING MEDICINALS: all herbs except for Cynanchi stauntonii Rhizoma *(bái qián)*

MOISTENING MEDICINALS: Mori Folium *(sāng yè)*, Eriobotryae Folium *(pí pá yè)*, Fritillariae cirrhosae Bulbus *(chuān bèi mǔ)*, Trichosanthis Pericarpium *(guā lóu pí)*, Eleocharitis Rhizoma *(bí qi)*, and White Chrysanthemi Flos *(bái jú huā)*

COUGH-ALLEVIATING MEDICINALS: Eriobotryae Folium *(pí pá yè)*, Fritillariae thunbergii Bulbus *(zhè bèi mǔ)*, Fritillariae cirrhosae Bulbus *(chuān bèi mǔ)*, Trichosanthis Pericarpium *(guā lóu pí)*, and Cynanchi stauntonii Rhizoma *(bái qián)*

INDIVIDUAL CHARACTERISTICS

- Mori Folium *(sāng yè)* is slightly acrid, slightly bitter, slightly sweet, and lightweight. It can clear and vent heat as well as expel wind-heat from the exterior and especially from the head and eyes. It also can moisten dryness and protect the fluids.

- White Chrysanthemi Flos *(bái jú huā)* is bitter, sweet, clears Lung heat, and nourishes the fluids of the Lungs. It is indicated for thirst with dry mouth.

- Eriobotryae Folium *(pí pá yè)* is bitter, clears Lung heat, transforms phlegm (by its ability to make phlegm thinner, less dry, and less sticky), and stops coughing by directing the Lung qi downward. Consider honey-prepared Eriobotryae Folium *(mì zhì pí pá yè)* for a later stage cough.

- Fritillariae thunbergii Bulbus *(zhè bèi mǔ)* and Fritillariae cirrhosae Bulbus *(chuān bèi mǔ)* both transform phlegm, clear Lung heat, and alleviate coughing. Fritillariae thunbergii Bulbus *(zhè bèi mǔ)* is better at expelling the pathogen and thus circulating Lung qi and is used more for acute situations. Fritillariae cirrhosae Bulbus *(chuān bèi mǔ)* tonifies the Lung yin and is best for chronic stage presentations. Three grams of powdered Fritillariae cirrhosae Bulbus *(chuān bèi mǔ)*, dissolved into the strained decoction, can be used instead of the 6g suggested above.

- Trichosanthis Pericarpium *(guā lóu pí)* clears Lung heat, diffuses the Lungs, transforms phlegm, clears dryness, and generates fluids, rendering the phlegm more slippery and easier to expectorate, and thereby alleviating the cough. In addition, it unblocks the Large Intestine by both facilitating the proper flow the Lung qi and softening the stools.

- Cynanchi stauntonii Rhizoma *(bái qián)* is neutral and directs Lung qi downward, stops coughing, and moistens the fluids. It is best for chronic stages with no exterior involvement. (Please refer to question no. 5 below for more details.)

- Eleocharitis Rhizoma *(bí qí)* is sweet and slightly cold and able to transform phlegm and clear heat. It is especially effective for cough and sore throat. It also has a moistening quality to help protect (or nourish) the fluids and loosen phlegm, aiding in expectoration. One should cut it into small pieces before decocting. If it is not available, one can substitute canned water chestnuts. If these are not available, one can use Phragmitis Rhizoma recens *(xiān lú gēn)* 20-30g, Phragmitis Rhizoma *(lú gēn)* 6-9g, or Pyri Exocarpium *(lí pí)* 1 peel (cleaned and cut into pieces).

This formula should only be cooked for 10-15 minutes. Dr. Qin's formula is based on Mulberry Leaf and Chrysanthemum Drink *(sāng jú yǐn)*:

Mulberry Leaf and Chrysanthemum Drink *(sāng jú yǐn)*

SOURCE: *Systematic Differentiation of Warm Pathogen Diseases* (1798)

Mori Folium *(sāng yè)* 7.5g
Chrysanthemi Flos *(jú huā)* 3g
Forsythiae Fructus *(lián qiào)* 4.5g
Menthae haplocalycis Herba *(bò hé)* 2.4g
Platycodi Radix *(jié gěng)* 6g
Armeniacae Semen *(xìng rén)* 6g
Phragmitis Rhizoma *(lú gēn)* 6g
Glycyrrhizae Radix *(gān cǎo)* 2.4g

MODIFICATIONS OF DR. QIN'S FORMULA

Dull headache (*tài yáng* topography—back and sides of head):

Menthae haplocalycis Herba *(bò hé)* 3g

Viticis Fructus *(màn jīng zǐ)* 4.5g

Severe cough (especially if acute):

Peucedani Radix *(qián hú)* 4.5g

Phlegm that is very sticky yellow with a strong odor:

Houttuyniae Herba *(yú xīng cǎo)* 6g

Hedyotis diffusae Herba *(bái huā shé shé cǎo)* 9g

Dry and sore throat:

Scrophulariae Radix *(xuán shēn)* 6g

Physalis Calyx seu Fructus *(guà jīn dēng)*[6] 3g

Oroxyli Semen *(mù hú dié)* 1.5g

---

6. Physalis Calyx seu Fructus (挂金灯 *guà jīn dēng*; also known as 锦灯笼 *jīn dēng lóng*) enters the Lungs and Kidneys and clears heat while resolving toxicity. It clears the Lungs, promotes the ability to swallow, transforms dysenteric disorders, and promotes urination. It is primarily used for cough from phlegm-heat with a swollen and painful throat, as well as painful urinary dribbling disorder.

Galli Membrana Ovi *(fēng huáng yī)*[7] 1.5g

Cicadae Periostracum *(chán tuì)* 2-3g

Increased severity with such problems as high fever and coughing with chest pain:

Clear and drain the Lungs with Drain the White Powder *(xiè bái sǎn)*

consisting of Mori Cortex *(sāng bái pí)*, Lycii Cortex *(dì gǔ pí)*,

Glycyrrhizae Radix *(gān cǎo)*, and Nonglutinous rice *(jīng mǐ)*

. . . . 10g per package placed in tea bag

Scutellariae Radix *(huáng qín)* 4-6g

Anemarrhenae Rhizoma *(zhī mǔ)* 6-9g

Gypsum fibrosum *(shí gāo)* 9-12g

QUESTIONS

1. *How can this formula be based on Mulberry Leaf and Chrysanthemum Drink (sāng jú yǐn) if this is not an exterior pattern?*

   Although Dr. Qin's formula is an adaptation of Mulberry Leaf and Chrysanthemum Drink *(sāng jú yǐn)*, it is not meant to release the exterior, because the pathogen is located in the interior. This is evidenced by his inclusion of Eriobotryae Folium *(pí pá yè)* and Cynanchi stauntonii Rhizoma *(bái qián)*. Such medicinals that stop coughing should only be used when the exterior has already been resolved. For example, Eriobotryae Folium *(pí pá yè)* is not appropriate in the early stages of an externally-contracted disease because it can lock in or retain the pathogen.

   Furthermore, one can notice that in the original prescription, Dr. Qin chooses 'frost mulberry leaves' *(shuāng sāng yè)*, which are less expelling than Mori Folium *(sāng yè)*, and hence are used more for conditions in the interior. In addition, combined with the other medicinals in the formula, it does not work to release the exterior but to clear heat, gently vent heat outward, and moisten. This follows Ye Tian-Shi's adage, "One should use light medicinals to clear the upper burner." This formula thus lies somewhere between Mulberry Leaf and Chrysanthemum Drink *(sāng jú yǐn)* and Clear the Qi and Transform Phlegm Pill *(qīng qì huà tán wán)*.

2. *If there is some exterior involvement, can one use this formula?*

   Yes, although one should modify it by removing Eriobotryae Folium *(pí pá yè)* and Cynanchi stauntonii Rhizoma *(bái qián)*, so as not to trap the pathogen. One can also choose regular Mori Folium *(sāng yè)*. See previous question as well.

3. *Doesn't a floating pulse indicate an exterior attack?*

   A floating pulse can surely correspond to an exterior attack. However, in this case, the

---

7. Galli Membrana Ovi (凤凰衣 *fēng huáng yī*) is the membrane of the chicken's egg and is similar in action to Oroxyli Semen *(mù hú dié)*. It is sweet, bland, and balanced, enters the Spleen, Stomach, and Lungs, and is useful for externally-contracted cough, wheezing, sore throat, loss of voice, hoarse voice, and hardened lymph nodes. Patients can prepare this for themselves. For example, ask them to boil one or two eggs, remove the shells, and use the thin, white membrane inside the shells.

floating pulse indicates heat in the upper burner. One must always evaluate a floating pulse within the context of the whole presentation. The more indicators that suggest an exterior condition, the more that one must address it. In this situation, the pathogen resides in the Lung, but it may also be located in other places simultaneously, such as the exterior. In addition, if this condition resulted from a wind-heat pathogen (versus internal generation), it is more probable that some remnant of an exterior condition would remain, but one would need to see signs and symptoms in order to confirm this.

4. *Why is understanding the etiology important if both of the above mentioned etiologies are treated with the same method?*

One can consider etiology in fine tuning the prescription. For example, knowing that a patient's phlegm-cough was triggered by eating too much greasy food, one might add a medicinal like Raphani Semen *(lái fú zǐ)* and reduce the dosage of expelling or exterior-related medicinals. If the phlegm-cough is the sole result of an external attack that progressed interiorly, one might add an extra wind-dispersing medicinal, or use Mori Folium *(sāng yè)* instead of frost mulberry leaves *(shuāng sāng yè)* and increase the dosage. Furthermore, if the patient has constitutional yin deficiency heat, one might add Cynanchi atrati Radix *(bái wéi)*, Polygonati odorati Rhizoma *(yù zhú)*, or Scrophulariae Radix *(xuán shēn)*. In all of these situations, though, one would have to see some manifestations related to the etiology.

5. *Why did Dr. Qin use Cynanchi stauntonii Rhizoma (bái qián) instead of Peucedani Radix (qián hú)?*

Peucedani Radix *(qián hú)* is too expelling and therefore best for acute stages. Cynanchi stauntonii Rhizoma *(bái qián)* is more moistening and better for chronic stages. Furthermore, it is an excellent symptomatic medicinal for coughs, and especially good for chronic coughs when paired with Farfarae Flos *(kuǎn dōng huā)* and Stemonae Radix *(bǎi bù)*, whereas Peucedani Radix *(qián hú)* is not.

3. Clarify the Qi and Transform Phlegm (肃气化痰 *sù qì huà tán*)

[PRESENTATION] Cold-phlegm congealing in the Lungs; asthma with phlegm and thin mucus

Inulae Flos *(xuán fù huā)*	4.5g
Pinelliae Rhizoma preparatum *(zhì bàn xià)*	4.5g
Prepared Perillae Fructus *(zhì zǐ sū zǐ)*	9g
Citri reticulatae Pericarpium *(chén pí)*	4.5g
Processed Polygalae Radix *(zhì yuǎn zhì)*	4.5g
Dry-fried Asteris Radix *(chǎo zǐ wǎn)*	6g
Pumex/Costaziae Os *(hǎi fú shí)*	9g

COMMENTARY

ADDITIONAL SIGNS AND SYMPTOMS

- Severe cough or wheezing that is very loud and worsens when lying down
- White phlegm (usually) of varying textures (e.g., large chunks or possibly thin and profuse, although the actual quality of the phlegm is not that important)
- Nausea and vomiting
- The pulse is floating, especially in the distal position, which will also be edgy
- The tongue is dark red, with a greasy, grey coating (if there is heat, the coating may be yellow)

DISCUSSION

PATHODYNAMIC AND ETIOLOGY: This is Lung qi rebellion or severe counterflow (ascent) of qi, stemming from cold congealing phlegm, which inhibits the normal function of the Lungs. This pattern may occur after a wind-cold attack enters the Lung, due to incorrect treatment, or various internal causes. One likely internal cause is Spleen yang deficiency unable to transform dampness, allowing dampness to accumulate and generate phlegm, which influences the clarifying and descending function of the Lungs.

This is an excessive, somewhat acute presentation. While there may be an underlying pattern of deficiency, at this point one needs to focus on the excess. This presentation may be an exacerbation of a chronic problem or an acute manifestation of a progressing situation (as in a wind-cold pathogen that enters the Lungs). Depending on the history and severity, one will decide what kind of follow-up is necessary. After the acute presentation is resolved, one should treat the root of the phlegm and thin mucus by addressing the Spleen and Kidney.

TREATMENT PRINCIPLE: Direct the Lung qi downward to treat the branch, and warm, disperse, and transform congealed cold-phlegm to treat the root.

MEDICINAL ANALYSIS

- Inulae Flos *(xuán fù huā)* is salty and alleviates cough, nausea, and vomiting. It is one of the few flowers that descends. Unprocessed Inulae Flos *(xuán fù huā)* is best here.

- Prepared Perillae Fructus *(zhì zǐ sū zǐ)* is acrid, disperses phlegm, opens the Lungs, and redirects qi downward. It is especially good if there is profuse mucus in the throat and Lungs with an inability to lie flat.

- Pinelliae Rhizoma preparatum *(zhì bàn xià)* is acrid, bitter, and disperses and dries phlegm. It is excellent for nausea and vomiting, as well as for thin or thick phlegm in the Lungs. It acts mostly on the Spleen and Stomach, but also the Lungs.

- Citri reticulatae Pericarpium *(chén pí)* dries dampness and is especially effective for cold thin mucus, and promotes the movement of qi to disperse congealed cold phlegm. It acts mostly on the Spleen and Stomach, but also the Lungs.

- Processed Polygalae Radix *(zhì yuǎn zhì)* calms the spirit, warms the Lungs, and expels phlegm. It is very useful in serious situations where the patient cannot sleep because of stress from a severe cough or else cannot lie flat without a serious exacerbation of the breathing problems. It can relax the mind to help the cough.

- Dry-fried Asteris Radix *(chǎo zǐ wǎn)* is best for chronic coughs and should not be used in acute cough because it is astringing and can lock in the pathogen. If not available, Asteris Radix *(zǐ wǎn)* is a suitable substitute.

- Pumex/Costaziae Os *(hǎi fú shí)* is slightly cool to neutral, salty, and guides qi downward. It has the ability to transform phlegm and eases the expectoration of phlegm. Its slightly astringent nature allows watery phlegm to thicken enough to be coughed up.

Overall, the medicinals in this formula are slightly warm, have a descending action, and transform phlegm, thereby quieting the Lungs. Dr. Qin's formula is based on Perilla Fruit Decoction for Directing Qi Downward *(sū zǐ jiàng qì tāng)* and Inula and Haematite Decoction *(xuán fù dài zhě tāng)*.

Perilla Fruit Decoction for Directing Qi Downward *(sū zǐ jiàng qì tāng)*
SOURCE: *Formulary of the Pharmacy Service for Benefiting the People in the Taiping Era* (1078)

Perillae Fructus *(zǐ sū zǐ)*	9-12g
Pinelliae Rhizoma preparatum *(zhì bàn xià)*	6-9g
Angelicae sinensis Radix *(dāng guī)*	6-9g
Glycyrrhizae Radix *(gān cǎo)*	3-4.5g
Magnoliae officinalis Cortex *(hòu pò)*	3-6g
Peucedani Radix *(qián hú)*	6-9g
Cinnamomi Cortex *(ròu guì)*	1.5-3g

Inula and Haematite Decoction *(xuán fù dài zhě tāng)*
SOURCE: *Discussion of Cold Damage* (c. 220)

Inulae Flos *(xuán fù huā)*	9g
Haematitum *(dài zhě shí)*	3g (9-15g)
Pinelliae Rhizoma preparatum *(zhì bàn xià)*	9g
Zingiberis Rhizoma recens *(shēng jiāng)*	15g (6g)
Ginseng Radix *(rén shēn)*	6g
Glycyrrhizae Radix preparata *(zhì gān cǎo)*	9g (3g)
Jujubae Fructus *(dà zǎo)*	12p (4p)

(Most commonly used dosage shown in parentheses)

MODIFICATIONS OF DR. QIN'S FORMULA

Chronic cough with no exterior involvement:

Armeniacae Semen dulce *(tián xìng rén)* 9g, or Pruni Amygdali
Semen *(bā dàn xìng rén)*, also known as almonds . . . . 9g (crushed)

Severe cough:

Honey-prepared Farfarae Flos *(mì zhì kuǎn dōng huā)* . . . . 6g[8]

---

8. The honey preparation slightly increases its moistening and cough-alleviating qualities. It is not cloying or sticky.

Severe cough in robust patient:

Lepidii/Descurainiae Semen *(tíng lì zǐ)* 6g

Sticky and difficult to expectorate phlegm:

Benincasae Semen *(dōng guā zǐ)* . . . . 9g (crushed)

Glue-like phlegm:

Coicis Semen *(yì yǐ rén)* 9g

Strong cold in the Lungs:

Asteris Radix *(zǐ wǎn)* 4-6g

Farfarae Flos *(kuǎn dōng huā)* 4-6g

Bloating and gas:

Dry-fried Raphani Semen *(chǎo lái fú zǐ)* 9g

Severe dampness:

Pinelliae massa fermentata *(bàn xià qū)* 9g

Congealed phlegm:

Meretricis/Cyclinae Concha *(gé qiào)* 6-9g

QUESTIONS

1. *Does the floating pulse show some bit of exterior involvement?*

   No, here the floating quality just indicates that the qi is ascending.

2. *Can this prescription be used if there is some exterior involvement?*

   Fundamentally, this prescription is not appropriate when there are exterior signs and symptoms. However, with appropriate modifications, it can be used to address a pattern with some exterior involvement. For example:

   - Use Perillae Folium *(zǐ sū yè)* instead of Perillae Fructus *(zǐ sū zǐ)*.
   - Add Armeniacae Semen amarum *(kǔ xìng rén)* 9g (crushed, full cook).
   - Do not use medicinals such as Farfarae Flos *(kuǎn dōng huā)*.[9]

   For a more significant external pattern, see the method "warm and transform phlegm and thin mucus" on p. 21.

---

4. Dry Dampness and Transform Phlegm (燥湿化痰 *zào shī huà tán*)

[PRESENTATION] Dampness collects and phlegm congeals; brim-over nausea[10] and cough

Prepared Atractylodis Rhizoma *(zhì cāng zhú)* 3g

Pinelliae Rhizoma preparatum *(zhì bàn xià)* 4.5g

---

9. It should be noted that raw Farfarae Flos *(kuǎn dōng huā)* can be harsh and can cause an itchy throat.

10. Brim-over nausea (泛恶 *fàn è*) is a desire to vomit either without vomiting or with upflow of clear drool into the mouth.

Magnoliae officinalis Cortex *(hòu pò)*	2.4g
Citri reticulatae Exocarpium rubrum *(jú hóng)*	2.4g
Bland Zingiberis Rhizoma *(dàn gān jiāng)*	1.5g
Dry-fried Aurantii Fructus *(chǎo zhǐ ké)*	4.5g
Dry-fried Coicis Semen *(chǎo yì yǐ rén)*	3g

COMMENTARY

ADDITIONAL SIGNS AND SYMPTOMS

- Cough is not very severe. The phlegm is thin and bubbly, and can be heard when the patient coughs.
- Nausea
- Hiccough and frequent belching
- Stifling sensation in the chest
- Indigestion, poor appetite, sensation of bloating, and a stuck feeling in the epigastrium
- Feeling of water moving in the stomach, or borborygmus
- Diarrhea
- Feeling of mucus in the throat
- Puffy face or puffiness under eyes
- Symptoms will increase when the weather is humid or the patient drinks too much (e.g. water or beer).
- Pulse is soggy and deeper in the right middle position
- Tongue body is pale/dark pale, puffy, and swollen with teeth marks. The coating is white, moist, thick, and greasy.

DISCUSSION

LOCATION AND PATHOGEN: Congealing cold-dampness and phlegm in the Spleen, Stomach, and Lungs

DURATION: This is usually a chronic presentation but may be acute.

ETIOLOGY: This pattern usually has some underlying Spleen qi deficiency; however, the dampness can accumulate over time due to diet, humid weather, living near the water, etc. Acute situations can come about from being caught in the rain, falling in a river, etc. Yet even acute cases should not manifest with exterior symptoms.

TREATMENT STRATEGY: For congealed cold-phlegm in the Lungs, one should transform phlegm, regulate the qi, and warm the Lungs. For damp-phlegm congealing and gathering in the Spleen and Stomach, one should warm and tonify the Spleen, regulate the qi, and dry and leach out dampness. Regulating the qi is essential to this method because the nature of dampness is to congeal and cause qi stagnation. Promoting the movement of qi facilitates the movement of dampness.

MEDICINAL ANALYSIS

SUMMARY

All medicinals in the prescription are warm except for dry-fried Coicis Semen *(chǎo yì yǐ rén)* and dry-fried Aurantii Fructus *(chǎo zhǐ ké)*.

INDIVIDUAL CHARACTERISTICS

• Prepared Atractylodis Rhizoma *(zhì cāng zhú)* eliminates turbid dampness and strengthens the Spleen. Preparing the Atractylodis Rhizoma *(cāng zhú)* tempers its acrid and drying nature, rendering it more gentle and tonifying for the Spleen, as well as reducing its exterior-releasing properties. Unprocessed Atractylodis Rhizoma *(cāng zhú)* is oily and can cause nausea. However, if there is exterior involvement or sweating, unprocessed Atractylodis Rhizoma *(cāng zhú)* is best.

• Bland Zingiberis Rhizoma *(dàn gān jiāng)* and Pinelliae Rhizoma preparatum *(zhì bàn xià)* are acrid, warm, and transform phlegm.

• Pinelliae Rhizoma preparatum *(zhì bàn xià)* is bitter, directs qi downward, opens, expels, disperses, and dries phlegm and dampness. It is excellent for nausea, vomiting, and coughing. It can transform thin or thick phlegm in the Lungs as well as dampness, water, or phlegm in the Stomach. It is not as drying as Magnoliae officinalis Cortex *(hòu pò)*, Citri reticulatae Exocarpium rubrum *(jú hóng)*, and Atractylodis Rhizoma *(cāng zhú)*; however, when combined with these medicinals, it becomes more drying.

• Bland Zingiberis Rhizoma *(dàn gān jiāng)* is hot and has an affinity for the Spleen. It warms the yang and eliminates cold. It is indicated for symptoms such as diarrhea, nausea, vomiting, cough, and wheezing. Bland Zingiberis Rhizoma *(dàn gān jiāng)* is more mild than Zingiberis Rhizoma *(gān jiāng)*.

• Magnoliae officinalis Cortex *(hòu pò)*, Citri reticulatae Exocarpium rubrum *(jú hóng)*, and dry-fried Aurantii Fructus *(chǎo zhǐ ké)* all promote the movement of qi.

• Magnoliae officinalis Cortex *(hòu pò)* is acrid and bitter, directs qi downward, disperses fullness, dries dampness, and reduces phlegm.

• Citri reticulatae Exocarpium rubrum *(jú hóng)* dries dampness, transforms phlegm, and regulates and directs the qi downward.

• Aurantii Fructus *(chǎo zhǐ ké)* is acrid, neutral, and tonifies the Spleen's circulation (regulates and harmonizes the Spleen and Stomach qi), which helps transform and move dampness.

• Dry-fried Coicis Semen *(chǎo yì yǐ rén)* is sweet, bland, and neutral. It strengthens the Spleen and resolves dampness by regulating, draining, and drying. Dry frying moderates the cold nature of this medicinal and improves its ability to strengthen the Spleen and harmonize the middle as well as enabling it to dry dampness. Therefore, dry frying should be used when aromatic medicinals that dry dampness are also used. Conversely, the raw form is better at opening the channels and collaterals, enabling it to treat painful obstruction and atrophy, expel pus, and reduce swelling.

Dr. Qin's formula is based on Calm the Stomach Powder *(píng wèi sǎn)* and Two-Aged [Herb] Decoction *(èr chén tāng)*.[11]

Calm the Stomach Powder *(píng wèi sǎn)*

SOURCE: *Formulary of the Pharmacy Service for Benefiting the People in the Taiping Era* (1078)

Atractylodis Rhizoma *(cāng zhú)* 12-15g
Magnoliae officinalis Cortex *(hòu pò)* 9-12g
Citri reticulatae Pericarpium *(chén pí)* 9-12g
Glycyrrhizae Radix preparata *(zhì gān cǎo)* 3-6g

---

Two-Aged [Herb] Decoction *(èr chén tāng)*

SOURCE: *Formulary of the Pharmacy Service for Benefiting the People in the Taiping Era* (1078)

Pinelliae Rhizoma preparatum *(zhì bàn xià)* 15g
Citri reticulatae Exocarpium rubrum *(jú hóng)* 15g
Poria *(fú líng)* 9g
Glycyrrhizae Radix preparata *(zhì gān cǎo)* 4.5g

---

MODIFICATIONS OF DR. QIN'S FORMULA

Nausea:

Substitute 2 pieces of Zingiberis Rhizoma recens *(shēng jiāng)* for Zingiberis Rhizoma *(gān jiāng)*.

Bloating and gas (lower abdomen):

Dry-fried Aurantii Fructus immaturus *(chǎo zhǐ shí)*

Digestive issues (e.g., no appetite, or sensation of fullness in the epigastrium and abdomen):

— If the Stomach is more affected (e.g., lack of appetite, nausea, and stomach distention): Amomi Fructus *(shā rén)* 3g

— If the Spleen is more affected (for example, appetite is good, but after eating there is bloating, gas, and blocked sensation. There may also be alternating constipation and diarrhea with difficult to pass stools. This is a 'strong Stomach, weak Spleen'.): Amomi Fructus rotundus *(bái dòu kòu)* 3g

— If both the Spleen and Stomach are impaired: Amomi Fructus *(shā rén)* and Amomi Fructus rotundus *(bái dòu kòu)* 3g each

Very poor digestion:

Dry-fried Atractylodis macrocephalae Rhizoma *(chǎo bái zhú)* 9g

---

11. When combined, these two formulas are called Calm and Aged Decoction *(píng chén tāng)* and consists of Atractylodis Rhizoma *(cāng zhú)*, Pinelliae Rhizoma preparatum *(zhì bàn xià)*, Glycyrrhizae Radix *(gān cǎo)*, Magnoliae officinalis Cortex *(hòu pò)*, Citri reticulatae Pericarpium *(chén pí)*, and Poria rubra *(chì fú líng)*. Source: Dr. Qin Bo-Wei.

Dark urine, with urinary difficulty, dribbling, or hesitant urinary flow (as in prostatitis), or dampness in urine (cloudy, or some mucus discharge after urination):

Poria *(fú líng)* 9g
  (if there is some Spleen impairment/deficiency)

Alismatis Rhizoma *(zé xiè)* 4.5g
  (more heat, but no Spleen deficiency)

Tetrapanacis Medulla *(tōng cǎo)* 1-1.5g
  (can also facilitate fluid metabolism of the Lungs)

QUESTIONS

1. *Can one use Zingiberis Rhizoma recens (shēng jiāng) instead of Zingiberis Rhizoma (gān jiāng) in the formula?*

   As mentioned in the modifications, Zingiberis Rhizoma recens *(shēng jiāng)* can be used if there is nausea. However, one should compare this formula with the one used in the method "diffuse and transform phlegm" (see p. 4). Zingiberis Rhizoma recens *(shēng jiāng)* has a much more expelling nature (compared to Zingiberis Rhizoma *(gān jiāng)*) and is thus appropriate when there is some exterior involvement. Thus, in this presentation, if there are signs of strong exterior dampness, one may choose Zingiberis Rhizoma recens *(shēng jiāng)*. By contrast, Zingiberis Rhizoma *(gān jiāng)* is less dispersing and focuses more on the interior. It is therefore the preferred choice in this presentation.

2. *Can this formula be used if there are exterior symptoms?*

   This method is generally not used for exterior patterns. However, as mentioned above, this can be used for an acute presentation with no exterior symptoms. If there are only minor exterior symptoms, one could add such medicinals as Pogostemonis/Agastaches Herba *(huò xiāng)* or Eupatorii Herba *(pèi lán)*.

3. *Why does Dr. Qin use Citri reticulatae Exocarpium rubrum (jú hóng) instead of Citri reticulatae Pericarpium (chén pí)?*

   Citri reticulatae Exocarpium rubrum *(jú hóng)* is more aromatic, warmer, more acrid, and drying, hence better for eliminating dampness than Citri reticulatae Pericarpium *(chén pí)*.

4. *Why are medicinals like Imperatae Rhizoma (bái máo gēn), Phragmitis Rhizoma (lú gēn), or Akebiae Caulis (mù tōng) not used when the patient presents with dark urine, urinary difficulty, dribbling, hesitant urinary flow, or dampness in the urine?*

   This condition is caused by dampness and phlegm and is thus primarily a yin-type disorder. Imperatae Rhizoma *(bái máo gēn)* and Phragmitis Rhizoma *(lú gēn)* are both too moist and cooling; here they will create more stagnation and increase the amount of phlegm. Akebiae Caulis *(mù tōng)* is too cold and harsh. Usually the patient will not have yellow burning urine, but cloudy and dark urine. This is caused by local stagnation secondary to either dampness and phlegm or from congealing of cold, as in prostatitis in elderly people. One should consider medicinals such as Plantaginis Semen *(chē qián zǐ)*, Alismatis Rhizoma *(zè xiè)*, and Tetrapanacis Medulla *(tōng cǎo)*, but not something like Pyrrosiae Folium *(shí wéi)*.

5. Warm and Transform Phlegm and Thin Mucus
(温化痰饮 *wēn huà tán yǐn*)

[PRESENTATION] Spleen and Kidney cold-phlegm ascending counterflow; urgent breathing with phlegm and thin mucus

Prepared Ephedrae Herba *(zhì má huáng)*	2.4g
Bland Zingiberis Rhizoma *(dàn gān jiāng)*	1.8g
Cinnamomi Ramulus *(guì zhī)*	2.4g
Schisandrae Fructus *(wǔ wèi zǐ)*	1.5g
Asari Radix et Rhizoma *(xì xīn)*	2.4g
Pinelliae Rhizoma preparatum *(zhì bàn xià)*	4.5g
Stalactite *(é guǎn shí)*	9g

COMMENTARY

ADDITIONAL SIGNS AND SYMPTOMS

- Cough and wheezing with phlegm and thin mucus
- Phlegm is profuse, watery, thin, clear, and easily expectorated
- Possible exterior presentation: aversion to cold, chills, fever, and absence of sweat
- A sense of heaviness or swelling in the limbs and face
- In general, there should not be a dry mouth, thirst, or sore throat. However, as discussed below, some patients may experience thirst.

Chronically, these patients may have:

- An aversion to cold on the back
- Dizziness
- Inability to lie down
- Flank pain
- This is mostly seen in elderly patients where their condition is usually worse in the autumn and winter, or with sudden cold.
- The pulse, with:
  — acute exacerbation with external component: thin, wiry, tight, floating, and/or rapid, especially in distal position
  — less serious condition (or more chronic stage): thin, deep, and slightly wiry
- Tongue is pale, slightly swollen with teeth marks, with a moist, thin, and white coating. There may be lots of saliva on the tongue.

DISCUSSION

ETIOLOGY AND PATHODYNAMIC: This method is for an acute exacerbation of a chronic problem (chronic wheezing due to phlegm and thin mucus); it is 'mutual contraction of two colds,' that is, (1) external contraction of wind-cold, and (2) underlying deficiency leading to cold.

This is a constitutional Spleen and Kidney (and secondarily Lung) yang deficiency and cold[12] with a possible simultaneous invasion of wind-cold. The deficiency cold leads to a chronic water metabolism issue that results in congested fluids/phlegm. However, this is coupled with a wind-cold pathogen that enters the protective level, which is connected to the Lungs.

The Lung qi travels upward to the protective level to counterattack the wind-cold pathogen. Consequently, the Lung qi is no longer able to fulfill its normal downward movement. It also brings the cold-phlegm up with it. This causes symptoms such as coughing and wheezing with urgent breathing, where one cannot lie flat. Since there is impairment of the Lung qi, this causes the already congested fluids to further accumulate, leading to more Lung counterflow. This type of acute exacerbation can easily occur if the patient catches a cold, or drinks or eats cold items such as ice cream or even an iced beverage. The wheezing is also caused by spasm (from cold), phlegm, and thin mucus.

In general, when there is not an acute exacerbation (such as from external contraction or overwork), the symptoms are not that severe. With proper modifications, this formula can address the chronic stage.

TREATMENT PRINCIPLE: There are two aspects. First, disperse the external pathogen. Second, warm the cold-phlegm and build up the Spleen and Kidneys by supporting the yang. One must adjust the formula based on the prevalence of the external pathogen and the acuteness of the counterflow.

MEDICINAL ANALYSIS

- Prepared Ephedrae Herba *(zhì má huáng)* (processed by water frying) is acrid, expelling, warming, and diffuses and opens the Lungs. Stir-frying it with water moderates the hot, acrid, and dispersing nature of this herb, making it better at calming the Lungs, and is best for sub-acute stages. Other forms of Ephedrae Herba *(má huáng)* may be considered. For example, unprocessed Ephedrae Herba *(má huáng)* is very pungent and is appropriate for very acute stages (aversion to cold, chills, fever, etc.) while honey-prepared Ephedrae Herba *(mì zhì má huáng)* is best for chronic asthma. While there is no real substitute for Ephedrae Herba *(má huáng)*, the following medicinals can be used to some effect if Ephedrae Herba *(má huáng)* is not available: Schizonepetae Herba *(jīng jiè)* for back pain, body pain, neck pain, headache, etc.; Perillae Folium *(zǐ sū yè)* for Lung issues (coughing, wheezing, chest pain).

---

12. This is usually a mixture of a genetic predisposition with an invasion of cold that damages the Spleen and thereby produces damp-turbidity.

- Cinnamomi Ramulus *(guì zhī)* is acrid, slightly sweet, and warm. It unblocks the yang, releases the muscle layer, and warms the middle burner.

- Together, prepared Ephedrae Herba *(zhì má huáng)* and Cinnamomi Ramulus *(guì zhī)* release the exterior and scatter cold. Ephedrae Herba *(má huáng)* works more on the protective layer/surface and Cinnamomi Ramulus *(guì zhī)* more on warming the nutritive and muscle layers and channels.

- Zingiberis Rhizoma *(gān jiāng)*, Asari Radix et Rhizoma *(xì xīn)*, and Schisandrae Fructus *(wǔ wèi zǐ)*, along with Pinelliae Rhizoma preparatum *(zhì bàn xià)*, transform internal phlegm and thin mucus.

  ⚠ Zhang Zhong-Jing often used the following three-herb synergistic combination for chronic cough and wheezing due to cold, thin mucus. One should be cautious about removing any of the ingredients so as not to disrupt the synergy.
  — Zingiberis Rhizoma *(gān jiāng)* enters the Spleen.
  — Asari Radix et Rhizoma *(xì xīn)* enters the Lung and Kidney.
  — Schisandrae Fructus *(wǔ wèi zǐ)* enters the Lung and Heart.

- Bland Zingiberis Rhizoma *(dàn gān jiāng)* is acrid and expelling, warms the yang, and eliminates cold in the middle burner. It is milder than Zingiberis Rhizoma *(gān jiāng)*, which may be too hot for this presentation.

- Schisandrae Fructus *(wǔ wèi zǐ)* is sour, slightly bitter, slightly warm, and moistens, astringes, and preserves the Lung qi. It balances the other dispersing and drying medicinals in the formula.

- Asari Radix et Rhizoma *(xì xīn)* is acrid, hot, and dry. It warms and disperses cold and dampness from the interior, tonifies the Kidney and Lung yang, and enters the organs as well as the deep collaterals. Unlike Ephedrae Herba *(má huáng)* and Cinnamomi Ramulus *(guì zhī)*, it does not really enter the muscle layer and superficial aspects, but assists them in expelling the cold, mainly from the deep regions outward. Usually 0.5-1.5g is enough.

- Pinelliae Rhizoma preparatum *(zhì bàn xià)* is bitter and acrid and directs the qi downward. It opens, expels, disperses, and dries.

- Stalactite *(é guǎn shí)*[13] warms the Lungs, quiets the Lung qi, and transforms phlegm and thin mucus. For example, it can firm up watery phlegm or moisten thick, glue-like phlegm, allowing the body to expectorate or transform it, as well as reduce the overall production of phlegm. From a biomedical perspective, it relaxes the bronchioles and spasms. If unavailable, one can substitute Stalactitum *(zhōng rǔ shí)* or White Quartz *(bái shí yīng)*. All three medicinals should be crushed and pre-cooked for 45 minutes.

Dr. Qin's formula is based on Minor Bluegreen Dragon Decoction *(xiǎo qīng lóng tāng)*. It should not be used for an extended period. One should switch to a less dispersing formula when the acute exacerbation is under control (see discussion below).

---

13. Nature: sweet, salty, warm, and nontoxic. Channels: Lung, Kidney, and Stomach.

Minor Bluegreen Dragon Decoction *(xiǎo qīng lóng tāng)*

SOURCE: *Discussion of Cold Damage* (c. 220)

Ephedrae Herba *(má huáng)* 9g
Cinnamomi Ramulus *(guì zhī)* 9g
Zingiberis Rhizoma *(gān jiāng)*. 9g
Asari Radix et Rhizoma *(xì xīn)* 9g
Schisandrae Fructus *(wǔ wèi zǐ)* 9g
Paeoniae Radix alba *(bái sháo)* 9g
Pinelliae Rhizoma preparatum *(zhì bàn xià)* 9g
Glycyrrhizae Radix preparata *(zhì gān cǎo)*. 9g

---

MODIFICATIONS OF DR. QIN'S FORMULA

Fullness in the chest:

Dry-fried Citri reticulatae Pericarpium *(chǎo chén pí)* 3-5g

Dry-fried Aurantii Fructus *(chǎo zhǐ ké)*. 4-6g

Severe asthma, unable to lie flat:

Prepared Perillae Fructus *(zhì zǐ sū zǐ)* 4-5g

Sinapis Semen *(bái jiè zǐ)* . . . . 3g (only a small dose)

Internal heat (e.g., irritability, thirst) with sweating or no sweating:

Gypsum fibrosum *(shí gāo)* . . . . 9-12g[14]

NOTES

- For pneumonia with bad cough and blood expectoration, one can use Ephedra, Apricot Kernel, Gypsum, and Licorice Decoction *(má xìng shí gān tāng)*. Do not use Cinnamomi Ramulus *(guì zhī)* because it works more interiorly and can cause more bleeding.

- Strong medicinals like Aconiti Radix lateralis preparata *(zhì fù zǐ)* should be avoided.

- These patients need to pay special attention to the weather, living conditions, and food choices. Their houses should face the sun, and the living environment should be warm and peaceful. When the weather changes, they should take extra measures to stay warm. They should avoid cold and uncooked foods, greasy and oily foods, seafood, and rich foods. They should eat foods that warm the stomach, such as fresh ginger and pepper (Piperis Fructus *[hú jiāo]*). They should also make great efforts to avoid the common cold and flu and give themselves proper opportunity to recover if they get sick.

QUESTIONS

1. Is this formula only suitable if there is a simultaneous external attack?

---

14. Gypsum fibrosum *(shí gāo)* is cold and acrid and is able to expel pathogens without locking them in, unlike other cold medicinals such as Gardeniae Fructus *(zhī zǐ)*, Coptidis Rhizoma *(huáng lián)*, Scutellariae Radix *(huáng qín)*, or Forsythiae Fructus *(lián qiào)*. Therefore, do not use the latter medicinals in this situation. One can add Gypsum fibrosum *(shí gāo)* whether or not there is sweating.

In general, this formula is for an acute presentation, but there does not have to be external contraction for its use. This is a very flexible formula that can be applied, with modifications, to very acute external contractions or to chronic cases with no acute presentation.

2. *Is this formula appropriate for deficient patients?*

This formula's presentation stems from an underlying pattern of yang deficiency. Furthermore, with the key principle of 'warming' phlegm and thin mucus, we know that it is suitable for deficient patients. However, the formula has a strong discharging and dispersing nature, and can damage the Lung and uproot the Kidney qi in the lower burner. One must measure the amount of deficiency against the formula's dispersing nature and adjust the dosages, choice of medicinals, and duration of use accordingly. In general, this formula is contraindicated for very deficient patients, especially without modification.

3. *The above modification mentioned that Gypsum fibrosum (shí gāo) can be used whether or not there is sweating. Why?*

Gypsum fibrosum *(shí gāo)* is used for a pattern of wind-cold with simultaneous internal heat. It has the unique ability to release pathogens from the muscle layer and to clear heat that is trapped within pathogenic fluids. Because of this, it can be used for conditions that involve either sweating or the absence of sweating. There are two pathodynamics worth understanding in regard to sweating in patterns of internal heat that combine with external cold:

A. SWEATING: There is heat in the muscle layer that is causing the sweating. Minor Bluegreen Dragon Decoction *(xiǎo qīng lóng tāng)* plus Gypsum fibrosum *(shí gāo)* eliminates the wind-cold pathogen plus the heat in the muscles. The sweating is thereby eliminated.

B. ABSENCE OF SWEATING: This is due to the heat blocking the body's ability to create a sweat. Minor Bluegreen Dragon Decoction *(xiǎo qīng lóng tāng)* plus Gypsum fibrosum *(shí gāo)* releases the heat and thereby causes a sweat, bringing about resolution.

4. *How can there be thirst in a condition coming from cold and phlegm and thin mucus?*

Chronic asthma patients, with phlegm and thin mucus, are generally not thirsty and do not like to drink. Nevertheless, some people will have a very wet, swollen, and greasy tongue, and also a dry mouth and thirst, and will only desire warm beverages. This is due to the phlegm/dampness/thin mucus (pathological fluids) blocking the body's normal fluid circulation. This thirst is not due to heat.

5. *Why is Stalactite (é guǎn shí) used instead of the usual Paeoniae Radix alba (bái sháo)?*

Minor Bluegreen Dragon Decoction *(xiǎo qīng lóng tāng)* usually contains Paeoniae Radix alba *(bái sháo)*, yet Dr. Qin decided to use Stalactite *(é guǎn shí)*. This demonstrates the urgency that may be present in this condition. Stalactite *(é guǎn shí)*, a stone, has a relatively strong effect in directing the qi downward, and thus quickly calms the situation. Of course, one must remain flexible, and if the patient has more damage to the yin and fluids, one may choose to use Paeoniae Radix alba *(bái sháo)* instead.

6. *After the branch is eliminated with this method, how should one proceed to address the chronic underlying pattern?*

After the branch is eliminated, one should switch to a more sustainable approach of tonifying the Spleen and Kidney yang, abiding by the adage from *Essentials from the Golden Cabinet:* "For patients with phlegm and thin mucus, use warm medicinals to harmonize." In general, diseases in the middle burner are relatively mild compared to those in the lower burner. Thus it is said, "For exterior thin mucus treat the Spleen. For interior thin mucus treat the Kidneys." The reference to exterior and interior here refers to the superficiality (lightness) or deepness of the disease, and not to external contraction and internal damage. Therefore, in mild conditions, warm the Spleen. In more severe conditions, warm the Kidneys.

One issue with treating phlegm and thin mucus patterns is that once you eliminate the pathogen, more is produced, because of the underlying yang deficiency. Thus, addressing the root, even while eliminating the pathogen, is essential. This brings up an important distinction between this type of condition and general coughing and wheezing diseases.

For example, although both conditions will have phlegm and possibly wheezing, their treatment strategies are different. In a phlegm and thin mucus condition, if one only transforms phlegm and thin mucus and normalizes the qi to stop the coughing and wheezing, the result will not be satisfactory. One must utilize a 'warming' strategy, which refers to addressing the root. Without this aspect, more phlegm and thin mucus will continue to be produced. Even if urgent, one must simultaneously treat the branch and root, thus incorporating a warming method.

Even after resolving an acute episode, such patients will frequently experience recurrent acute attacks. These may be due to external pathogens attacking or internal imbalances reaching a critical point, for example, an accumulation of severe and profuse phlegm congestion. The level of acute involvement must be carefully ascertained and the formula must be modified appropriately. Depending on the severity of the acute attack, there is a continuum of how much one needs to address the root (tonify) and branch (drain/expel). The more acute, the more drastic the modifications must be. For example, with clear signs of exterior wind-cold, one should switch to unprocessed Ephedrae Herba *(má huáng)*; with acute severe and profuse phlegm congestion (no exterior symptoms), one may add Three-Seed Decoction to Nourish One's Parents *(sān zǐ yǎng qīn tāng)*.

Here are a few considerations for the treatment of the more chronic stage.

A. One can modify the above formula:

    i. Be sure to use a processed form of Ephedrae Herba *(má huáng)*.

    ii. Remove Cinnamomi Ramulus *(guì zhī)* and add:
        Honey-prepared Farfarae Flos *(mì zhì kuǎn dōng huā)* 6g
        Gingko Semen *(bái guǒ)* 6g
        (crushed)

Mori Cortex *(sāng bái pí)* 6g
(if there is cough with sticky phlegm).

iii. Reduce the overall dose of the prescription or grind it into powder using a 2 tsp draft, twice a day.

iv. Add Citri reticulatae Pericarpium *(chén pí)* to rectify the qi and transform the phlegm.

B. An additional core formula to consider is Poria, Licorice, Schisandra, Ginger, and Asarum Decoction *(líng gān wǔ wèi jiāng xīn tāng).*[15] Key symptoms: thin and bubbly phlegm, chronic cough, wheezing.

Poria, Licorice, Schisandra, Ginger, and Asarum Decoction *(líng gān wǔ wèi jiāng xīn tāng)*

Poria *(fú líng)*
Glycyrrhizae Radix preparata *(zhì gān cǎo)*
Schisandrae Fructus *(wǔ wèi zǐ)*
Zingiberis Rhizoma *(gān jiāng)*
Asari Radix et Rhizoma *(xì xīn)*

MODIFICATIONS OF Poria, Licorice, Schisandra, Ginger, and Asarum Decoction *(líng gān wǔ wèi jiāng xīn tāng)*

Profuse phlegm, poor digestion, poor appetite:
add Pinelliae Rhizoma preparatum *(zhì bàn xià)* 6-9g
→ *this is then* Poria, Licorice, Schisandra, Ginger, Asarum, and Pinellia Decoction *(líng gān wǔ wèi jiāng xīn xià tāng).*

Frequent cough and clearing of throat:
add Armeniacae Semen *(xìng rén)* 6-9g
→ *this is then* Poria, Licorice, and Schisandra plus Ginger, Asarum, Pinellia, and Apricot Kernel Decoction *(líng gān wǔ wèi jiā jiāng xīn bàn xià xìng rén tāng).*

Constipation (from ascending Lung qi):
add steamed Rhei Radix et Rhizoma *(shú dà huáng)* 4-6g
→ *this is then* Poria, Licorice, and Schisandra plus Ginger, Asarum, Pinellia, Apricot Kernel, and Rhubarb Decoction *(líng gān wǔ wèi jiā jiāng xīn bàn xià xìng rén dà huáng tāng).*

Serious cough:
Inulae Flos *(xuán fù huā)* 4-6g

Stomach qi rebellion (i.e., hiccough):
Haematitum *(dài zhě shí)* 6-9g

---

15. Also consider the simple formula Poria, Cinnamon Twig, Atractylodes, and Licorice Decoction *(líng guì zhú gān tāng)*: Poria *(fú líng)*, Cinnamomi Ramulus *(guì zhī)*, Atractylodis macrocephalae Rhizoma *(bái zhú)*, and Glycyrrhizae Radix *(gān cǎo)*.

C. A formula like Kidney Qi Pill *(shèn qì wán)*[16] can be used.

D. If the chronic pattern is hotter in nature, consider using a modified Arrest Wheezing Decoction *(dìng chuǎn tāng).*[17]

7. *How do inhalers impact the presentation?*

Most inhalers are warm to hot, drying, and dispersing. Consequently, patients using inhalers may not present with the above presentation, even when they fit this pattern. That is, there may not be clear profuse phlegm, wet tongue, etc. Instead, their tongues may become dark pale or dark red on the tips and sides. However, since phlegm and thin mucus is essentially a Spleen and Kidney yang deficiency, one should still treat the root pattern even when the presentation might not match as clearly as someone who is not on inhalers. Although the inhalers may add some 'heat' signs and symptoms, they do not have to be addressed. Of course, if severe, one can include medicinals such as dry-fried Scutellariae Radix *(chǎo huáng qín)*, Lilii Bulbus *(bǎi hé)*, or Hedyotis diffusae Herba *(bái huā shé shé cǎo)*, but in general, one can ignore the mild heat presentation that may occur in such a situation.

8. *What is the difference between the previous treatment strategy—dry dampness and transform phlegm—and the treatment for the root of phlegm and thin mucus outlined above?*

Both situations are due to cold-dampness and phlegm. Thus both methods utilize warming strategies. However, while the dry dampness and transform phlegm method can be used for chronic presentations, it is usually used for transient situations where merely transforming dampness and eliminating phlegm achieves a result. On the other hand, phlegm and thin mucus is a chronic disease from Spleen yang weakness that has a chief symptom of wheezing. One must therefore strengthen the Spleen and support the yang in order stop the production of the turbid phlegm, and no temporary treatment of transforming phlegm will be able to resolve it.

---

6. Clear and Cause Phlegm-Heat to Descend (清降痰热 *qīng jiàng tán rè*)

[PRESENTATION] Ascending counterflow of phlegm-heat; the spirit is confounded and the qi is stopped up.[18]

Prepared Mori Cortex *(zhì sāng bái pí)*	2.4g
Aurantii Fructus immaturus *(zhǐ shí)*	4.5g
Bambusae Concretio silicea *(tiān zhú huáng)*	4.5g

---

16. Aconiti Radix lateralis preparata *(zhì fù zǐ)*, Cinnamomi Cortex *(ròu guì)*, Rehmanniae Radix preparata *(shú dì huáng)*, Dioscoreae Rhizoma *(shān yào)*, Corni Fructus *(shān zhū yú)*, Poria *(fú líng)*, Moutan Cortex *(mǔ dān pí)*, and Alismatis Rhizoma *(zé xiè)*.

17. Dry-fried Gingko Semen *(chǎo bái guǒ)*, Ephedrae Herba *(má huáng)*, Perillae Fructus *(zî sū zǐ)*, Glycyrrhizae Radix *(gān cǎo)*, Farfarae Flos *(kuǎn dōng huā)*, Armeniacae Semen *(xìng rén)*, prepared Mori Cortex *(zhì sāng bái pí)*, dry-fried Scutellariae Radix *(chǎo huáng qín)*, and Pinelliae Rhizoma preparatum *(zhì bàn xià)*.

18. This is a blockage that manifests physically. One can palpate the chest and the patient will report a sense of blockage.

Bambusae Succus *(zhú lì)*	10cc
Arisaema cum Bile *(dǎn nán xīng)*	4.5g
Trichosanthis Semen *(guā lóu rén)*	9g
Acori tatarinowii Rhizoma *(shí chāng pǔ)*	2.4g

COMMENTARY

ADDITIONAL SIGNS AND SYMPTOMS

- Headache
- Dizziness
- Blocked ears
- Cough and wheezing
- Intense emotions
- Restlessness
- Insomnia
- Constipation
- Dark urine with a strong odor
- Twitches or spasms of the face, scalp, lips, or eyes
- High blood pressure, especially after ingesting alcohol or spicy foods
- Pre-stroke conditions
- Epilepsy or Tourette's syndrome
- The pulse is floating, forceful, and slippery, especially in the distal position
- The tongue is fresh red with a thick and yellow or brown coating (like chocolate)

DISCUSSION

Symptoms primarily manifest in the upper burner and are less likely to manifest in the abdominal region. This is a potentially serious presentation and one should approach it with caution.

The previous methods (nos. 1-5) focus on the Lungs and Spleen with patterns that essentially manifest with some type of cough, wheezing, phlegm, or thin mucus. By contrast, this method treats phlegm-heat that combines with wind and gushes upward, harassing the head, eyes, and the mansion of the spirit radiance.

MEDICINAL ANALYSIS

- Prepared Mori Cortex *(zhì sāng bái pí)* and Arisaema cum Bile *(dǎn nán xīng)* are quick, moving, and fluid (smooth). They flush phlegm and transform heat. Prepared Mori Cortex *(zhì sāng bái pí)* is sweet, bitter, and cold, directs both qi and phlegm downward, alleviates cough, clears heat, promotes urination, and moistens the yin of the Lungs. Arisaema cum Bile *(dǎn nán xīng)* is bitter and cool, scatters wind, and clears phlegm and heat from the deep collaterals, making it appropriate for many entrenched problems such as stroke, seizures, epilepsy, mental disease, as well as menopause.

- Bambusae Concretio silicea *(tiān zhú huáng)* and Bambusae Succus *(zhú lì)* are cool (to cold), slippery, sweet, transform and scour out phlegm, cause phlegm heat to descend, stop cough, open the orifices, and enter the collaterals of the Lung. Although similar in function, both are selected because they form a powerful combination. Bambusae Concretio silicea *(tiān zhú huáng)* (bamboo sugar), slightly bitter, is able to dislodge phlegm, facilitating the expulsion of dry and difficult-to-remove phlegm. It also moistens the bowels and opens the orifices, removing phlegm-heat obstruction. Bambusae Succus *(zhú lì)* is colder and stronger than Bambusae Concretio silicea *(tiān zhú huáng)*, and thus one must be cautious because it can cause Stomach pain in patients with Spleen deficiency. It is more moving and better at penetrating the channels and collaterals. It is also better at facilitating the bowels. If unavailable, one might consider Lophatheri Herba *(dàn zhú yè)*.

- Acori tatarinowii Rhizoma *(shí chāng pǔ)* is warm, aromatic, mobile, and piercing and is good at transforming damp-turbidity, dislodging phlegm, diffusing congestion, opening the orifices, and clearing the mind.

- Aurantii Fructus immaturus *(zhǐ shí)* and Trichosanthis Semen *(guā lóu rén)* facilitate the functions of the Large Intestine in order to clear phlegm-heat through the bowels. Aurantii Fructus immaturus *(zhǐ shí)* directs qi downward. If the qi descends, the phlegm will also descend. Trichosanthis Semen *(guā lóu rén)* is moist and slippery and should be crushed.

Dr. Qin's formula is based on Guide Out Phlegm Decoction *(dǎo tán tāng)*.

Guide Out Phlegm Decoction *(dǎo tán tāng)*
SOURCE: *Formulas to Aid the Living* (1253)

Citri reticulatae Exocarpium rubrum *(jú hóng)* 3g
Pinelliae Rhizoma preparatum *(zhì bàn xià)* 6g
Poria *(fú líng)*. 3g
Glycyrrhizae Radix *(gān cǎo)*. 1.5g
Aurantii Fructus immaturus *(zhǐ shí)*. 3g
Arisaematis Rhizoma preparatum *(zhì tiān nán xīng)*
 or Arisaema cum Bile *(dǎn nán xīng)* 3g

---

MODIFICATIONS OF DR. QIN'S FORMULA

Constipation:

Steamed Rhei Radix et Rhizoma *(shú dà huáng)* 4.5g

Chloriti Lapis/Micae Lapis aureus *(méng shí)* 9g

Qi constraint/intense emotions (e.g., stress, sadness, or depression):

Curcumae Radix *(yù jīn)* 6g

Fritillariae cirrhosae Bulbus *(chuān bèi mǔ)* 3g

Bloating and gas:

Increase the dosage of Aurantii Fructus immaturus *(zhǐ shí)* to 9g

Pharbitidis Semen *(qiān niú zǐ)*. 6g
(especially for fullness in the chest and abdomen)

Gurgling sound of phlegm:

Fritillariae cirrhosae Bulbus *(chuān bèi mǔ)* . . . . 2-3g (powder)

Channels and collaterals are blocked:

Luffae Fructus Retinervus *(sī guā luò)*. 4-6g

---

7. Attack and Drive Out Phlegm Accumulation (攻逐痰积 *gōng zhú tán jī*)

[PRESENTATION] Phlegm and thin mucus twist together and accumulate; suspended thin mucus and propping thin mucus

Lepidii/Descurainiae Semen *(tíng lì zǐ)* 2.4g
Dry-fried Aurantii Fructus immaturus *(chǎo zhǐ shí)* 3g
Processed Genkwa Flos *(zhì yuán huā)* 2.4g
Dry-fried Plantaginis Semen *(chǎo chē qián zǐ)* 9g
Processed Kansui Radix *(zhì gān suì)* 2.4g
Alismatis Rhizoma *(zé xiè)*. 9g
Control Mucus Special Pill *(kòng xián dān)* . . . . 0.9g (swallowed)

COMMENTARY

This is a serious presentation with key manifestations of ascites, serious edema, or water accumulating under the ribs (pleurisy). A strong formula is therefore needed. This formula is a strong purgative that can bring about intense, watery diarrhea as well as promote urination.

Due to the potential toxicity of processed Kansui Radix *(zhì gān suì)* and processed Genkwa Flos *(zhì yuán huā)*, the forceful action of the formula, and the fact that these patients are usually under biomedical care, this formula is not commonly used in the West. In general, it is contraindicated for deficient or weak patients.

If, after administering this formula, there is severe diarrhea, cold rice porridge should be given. This formula should not be used long term.

MEDICINAL ANALYSIS

- Lepidii/Descurainiae Semen *(tíng lì zǐ)* is bitter and cold, forcefully descends and drains, moves water, dampness, and phlegm downward and out. It also has some ability to loosen the stool. This medicinal should only be used for an excess presentation. However, most pharmacies carry a processed version (often dry-fried), which moderates its effect.

- Dry-fried Aurantii Fructus immaturus *(chǎo zhǐ shí)* is bitter and descending, acrid and dispersing, and is able to transform phlegm by draining it. It also unblocks the bowels.

- Processed Kansui Radix *(zhì gān suì)* and processed Genkwa Flos *(zhì yuán huā)* fiercely drive out thin mucus. Both are toxic and should be used with caution.

- Dry-fried Plantaginis Semen *(chǎo chē qián zǐ)* is sweet and cold and facilitates the removal of dampness (and heat) through the urine.

- Alismatis Rhizoma *(zé xiè)* promotes urination and causes the pathogenic thin mucus to exit via the urine.

- Control Mucus Special Pill *(kòng xián dān)* is taken with the decoction and is very effective at attacking and driving out stubborn phlegm and suspended thin mucus. It contains Kansui Radix *(gān suì)*, Sinapis Semen *(bái jiè zǐ)*, and Euphorbiae pekinensis Radix *(jīng dà jǐ)*.

All of the above processing methods moderate the herbs, and reduce their toxicity.

Dr. Qin's formula is based on Ten-Jujube Decoction *(shí zǎo tāng)* and Descurainia and Jujube Decoction to Drain the Lungs *(tíng lì dà zǎo xiè fèi tāng)*.

Ten-Jujube Decoction *(shí zǎo tāng)*

SOURCE: *Discussion of Cold Damage* (c. 220)

▶ Grind equal amounts of the following into powder and take in 0.5-1g doses:

Kansui Radix *(gān suì)*
Euphorbiae pekinensis Radix *(jīng dà jǐ)*
Genkwa Flos *(yuán huā)*
Jujubae Fructus *(dà zǎo)*

Descurainia and Jujube Decoction to Drain the Lungs *(tíng lì dà zǎo xiè fèi tāng)*

SOURCE: *Essentials from the Golden Cabinet* (c. 220)

Lepidii/Descurainiae Semen *(tíng lì zǐ)* 9-12g
Jujubae Fructus *(dà zǎo)* 12p

ADDITIONAL CONSIDERATIONS

- If the condition is mild, one may consider using a Flushing Away Roiling Phlegm Pill *(gǔn tán wán)*[19] type of formula.

- If the phlegm and thin mucus are mild, simply use Lepidium/Descurainia and Jujube Decoction to Drain the Lungs *(tíng lì dà zǎo xiè fèi tang)*.

- If more serious, use Ten-Jujube Decoction *(shí zǎo tāng)*.

---

19. Chloriti Lapis *(qīng méng shí)*, Aquilariae Lignum resinatum *(chén xiāng)*, Rhei Radix et Rhizoma *(dà huáng)*, and Scutellariae Radix *(huáng qín)*.

8. **Disperse and Grind Away Phlegm Nodules** (消磨痰核 *xiāo mó tán hé*)

[PRESENTATION] Moveable subcutaneous phlegm nodules[20]

Bland Sargassum (*dàn hǎi zǎo*)	4.5g
Sinapis Semen (*bái jiè zǐ*)	4.5g
Bland Eckloniae Thallus (*dàn kūn bù*)	4.5g
Fritillariae thunbergii Bulbus (*zhè bèi mǔ*)	9g
Cremastrae/Pleiones Pseudobulbus (*shān cí gū*)	1.5g
Processed Bombyx batryticatus (*zhì bái jiāng cán*)	9g
Rhopilemae Umbrella (*hǎi zhé pí*)	30g
(pre-cook, discard medicinal, and use strained liquid)	

COMMENTARY

ADDITIONAL SIGNS AND SYMPTOMS

This method may be used for just phlegm nodules. However, there may also be other symptoms that relate to phlegm, as listed in the above methods. For example, many times there will also be:

- Symptoms related to poor Spleen circulation (such as poor appetite, or a good appetite with a feeling of blockage after eating)[21]
- Dark face
- Puffiness/edema
- Cloudy urine
- Mucus in the throat
- Incomplete bowel movements
- The pulse is soggy
- The tongue has a greasy coating

DISCUSSION

This method is suitable for phlegm qi that congeals leading to substantial phlegm nodules that can be located internally or on the skin. This can manifest in many ways, such as lipomas, goiter, scrofula, or even uterine myomas.

TREATMENT PRINCIPLE: This formula focuses primarily on the manifestation (branch), but many times there is an underlying root cause that must also be addressed. For example, scrofula can come about from turbid phlegm constraint and clumping coupled with Liver and Gallbladder qi constraint leading to fire. In that situation, one may modify the formula

---

20. A more literal translation of the original text is "flowing phlegm nodules that are located inside the skin and outside the membrane." This refers to a location that is not on the surface and not in the organs. It is in-between, for example, in the muscles, tissues (as in breast tissue), or lymph.

21. Poor Spleen circulation describes a general condition that can arise from multiple patterns such as Spleen yang, yin, or qi deficiency.

to treat both root and branch simultaneously. Therefore, one would soften hardness and disperse and grind down nodules, as well as dredge the Liver and regulate the qi. The phlegm nodule is the branch and Liver and Gallbladder qi constraint and fire is the root. There is often Liver involvement in this pattern; if so, one can add Bupleuri Radix *(chái hú)* or Prunellae Spica *(xià kū cǎo)*.

In general, this problem is difficult to cure with Chinese medicine and takes a minimum of six months of treatment.

MEDICINAL ANALYSIS

All of these medicinals are specific for eliminating nodules.

- Sargassum *(hǎi zǎo)* and Eckloniae Thallus *(kūn bù)* soften hardness and disperse clumping. Both are salty, cool, and are able to disperse phlegm. Bland Eckloniae Thallus *(dàn kūn bù)* works more on the qi aspect and Bland Sargassum *(dàn hǎi zǎo)* more on the blood aspect.

- Sinapis Semen *(bái jiè zǐ)* is very acrid, bitter, and warm, disperses phlegm, and breaks up stagnation of qi to dislodge phlegm. It may be too warm for long-term use. Therefore, after 1-2 months, one should substitute others herbs such as Arcae Concha *(wǎ léng zǐ)* 6-9g, Prunellae Spica *(xià kū cǎo)* 4-6g, or Gleditsiae Spina *(zào jiǎo cì)* 3-5g.

- Fritillariae thunbergii Bulbus *(zhè bèi mǔ)* and Cremastrae/Pleiones Pseudobulbus *(shān cí gū)* disperse and transform phlegm. Fritillariae thunbergii Bulbus *(zhè bèi mǔ)* is bitter, cool, and promotes the movement of qi. Cremastrae/Pleiones Pseudobulbus *(shān cí gū)* is bitter, cool, and toxic yet is able to remove toxins. However, it should not be taken for an extended period of time. It can cause nausea and vomiting in some people.

- Bombyx batryticatus *(bái jiāng cán)* is salty, slightly cool, transforms phlegm, and opens the channels and deep collaterals.

- Rhopilemae Umbrella (海蜇皮 *hǎi zhé pí*—jellyfish) is cold, acrid, salty, and enters the Lungs and Kidneys. It softens hardness, scatters clumps, moves through stasis, transforms phlegm, and transforms accumulation. If not available, one may substitute Arisaema cum Bile *(dǎn nán xīng)* 4.5g.
    —*Preparation:* Cut into small pieces, fry in water for 15-20 minutes, discard jellyfish, and then use the water to decoct the remaining herbs.

- Bombyx batryticatus *(bái jiāng cán)* is acrid, salty, and neutral. It transforms phlegm, disperses clumping, softens hardness, and dissipates nodules, and is specifically used for scrofula and phlegm nodules.

MODIFICATIONS OF DR. QIN'S FORMULA

**Breast nodules especially evident before the menstrual period
(caused by Liver qi constraint):**

   Dry-fried Bupleuri Radix *(chǎo chái hú)* 3g

"Stressed out," angry, or intense emotions:

Prunellae Spica *(xià kū cǎo)*. 6g

Poor digestion:

Unprocessed Gigeriae galli Endothelium corneum *(jī nèi jīn)*[22]. 6g

Immobile nodules:

Arcae Concha *(wǎ léng zǐ)*. 6g

Internal nodules (such as uterine myoma):

Trogopterori Faeces *(wǔ líng zhī)*[23]. 6g

Angelicae sinensis radicis Cauda *(dāng guī wěi)*[24]. 4.5g

Aid in dissolving nodules:

Gleditsiae Spina *(zào jiǎo cì)*. 4.5g

Liquidambaris Fructus *(lù lù tōng)*. 4.5g

Vaccariae Semen *(wáng bù liú xíng)*. 6g

---

22. Unprocessed Gigeriae galli Endothelium corneum *(jī nèi jīn)* also dissolves nodules.

23. For phlegm and blood stasis mixed together.

24. Enters the collaterals.

2

Treatment Guidelines for

Food Stagnation 食 *(shí)*

ETIOLOGY Loss of dietary restraint, inability of the Spleen and Stomach to digest, and/or accumulation and stagnation in the middle

Many Westerners are prone to food stagnation due to such factors as poor dietary choices, irregular eating times, eating too quickly, and overeating. Many times there is accompanying difficulty in the ability of the Spleen and Stomach to properly digest food, stemming from Spleen deficiency. The combination of these two factors leads to a blockage and stagnation in the middle burner. Therefore, most sufferers, in addition to having an obvious food component, will have some internal disharmony allowing the problem to manifest.

MANIFESTATIONS Chest and diaphragm focal distention and fullness, acid regurgitation, belching up a rotten egg smell, aversion to food, and headache

Other typical symptoms include tenderness at CV-12 *(zhōng wǎn)* (see below), gas, constipation, nausea or vomiting, heartburn, relatively thick tongue coating (almost always present), or no desire to eat.

Diagnosing food stagnation is usually relatively clear-cut because of the unambiguous disease causes (listed above). However, some people will not present with the typical picture and may not report any abdominal symptoms. Instead, they may have a chief complaint such as sore throat or cough, or either headaches or dizziness after eating. The latter two complaints are special diagnostic symptoms caused by a middle burner blockage, as originally discussed by Li Dong-Yuan. Therefore, one must thoroughly investigate accompanying signs, symptoms, and etiology.

PALPATION

Upon palpation, almost all people with food stagnation will have an uncomfortable or painful sensation at CV-12 (*zhōng wǎn*) and sometimes at CV-8 *(shén què)*. The location that is more tender will help determine where the stagnation is located. For example, a tender CV-12 (*zhōng wǎn*) will suggest stagnation occurring predominantly in the upper abdomen (Stomach), while tenderness at CV-8 *(shén què)* points to stagnation occurring more in the lower burner (Intestines). This differentiation helps determine the correct method of treatment as well as helping to fine tune herb choices.

Furthermore, when pressing on CV-12 (*zhōng wǎn*) there may be a sensation of radiating pain or movement from the palpated area to the throat, back, chest, or different areas of the abdomen. This represents qi stagnation Stomach pain, where food stagnation has led to qi stagnation. Many times, there will be some acid regurgitation with this presentation. This demonstrates a more serious condition compared to a nonradiating, local sensation.

> **PULSE MANIFESTATIONS**
> * Floating and large, but choppy when pressed; or slippery and rapid; or, for long-standing food stagnation, slippery and slow

While this is an acute presentation with a floating pulse, it is not an externally-contracted disease. In an acute food stagnation pattern one may see a slight headache, slight nausea, slight aversion to wind, and possibly a low fever (below 38°C or 100.4°F) with a floating pulse. This is not an external attack. One may rule out an external attack based upon the following:

* Recent eating habits

* With external contraction the distal position is more floating, and with acute food stagnation the distal position should be relatively normal and the middle position will be more floating.

* In addition, one will observe other signs and symptoms such as those listed above. For example, tenderness at CV-12 (*zhōng wǎn*), thick tongue coating, and bad breath can confirm a diagnosis of food stagnation. These signs are especially useful in children.

NOTE: Sometimes there will be a floating pulse in chronic stages of food stagnation. However, this will usually only occur in the middle position.

> * A tight pulse reflects cold-food stoppage and stagnation.

This may be acute or chronic. Acute situations are often preceded by excessive consumption of cold foods. The pulse will also be floating and there is usually pain at CV-12 (*zhōng wǎn*).

> * A deep, tight, and thin pulse reflects long-standing food adhering and stagnating such that the Stomach qi cannot properly move.

There is usually long-term Spleen cold with cold food stagnation and deep pain when palpating CV-12 *(zhōng wǎn)*.

> • A choppy pulse reflects Spleen deficiency, where the Spleen is unable to rally its essence. It may also correspond to Stomach deficiency where the Stomach is unable to decompose water and grains.

OTHER IMPORTANT PULSE QUALITIES

If the pulse is soggy or blurred[1] there are usually complicating factors such as food stagnation, qi stagnation, dampness, and/or phlegm mixed together.

> **TREATMENT METHOD**
> Induction of vomiting, reduction, or purge

1. **Vomiting** eliminates pathogenic substances via the upper digestive tract. This is used for stagnation in the upper part of the body. One of the two commonly-used formulas is Melon Pedicle Powder *(guā dì sǎn)*, which is given when something substantial is in the Stomach cavity, such as deep-seated stagnant food, phlegm, or congested fluids. The other is Gardenia and Prepared Soybean Decoction *(zhī zǐ chǐ tāng)*, which is used to treat symptoms that are primarily due to emotional considerations. If these are not available, one may instruct the patient to drink rice milk or 9% salted water[2]. Then use a chicken feather coated with olive oil to touch the throat so as to induce vomiting.

2. **Reduction** breaks up and removes stagnation such as food, dampness, phlegm, qi, blood, mucus, etc. This is an important step, because without first removing the stagnation, one cannot tonify the Spleen.

3. **Purging** eliminates pathological substances via the bowels and is used in food stagnation patterns with high fever, constipation, etc. The Order the Qi Decoction *(chéng qì tāng)* family of formulas is useful here.

Note: Vomiting and purging methods are not used that often. Reduction is the most commonly used method in the clinic.

This chapter essentially deals with various patterns of food stagnation. However, these methods may be combined with other methods to treat other causes of stagnation (e.g. dampness), where removing stagnation from the Intestines is a necessary first step.

---

1. Blurred pulse (模糊 *mó hu*) is a description used by Dr. Qin. It feels soft, soggy, and difficult to move. It feels like the surface of the vessel is covered by a tissue and thus one is unable to feel the surface of the pulse clearly. It also can mean that sometimes the pulse is clear and sometimes it is difficult to find. It is usually caused by a combination of etiological factors that are stagnating together, such as qi, dampness, food, and phlegm. A soggy pulse is usually just dampness.

2. This is to guard against fluid depletion, hardening of undigested food, heat-phlegm becoming sticky and stagnating, and impeded dry retching. Rice milk specifically protects the gastric mucosa from damage and salt water can dilute heat-phlegm and undigested food in order to facilitate vomiting.

1. Reduce[i] Food [Stagnation] and Transform Accumulation
(消食化积 *xiāo shí huà jī*)

[PRESENTATION] Stoppage by food stagnation; focal distention in the gastric cavity with aversion to food

Raphani Semen *(lái fú zǐ)* 9g
dry-fried Aurantii Fructus *(chǎo zhǐ ké)* 4.5g
scorched Crataegi Fructus *(jiāo shān zhā)* 9g
Citri reticulatae viride Pericarpium *(qīng pí)* 4.5g
Massa medicata fermentata *(shén qū)* 9g
scorched Hordei Fructus germinatus *(jiāo mài yá)* 9g
Chrysomyiae Larva *(wǔ gǔ chóng)* 4.5g

COMMENTARY

ADDITIONAL SIGNS AND SYMPTOMS

- Bad breath
- Belching and nausea
- There is usually a subjective feeling of fullness and pain in the epigastrium.
- The tongue has a red body with a yellow coating
- The pulse is floating (especially in the middle), edgy (distal), and rapid

DISCUSSION

PALPATION: The area around CV-12 *(zhōng wǎn)* usually has obvious discomfort, while CV-8 *(shén què)* does not. This presentation shows that stagnation is only in the middle burner, specifically the Stomach.

ETIOLOGY: There is usually a clear history of overeating or eating too many types of foods at one time, such as at holidays or banquets.

DURATION: This is usually an acute presentation; however, this method can be used for some chronic situations.

LOCATION: Stomach/epigastrium

TREATMENT PRINCIPLE: One aspect is to reduce and guide out food accumulation, another is to regulate the qi and build up the Stomach.

This formula can be taken prophylactically, for example, before one goes to a party.

MEDICINAL ANALYSIS

- Dry-fried Aurantii Fructus *(chǎo zhǐ ké)* and Citri reticulatae viride Pericarpium *(qīng pí)* both regulate the qi and build up the Stomach.

1. Reduce Food (Stagnation) and Transform Accumulation

- Citri reticulatae viride Pericarpium *(qīng pí)* is acrid, bitter, and warms and regulates the Stomach and Intestines. It is especially good if there is flank distention or discomfort, although this symptomology is not necessary for its use. Dry-fried Aurantii Fructus *(chǎo zhǐ ké)* is acrid, neutral, and tonifies the Spleen's circulation (regulates and harmonizes the Spleen and Stomach qi) and can directly reduce food stagnation.

- Raphani Semen *(lái fú zǐ)*, scorched Crataegi Fructus *(jiāo shān zhā)*, dry-fried Massa medicata fermentata *(chǎo shén qū)*, scorched Hordei Fructus germinatus *(jiāo mài yá)*, and Chrysomyiae Larva *(wǔ gǔ chóng)* all reduce food stagnation. Raphani Semen *(lái fú zǐ)* is slightly acrid, slightly warm, and guides the qi downward and out (especially if dry-fried). Scorched Crataegi Fructus *(jiāo shān zhā)* is sour, slightly warm, and reduces food stagnation, especially from meat and protein. Although it strengthens the Spleen's circulation, it does not promote the movement of qi.

- Massa medicata fermentata *(shén qū)* is acrid, bitter, warm, and reduces food stagnation. However, Dr. Wu prefers dry-fried Massa medicata fermentata *(chǎo shén qū)*, which is best for this situation, and is better at aiding digestion, regulating the Liver qi, and tonifying the Spleen. Dry-frying enables it to work more internally, whereas unprocessed Massa medicata fermentata *(shén qū)* is best if there is some exterior involvement. Consider wrapping it in a filter if the unprocessed form is used.

- Scorched Hordei Fructus germinatus *(jiāo mài yá)* raises the Spleen qi.

- Chrysomyiae Larva *(wǔ gǔ chóng)*[ii] is especially good for children with food accumulation. One may consider grinding it into a powder so as not to offend the patient and then boiling the powder together with the other herbs. If this is unavailable, then Aspongopus *(jiǔ xiāng chóng)* 4.5g can be substituted. If that is also not available, then the next best is prepared Gigeriae galli Endothelium corneum *(zhì jī nèi jīn)* 4.5g.

Summary of common food stagnation herbs that can be used for individualized modifications

Crataegi Fructus (*shān zhā*)	for meat/protein stagnation
Hordei Fructus germinatus (*mài yá*)	for rice/grain/bread/noodle stagnation
Massa medicata fermentata (*shén qū*)	for vegetable or fruit stagnation
Gigeriae galli Endothelium corneum (*jī nèi jīn*)	for all types of stagnation, but especially from oily foods
Arecae Semen (*bīng láng*)	to guide everything out, pass gas, and move downward

Dr. Qin's formula is based on Preserve Harmony Pill *(bǎo hé wán)*.

Preserve Harmony Pill *(bǎo hé wán)*

SOURCE: *Essential Teachings of [Zhu] Dan-Xi* (1481)

Crataegi Fructus *(shān zhā)* 180g (9-15g)
Massa medicata fermentata *(shén qū)* 60g (9-12g)
Raphani Semen *(lái fú zǐ)* 30g (6-9g)
Citri reticulatae Pericarpium *(chén pí)* 30g (6-9g)
Pinelliae Rhizoma preparatum *(zhì bàn xià)* 90g (9-12g)
Poria *(fú líng)* 90g (9-12g)
Forsythiae Fructus *(lián qiào)* 30g (3-6g)

MODIFICATIONS OF DR. QIN'S FORMULA

Nausea (from cold):

Zingiberis Rhizoma recens *(shēng jiāng)*

. . . . 2 slices or add ginger liquid to decoction

Nausea (from heat):

Bambusae Caulis in taeniam *(zhú rú)* 4-6g

Abdominal distention and fullness:

Arecae Pericarpium *(dà fù pí)* 6-9g

Arecae Semen *(bīng láng)* 6-9g

Dry-fried Pharbitidis Semen *(chǎo qiān niú zǐ)* 6-9g

**Sensation of feeling stuck (CV-12 [*zhōng wǎn*] area) and
difficulty belching (with dampness)**

Magnoliae officinalis Cortex *(hòu pò)* . . . . 4-6g (see Questions below)

Citri sarcodactylis Fructus *(fó shǒu)* 3-5g

Prepared medicines:

• Scorched Three Immortals *(jiāo sān xiān)* [scorched Crataegi Fructus *(jiāo shān zhā)*, scorched Hordei Fructus germinatus *(jiāo mài yá)*, scorched Massa medicata fermentata *(jiāo shén qū)*]

• Scorched Four Immortals *(jiāo sì xiān)* [Scorched Three Immortals *(jiāo sān xiān)* + Gigeriae galli Endothelium corneum *(jī nèi jīn)*] — used when a stronger formula is needed, or more emphasis on oily foods is necessary

• Scorched Five Immortals *(jiāo wǔ xiān)* [Scorched Four Immortals *(jiāo sì xiān)* + dry-fried Arecae Semen *(chǎo bīng láng)*] — used when there is more qi stagnation, with fullness and gas

PREPARATION AND DOSAGE: Grind into powder (equal amount of all ingredients) 1 teaspoon in ½ cup of warm water, steep for 5-7 minutes. Drink 30-40 minutes before eating, 2-3x/day.

1. Reduce Food (Stagnation) and Transform Accumulation

FORMULAS' SOURCE: To our knowledge, these formulas are not recorded in any major formulary. They can be considered folk remedies used by Drs. Qin and Wu.

This approach can be used either as a preventative (e.g., before a big holiday dinner) or as a treatment. One should modify ingredients and dosage based on the individual's particular diet and presentation. These are especially good for kids, the elderly, cancer patients, and post-surgery, although they can be added into anyone's regimen.

QUESTIONS

1. *Could one also add Magnoliae officinalis Cortex (hòu pò) as a modification for abdominal distention and fullness?*

   Using Magnoliae officinalis Cortex *(hòu pò)* in this situation is not appropriate. It is too light and best suited for dampness (e.g., greasy tongue coating and stifling sensation in the chest), not for food stagnation, and in general is best for deficiency distention (soft pulse, pale, swollen tongue). If combined with Aurantii Fructus immaturus *(zhǐ shí)* (4-6g), it may be more suitable. The above modifications—(Arecae Pericarpium *(dà fù pí)*, Arecae Semen *(bīng láng)*, and dry-fried Pharbitidis Semen *(chǎo qiān niú zǐ)*—are stronger than Magnoliae officinalis Cortex *(hòu pò)* and are more appropriate here.

2. *Why does Dr. Qin choose to use Citri reticulatae viride Pericarpium (qīng pí) instead of Citri reticulatae Pericarpium (chén pí)?*

   Citri reticulatae Pericarpium *(chén pí)* circulates and regulates the qi while Citri reticulatae viride Pericarpium *(qīng pí)* is stronger and is able to break up qi stagnation. This is very important for the elimination of food stagnation in this pattern. Although Citri reticulatae Pericarpium *(chén pí)* focuses on the middle burner and one could add this to the prescription, it would be incorrect to use it instead of Citri reticulatae viride Pericarpium *(qīng pí)* here.

3. *Are there any additional preparation methods to consider for this pattern?*

   Yes. One could use a dry-frying method for Raphani Semen *(lái fú zǐ)*, Massa medicata fermentata *(shén qū)*, and Citri reticulatae viride Pericarpium *(qīng pí)*. In general, dry-frying or scorching can enhance the ability of these herbs to work on the digestion and reduce food stagnation.

4. *It is noted above that Dr. Qin's formula, as well as the above-mentioned patents, can be taken prophylatically before a large meal. Why?*

   Actually, one can take this formula before eating, during meals, or even after eating. Taking it beforehand helps the digestion prepare for the food, by increasing the body's ability to produce enzymes when needed. Taking it with food, or after, will allow the herbs to directly work on the food, picking up the slack of the body's own digestive ability.

2. Purging Food Accumulation (攻下食积 *gōng xià shí jī*)

[PRESENTATION] Food stagnation in the Intestines and Stomach; abdominal pain and constipation

Dry-fried Aurantii Fructus immaturus *(chǎo zhǐ shí)*	4.5g
Sennae Folium *(fān xiè yè)*	2.4g
Natrii Sulfas siccatus *(xuán míng fěn)*	2.4g
Raphani Semen *(lái fú zǐ)*	9g
Arecae Semen *(bīng láng)*	4.5g
Scorched Crataegi Fructus *(jiāo shān zhā)*	9g
Citri reticulatae Pericarpium *(chén pí)*	4.5g

COMMENTARY

ADDITIONAL SIGNS AND SYMPTOMS

• Bloating and gas (with or without an inability to pass gas)

• Abdominal tightness, distention, and fullness

• Constipation that may persist for 3-7 days, or passing only a small amount of sticky or smelly stool

• Constitutionally, these patients have a propensity toward constipation or sticky stools.

• May have frequent urination, urinary blockage,[iii] or strong-smelling urine.

• Typically, symptoms such as nausea and vomiting are not present.

• The pulse is forceful and floating in middle positions

• The tongue body is red or dark red with a brown coating, which may be a little black on the surface, showing that the food stagnation has created toxins.

DISCUSSION

This is an excess presentation and is more severe than the one for which the previous method was indicated. The simple method of reducing and guiding out is not sufficient. One must reduce and guide out while simultaneously purging. This will assist in directing the qi downward to eliminate the fullness. Thus, compared with the previous method, stronger medicinals are required.

PALPATION: CV-8 *(shén què)* is more painful than CV-12 *(zhōng wǎn)*.

LOCATION: Lower abdomen (Intestines)

DURATION: While this formula is primarily used for chronic conditions, it can also be used for acute problems.

MEDICINAL ANALYSIS

- Dry-fried Aurantii Fructus immaturus *(chǎo zhǐ shí)* is bitter, acrid, and promotes the movement of qi downward, unblocking the bowels, and reduces food stagnation.

- Sennae Folium *(fān xiè yè)* is bitter, cold, and mildly promotes the bowels and guides the qi downward.

- Natrii Sulfas siccatus *(xuán míng fěn)* is salty and cold and draws fluids into the Intestines, making the stool more slippery. It should be dissolved into the strained decoction. If not available, one can substitute powdered Natrii Sulfas *(máng xiāo)*; however, Natrii Sulfas siccatus *(xuán míng fěn)* is best for food stagnation.

- Raphani Semen *(lái fú zǐ)* is slightly acrid, slightly warm, reduces food stagnation, and guides the qi downward and out.

- Arecae Semen *(bīng láng)* promotes the movement of qi downward and unblocks the bowels. It is especially important if there is abdominal fullness, distention, and gas.

- Scorched Crataegi Fructus *(jiāo shān zhā)* is sour, slightly warm, and reduces food stagnation, especially from meat and protein. Although it strengthens the Spleen's circulation, it does not promote the movement of qi.

- Citri reticulatae Pericarpium *(chén pí)* promotes the movement of qi in the Spleen and Stomach.

Dr. Qin's formula is based on Major Order the Qi Decoction *(dà chéng qì tāng)* and Unripe Bitter Orange Pill to Guide Out Stagnation *(zhǐ shí dǎo zhì wán)*.

Major Order the Qi Decoction *(dà chéng qì tāng)*
SOURCE: *Discussion of Cold Damage* (c. 220)

Rhei Radix et Rhizoma *(dà huáng)* 12g
Natrii Sulfas *(máng xiāo)* 9-12g
Aurantii Fructus immaturus *(zhǐ shí)*. 12-15g
Magnoliae officinalis Cortex *(hòu pò)* 24g

---

Unripe Bitter Orange Pill to Guide Out Stagnation *(zhǐ shí dǎo zhì wán)*
SOURCE: *Clarifying Doubts about Damage from Internal and External Causes* (1247)

Dry-fried Aurantii Fructus immaturus *(chǎo zhǐ shí)* 15g
Rhei Radix et Rhizoma *(dà huáng)* 30g (6-9g)
Dry-fried Massa medicata fermentata *(chǎo shén qū)* 15g
Poria *(fú líng)*. 9g
Scutellariae Radix *(huáng qín)*. 9g
Coptidis Rhizoma *(huáng lián)*. 9g
Atractylodis macrocephalae Rhizoma *(bái zhú)* 9g
Alismatis Rhizoma *(zé xiè)* 6g

MODIFICATIONS OF DR. QIN'S FORMULA

Severe constipation:

Steamed Rhei Radix et Rhizoma *(shú dà huáng)* 4.5g

   (instead of, or in addition to, Sennae Folium *(fān xiè yè)*)

Arecae Pericarpium *(dà fù pí)* 6-9g

Dry-fried Pharbitidis Semen *(chǎo qiān niú zǐ)* (crushed) 9g

If the bowels are sticky and smelly:

Charred Rhei Radix et Rhizoma *(dà huáng tàn)* 6g

Severe abdominal fullness:

Arecae Pericarpium *(dà fù pí)* 4-6g

Abdominal fullness with no desire to eat:

Aucklandiae Radix *(mù xiāng)* 4-6g

QUESTIONS

1. Why does Dr. Qin use Citri reticulatae Pericarpium (chén pí) in this formula while using the stronger Citri reticulatae viride Pericarpium (qīng pí) in the previous one?

This prescription contains other strong medicinals for breaking and removing, so the additional strength of Citri reticulatae viride Pericarpium *(qīng pí)* is not needed here. Furthermore, not using Citri reticulatae viride Pericarpium *(qīng pí)* (as well as other harsher herbs) keeps the formula more mild. Obviously, any formula that purges must use stronger herbs, but the herbs in this case are chosen very specifically so that the formula will be well-balanced and therefore appropriate for weaker or elderly patients. Citri reticulatae Pericarpium *(chén pí)* performs the function of circulating qi without breaking up areas of qi stagnation. Citri reticulatae viride Pericarpium *(qīng pí)* is simply not necessary here.

2. If this formula is based on Major Order the Qi Decoction (dà chéng qì tāng), then why does Dr. Qin choose not to use Rhei Radix et Rhizoma (dà huáng), especially when the chief manifestation is constipation?

Dr. Qin chooses to use Sennae Folium *(fān xiè yè)* instead of Rhei Radix et Rhizoma *(dà huáng)* because it is milder, thus keeping the formula from being overly harsh. Consequently, it can be used for the elderly, children, cancer patients, etc. Of course, one could add Rhei Radix et Rhizoma *(dà huáng)* to increase the strength of the formula, if necessary.

3. Could one use medicinals like Hordei Fructus germinatus (mài yá) and Setariae (Oryzae) Fructus germinatus (gǔ yá)?

This class of medicinals is too mild for this presentation. Even though they treat food stagnation, the method here is to move things out as quickly as possible. These herbs do not have a moving function, which is necessary for this method.

3. Reinforce the Spleen and Reduce Food Stagnation
(助脾消食 *zhù pí xiāo shí*)

[PRESENTATION] Spleen and Stomach weakness; food accumulation, difficult digestion, dull Stomach, and absence of hunger

Unripe Bitter Orange and Atractylodes Pill *(zhǐ zhú wán)* 9g
    [Atractylodis macrocephalae Rhizoma *(bái zhú)* plus
    Aurantii Fructus immaturus *(zhǐ shí)*]
Pinelliae Rhizoma preparatum *(zhì bàn xià)* 4.5g
Arecae Pericarpium *(dà fù pí)* 9g
Citri reticulatae Pericarpium *(chén pí)* 4.5g
Amomi Fructus *(shā rén)* 2.4g
Gigeriae galli Endothelium corneum *(jī nèi jīn)* 9g
Setariae (Oryzae) Fructus germinatus *(gǔ yá)* /
    Hordei Fructus germinatus *(mài yá)* . . . . 9g (each)

COMMENTARY

ADDITIONAL SIGNS AND SYMPTOMS

• Sensation of bloating and distention with the consumption of small amounts of food
• Little desire to eat with a sensation of something stuck in the stomach
• Other typical Spleen deficiency signs (e.g., fatigue, loose stools, etc.)
• The pulse is soft and deep in the right middle position; overall choppiness
• The tongue is swollen, pale, wet; teeth marks

DISCUSSION

The patient will be sensitive to small deviations in their normal diet or eating habits, stressful events, or to foods that are not problematic for people with normal digestive systems, such as slightly cool or greasy foods. Therefore, strengthening the Spleen is essential to remove the accumulation of food stagnation.

PALPATION: The area around CV-12 *(zhōng wǎn)* will feel soft or empty. However, the patient will often mention that they feel blocked in this area, even to the point of feeling as if there is a nodule there. In addition, after eating, this area will commonly be more painful on palpation.

LOCATION: Spleen and Stomach

DURATION: This is usually a chronic pattern.

PATHODYNAMIC: This is essentially a deficient pattern with some accumulated excess. There is Spleen qi deficiency, which leads to loss of ability to transport. This usually precedes the food stagnation. The food stagnation in this case is usually not from overeating, but from the inability of the Spleen and Stomach to digest and transport.

ETIOLOGY: Many times there is a genetic component and parents will have a similar presentation. Also, some problems such as parasites, bacteria, or food poisoning can damage the Spleen and lead to this type of chronic pattern.

TREATMENT PRINCIPLE: The primary focus is to tonify the Spleen, but as food stagnation has already developed, one should also gently reduce and guide it out. However, harsh methods such as breaking up areas of qi stagnation should not be used.

MEDICINAL ANALYSIS

SUMMARY

This formula has four functions:

1. Tonify the Spleen
2. Dry dampness
3. Mobilize food stagnation
4. Regulate the Spleen qi

INDIVIDUAL CHARACTERISTICS

- Atractylodis macrocephalae Rhizoma *(bái zhú)* and Aurantii Fructus immaturus *(zhǐ shí)* work together to tonify the Spleen and guide out food stagnation.

- Pinelliae Rhizoma preparatum *(zhì bàn xià)* is acrid, bitter, warm, and dries dampness. It also restores the normal movement of Stomach qi, which often starts to rebel upward when accumulation (e.g., dampness, food stagnation, qi stagnation) occurs in the middle burner.

- Arecae Pericarpium *(dà fù pí)* is bitter, acrid, and warm, guides qi, food, water, and dampness downward (as it helps promote bowel movements), and is especially good for bloating, gas, and distention. It has no tonifying ability.

- Citri reticulatae Pericarpium *(chén pí)* is acrid and bitter. It circulates and regulates qi in the middle.

- Amomi Fructus *(shā rén)* is acrid and slightly warm. It regulates the qi and opens the Stomach.

- Gigeriae galli Endothelium corneum *(jī nèi jīn)*, Setariae (Oryzae) Fructus germinatus *(gǔ yá)*, and Hordei Fructus germinatus *(mài yá)* all reduce food stagnation.

- In their unprocessed form, Setariae (Oryzae) Fructus germinatus *(gǔ yá)* and Hordei Fructus germinatus *(mài yá)* have the additional ability to raise the Spleen qi, tonifying the Spleen qi and yin. When stir-fried, they are more effective in removing food stagnation.

- Gigeriae galli Endothelium corneum *(jī nèi jīn)* strengthens the Spleen and has a general ability to increase the digestion of all foods, especially oily foods. However, prepared Gigeriae galli Endothelium corneum *(zhì jī nèi jīn)* can be used to enhance its function of reducing food stagnation.

Note on dosage: Because the treatment course may take a long time, it is usually helpful to moderate the dosage. For example, instead of the standard decoction, one may choose to grind the formula into a powder, giving two teaspoons steeped in hot water twice a day, 30-40 minutes before meals. Another possibility is to make the herbs into cakes to be eaten. These methods are not only more manageable for long-term use, but easier on the Spleen.

Dr. Qin's formula is based on Scorched Four Immortals (*jiāo sì xiān*) and Unripe Bitter Orange and Atractylodes Pill (*zhǐ zhú wán*).[3]

Scorched Four Immortals (*jiāo sì xiān*)

SOURCE: To our knowledge, this formula is not recorded in any major texts. It is a folk remedy collected by Drs. Qin and Wu.

Crataegi Fructus (*shān zhā*)
Hordei Fructus germinatus (*mài yá*)
Massa medicata fermentata (*shén qū*)
Gigeriae galli Endothelium corneum (*jī nèi jīn*)

Unripe Bitter Orange and Atractylodes Pill (*zhǐ zhú wán*)

SOURCE: *Clarifying Doubts about Damage from Internal and External Causes* (1247)

Atractylodis macrocephalae Rhizoma (*bái zhú*) 4.5g
Aurantii Fructus immaturus (*zhǐ shí*) 4.5g
  (Made into pills with rice fried in Nelumbinis Folium [*hé yè*])

MODIFICATIONS OF DR. QIN'S FORMULA

Hot and burning sensation in the Stomach (i.e., acid reflux):

Left Metal Pill (*zuǒ jīn wán*)

  CAPSULE: Coptidis Rhizoma (*huáng lián*) 60g

  Evodiae Fructus (*wú zhū yú*) 10g

  (grind into powder and put 0.3g into each capsule)

  DECOCTION: Dry-fried Coptidis Rhizoma (*chǎo huáng lián*) 3g

  Evodiae Fructus (*wú zhū yú*) 0.5g

Severe distention and fullness:

Dry-fried Arecae Semen (*chǎo bīng láng*) 4-6g

(*note:* the unprocessed form is too strong)

Cold predominates:

Aucklandiae Radix (*mù xiāng*) 4-6g

Heat predominates:

Eupatorii Herba (*pèi lán*) 3-5g

---

3. Dr. Qin also liked Eight-Ingredient Pill to Regulate the Middle (*bā wèi lǐ zhōng wán*). Source: *Systematic Great Compendium of Medicine Past and Present*. Its ingredients are Ginseng Radix (*rén shēn*), Atractylodis macrocephalae Rhizoma (*bái zhú*), Zingiberis Rhizoma preparata (*páo jiāng*), Glycyrrhizae Radix (*gān cǎo*), Poria (*fú líng*), Hordei Fructus germinatus (*mài yá*), Massa medicata fermentata (*shén qū*), and Amomi Fructus (*shā rén*).

Other herbs to consider: Magnoliae officinalis Cortex *(hòu pò)*, scorched Crataegi Fructus *(jiāo shān zhā)*, scorched Massa medicata fermentata *(jiāo shén qū)*, dry-fried Raphani Semen *(chǎo lái fú zǐ)*, or Poria *(fú líng)*

ADDITIONAL CONSIDERATIONS

- If there is generally poor digestion, one can take Scorched Three Immortals *(jiāo sān xiān)* or Scorched Four Immortals *(jiāo sì xiān)* (see previous page).

- One can use dry-fried Atractylodis macrocephalae Rhizoma *(chǎo bái zhú)*, dry-fried Aurantii Fructus immaturus *(chǎo zhǐ shí)*, Prepared Gigeriae galli Endothelium corneum *(zhì jī nèi jīn)*, dry-fried Hordei Fructus germinatus *(chǎo mài yá)*, and dry-fried (Oryzae) Fructus germinatus *(chǎo gǔ yá)* to increase the efficacy of these herbs for this treatment principle (i.e., enhance digestion, tonify the Spleen qi, and strengthen the Spleen's circulation.) However, Dr. Qin does not start with these prepared medicinals because they may create an overly drying formula that can aggravate Spleen yin deficiency, which can commonly occur with this pattern. Not to oversimplify the distinction, but the tongue is an important sign when deciding whether or not to use these prepared herbs. For example, they are appropriate with a very wet and sticky tongue coating, but not if the tongue is tender with no coating.

QUESTIONS

1. *Could one use Amomi Fructus rotundus (bái dòu kòu) instead of Amomi Fructus (shā rén)?*

   In general, Amomi Fructus *(shā rén)* is better for food stagnation and is indicated if the appetite is poor, indicating that the Stomach is more involved. If, on the other hand, the appetite is good and there is a sensation of blockage after eating, then Amomi Fructus rotundus *(bái dòu kòu)* should be substituted. For long-term Spleen deficiency, a small dosage (e.g., 2-3g) of both can be used simultaneously.

2. *Why is Arecae Pericarpium (dà fù pí) used instead of Magnoliae officinalis Cortex (hòu pò)?*

   Both herbs are similar. However, Arecae Pericarpium *(dà fù pí)* can eliminate the pathogenic dampness (created from the weak Spleen) through the bowels and urine, thereby working more on the lower burner. On the other hand, Magnoliae officinalis Cortex *(hòu pò)* regulates the qi and is more appropriate for Spleen deficiency with distention. It also dries dampness but does not move water and dampness the way that Arecae Pericarpium *(dà fù pí)* does.

ADDITIONAL OPTIONS AND CONSIDERATIONS FOR FOOD STAGNATION

SUPPLEMENTARY PATTERNS

■ 1. Dual weakness of the Spleen and Stomach with deficiency heat in the Stomach

3. Reinforce the Spleen and Reduce Food Stagnation

INDICATIONS: This is a long-term problem presenting with a poor appetite, frequent sensation of feeling full or a stifling sensation after a meal (or small amounts of food), sallow face and emaciated flesh, aversion to heat, dry and hard bowel movements or sloppy stools. This is also said to treat patterns of Spleen qi and yin deficiency.

The formula below functions to warm and augment the Spleen yang, balance and enrich the Spleen yin, tonify the Spleen and raise the clear, clear heat and dry dampness, and harmonize the Stomach.

Aid Life Pill (zī shēng wán)

SOURCE: *Extensive Notes on Medicine from the First-Awakened Studio* (1613)

Ginseng Radix (rén shēn)	90g
Atractylodis macrocephalae Rhizoma (bái zhú)	90g
Poria (fú líng)	45g
Citri reticulatae Pericarpium (chén pí)	60g
Crataegi Fructus (shān zhā)	60g
Glycyrrhizae Radix preparata (zhì gān cǎo)	15g
Dry-fried Dioscoreae Rhizoma (chǎo shān yào)	45g
Dry-fried Coptidis Rhizoma (chǎo huáng lián)	9g
Dry-fried Coicis Semen (chǎo yì yǐ rén)	45g
Dry-fried Lablab Semen album (chǎo biǎn dòu)	45g
Amomi Fructus rotundus (bái dòu kòu)	10.5g
Pogostemonis/Agastaches Folium (huò xiāng yè)	15g
Dry-fried Nelumbinis Semen (chǎo lián ròu)	45g
Dry-fried Alismatis Rhizoma (chǎo zé xiè)	10.5g
Platycodi Radix (jié gěng)	15g
Dry-fried Euryales Semen (chǎo qiàn shí)	45g
Dry-fried Hordei Fructus germinatus (chǎo mài yá)	30g
[Massa medicata fermentata (shén qū)	30g]
[Amomi Fructus (shā rén)[iv]	45g]

■ 2. Forceful Stomach and weak Spleen:

This pattern implies the presence of some excess heat.

INDICATIONS: There will be a decent appetite, but the patient will readily feel full, bloated, gassy, or 'stuck' after eating. This is common in people who eat fast food, pizza, etc.

METHOD: This pattern requires the combination of bitter, descending and acrid, opening medicinals. For example:

A. Left Metal Pill (zuǒ jīn wán): Coptidis Rhizoma (huáng lián) and Evodiae Fructus (wú zhū yú)

B. Aucklandia and Coptis Pill (xiāng lián wán): Coptidis Rhizoma (huáng lián), Aucklandiae Radix (mù xiāng), and Evodiae Fructus (wú zhū yú)

C. Minor Decoction [for Pathogens] Stuck in the Chest (xiǎo xiàn xiōng tāng): Pinelliae Rhizoma preparatum (zhì bàn xià), Trichosanthis Fructus (guā lóu), and Coptidis Rhizoma (huáng lián)

In addition, one must also include herbs that tonify the Spleen such as dry-fried Atractylodis macrocephalae Rhizoma *(chǎo bái zhú)* and dry-fried Codonopsis Radix *(chǎo dǎng shēn)*.

SUPPLEMENTARY FORMULAS

■ 1. Nourish the Stomach Decoction with Aucklandia and Amomum
   (xiāng shā yǎng wèi tāng)

INDICATIONS: poor digestion, low appetite, nausea, vomiting, or stagnation due to overeating. Sometimes there will be aversion to wind, headache, and dizziness.[4]

LOCATION: Stomach/epigastrium

Nourish the Stomach Decoction with Aucklandia and Amomum
   (xiāng shā yǎng wèi tāng)
SOURCE: *Restoration of Health from the Myriad Diseases* (1587)

Dry-fried Atractylodis macrocephalae Rhizoma *(chǎo bái zhú)* . .	9g
Dry-fried Aurantii Fructus immaturus *(chǎo zhǐ shí)*	9g
Citri reticulatae Pericarpium *(chén pí)*	5g
Pinelliae Rhizoma preparatum *(zhì bàn xià)*	9g
Poria *(fú líng)*	9g
Clear-prepared Glycyrrhizae Radix *(qīng zhì gān cǎo)*[v]	5g
Pogostemonis/Agastaches Herba *(huò xiāng)*	6g
Cyperi Rhizoma *(xiāng fù)*	9g
Aucklandiae Radix *(mù xiāng)*	6g
Amomi Fructus *(shā rén)*	3g
Amomi Fructus rotundus *(bái dòu kòu)*	5g
Magnoliae officinalis Cortex *(hòu pò)*	6g

---

Note: Can make into capsules (1 capsule = 0.33g) and take two capsules twice a day before or after meals. One can take two or three capsules prophylatically before overeating and excessive drinking to prevent stagnation.

■ 2. Preserve Harmony Pill *(bǎo hé wán)* (available in prepared form)

INDICATIONS: Food stagnation, especially in children

LOCATION: Stomach/epigastrium

Note: Nourish the Stomach Decoction with Aucklandia and Amomum *(xiāng shā yǎng wèi tāng)* is preferred for adults.

Preserve Harmony Pill *(bǎo hé wán)*
SOURCE: *Essential Teachings of [Zhu] Dan-Xi* (1481)

Crataegi Fructus *(shān zhā)*	180g (9-15g)
Massa medicata fermentata *(shén qū)*	60g (9-12g)
Raphani Semen *(lái fú zǐ)*	30g (6-9g)
Citri reticulatae Pericarpium *(chén pí)*	30g (6-9g)

---

4. These are not signs of the common cold. See the discussion of the 'floating pulse' on p. 38 for an explanation.

Pinelliae Rhizoma preparatum *(zhì bàn xià)* 90g (9-12g)
Poria *(fú líng)*. 90g (9-12g)
Forsythiae Fructus *(lián qiào)* 30g (3-6g)

The two formulas above are for straightforward food stagnation. However, once food stagnation accumulates for some time, it can mix with or create other pathogens such as dampness, phlegm, and heat. Therefore, a multifaceted approach is needed to eliminate the pathology. These conditions are usually more entrenched and therefore are located in the Intestines rather than the Stomach.

▨ 3. Aucklandia and Betel Nut Pill *(mù xiāng bīng láng wán)*

INDICATIONS: Bloating and gas in the lower abdomen with constipation, and tenderness on pressure at CV-6 *(qì hǎi)* or CV-8 *(shén què)*

LOCATION: Lower burner/Large Intestine

Notes: Stagnation of food, heat, and dampness in the lower burner. This formula is from Zhang Zi-He, who specialized in removing toxins from the body. In this situation, it is food toxin.

Aucklandia and Betel Nut Pill *(mù xiāng bīng láng wán)*

SOURCE: *Confucians' Duties to Their Parents* (1228)

Aucklandiae Radix *(mù xiāng)*. 6g
Scorched Arecae Semen *(jiāo bīng láng)* 6g
Processed Cyperi Rhizoma *(zhì xiāng fù)* 6g
Dry-fried Citri reticulatae viride Pericarpium *(chǎo qīng pí)* 6g
Dry-fried Citri reticulatae Pericarpium *(chǎo chén pí)* 5g
Dry-fried Coptidis Rhizoma *(chǎo huáng lián)*. 5g
Dry-fried Phellodendri Cortex *(chǎo huáng bǎi)*. 5g
Steamed Rhei Radix et Rhizoma *(shú dà huáng)* 6g
Dry-fried Pharbitidis Semen *(chǎo qiān niú zǐ)*. . . . . 9g[5]

▨ 4. Unripe Bitter Orange Pill to Guide out Stagnation *(zhǐ shí dǎo zhì wán)*

INDICATIONS: Constipation, dark urine, hemorrhoids, burning sensation after bowel movements, bloating, and gas.

LOCATION: Lower burner/Large Intestine.

Note: Spleen deficiency with heat and damp stagnation

Unripe Bitter Orange Pill to Guide out Stagnation *(zhǐ shí dǎo zhì wán)*

SOURCE: *Clarifying Doubts about Damage from Internal and External Causes* (1247)

Scorched Atractylodis macrocephalae Rhizoma *(jiāo bái zhú)*. . . 9g
Aurantii Fructus immaturus *(zhǐ shí)* 9g
Dry-fried Massa medicata fermentata *(chǎo shén qū)* 9g

---

5. Dosage and preparation methods are slightly modified from the original.

Poria (fú líng). 9g
Charred Rhei Radix et Rhizoma (dà huáng tàn) 6g
Dry-fried Scutellariae Radix (chǎo huáng qín) 3g
Dry-fried Coptidis Rhizoma (chǎo huáng lián). 3g
Alismatis Rhizoma (zé xiè) . . . . 6g[6]

Note: Many times the above two formulas are used together.

■ 5. Regulate the Middle and Reduce the Four [Stagnations] Pill (tiáo zhōng sì xiāo wán)

When enduring phlegm and dampness lead to blood stasis, a more forceful approach to remove the sticky phlegm-stasis that inhibits the Intestines is needed.

INDICATIONS: Sticky stools, incomplete evacuation, or constipation (*not* constipation with dry stools), malodorous stools, bloating, gas, and a feeling of blockage in the lower abdomen. The pulse is soggy and the tongue is swollen, has teeth marks, with a tight coating (i.e., cannot scrape off) that may be oily or sticky. There is pain at CV-8 (shén què) on palpation as well as a tight nodule in the lower abdomen. This formula is especially appropriate for food stagnation from poor diets (low quality oils, dairy, fast food, etc.). One can also take this formula prophylatically.

LOCATION: Lower burner/Large Intestine

Notes: This formula regulates the middle and removes the four stagnations (food, phlegm, qi, and blood) that can arise from a poor diet. This is a patent formula made by the Beijing *Tongrentang* pharmacy and comes in 6g packets. The recommended dose is 1.5g two times a day (three times a day, if serious). One can also make their own powder (1 teaspoon/4-5g, 2 times a day), make a decoction, usually 1 bag over 4 days (or 1 bag over 2 days, if serious), drinking a small amount 3-4 times a day, or incorporate this formula into the above prescription ideas (see Modifications below). Usually, one takes this formula for only 3-5 days. After taking the formula there may be lots of mucus that comes out in the stools, one's tongue coating will lessen, and there will be reduced pain on palpation at CV-8 (shén què). If you take too much of the formula, you can create more blockage.

Regulate the Middle and Reduce the Four [Stagnations] Pill (tiáo zhōng sì xiāo wán)
SOURCE: *Beijing Tongrentang pharmacy* (c. 1810)

Processed Cyperi Rhizoma (zhì xiāng fù) 9g
Steamed Rhei Radix et Rhizoma (shú dà huáng) 6g
Gleditsiae Fructus (zào jiá) . . . . 6g[7]
Dry-fried Pharbitidis Semen (chǎo qiān niú zǐ) 9g
Vinegar-fried Trogopterori Faeces (cù líng zhǐ). 6g

---

Common modifications that can be added to Regulate the Middle and Reduce the Four [Stagnations] Pill (tiáo zhōng sì xiāo wán):

---

6. Dosage and preparation methods are slightly modified from the original.

7. Too high a dosage of Gleditsiae Fructus (zào jiá) can lead to nausea, thus Gleditsiae Spina (zào jiǎo cì) can be substituted here.

3. Reinforce the Spleen and Reduce Food Stagnation

Vinegar Curcumae Rhizoma *(cù é zhú)* 6g

Arecae Semen *(bīng láng)* 6-9g

Dry-fried Aurantii Fructus immaturus *(chǎo zhǐ shí)* 6-9g

Dry-fried Raphani Semen *(chǎo lái fú zǐ)* 6-9g

Scorched Hordei Fructus germinatus *(jiāo mài yá)* 4-6g

Dry-fried Gigeriae galli Endothelium corneum *(chǎo jī nèi jīn)* 4-6g

Arecae Pericarpium *(dà fù pí)* 4-6g

Aucklandiae Radix *(mù xiāng)* 4-6g

Magnoliae officinalis Cortex *(hòu pò)* 4-6g

3

Treatment Guidelines for

Qi Disorders 气 *(qì)*

All qi disorders are a result of the seven emotions.[i]

All qi disorders are caused by some mental and emotional imbalance or disturbance. However, different disturbances lead to varying types of changes in the qi circulation (see below). Note that the underlying concepts for the pathologies discussed below are derived from Ch. 39 of *Basic Questions.*

1. **Anger**: vomiting of blood, fullness in the chest, flank pain, boiling inversion, and sudden inversion[1]

Anger causes qi to counterflow and ascend. This can lead to headaches, migraines, a heavy or hot feeling in the head, belching, hiccough, or, when severe, even coughing of blood or stroke.

2. **Elation**: unceasing wild laughing, yang qi is unable to gather

Excess elation scatters and dissipates the qi, leading to palpitations and insomnia as well as fatigue.

3. **Sadness**: blurred vision, tingling or sore sensation in the nose, profuse uterine

$\rightarrow$

---

1. Boiling inversion (煎厥 *jiān jué*) is when there is an overabundance of Liver qi with irascibility leading to collapse. The manifestations are very similar to those of sudden inversion. Sudden inversion (薄厥 *bó jué*) is where one's essence-spirit becomes irritated and causes yang qi to become acutely hyperactive. The blood follows the qi inversion, which causes the blood to become constrained and accumulate in the head. This can lead to such symptoms as headache, dizziness, and sudden clouding collapse.

bleeding, vessel atrophy,[2] constant shortness of breath

Sadness causes qi to become constrained and dissipated, leading to a depletion of Lung qi.

4. **Fear**: aching bones and atrophy inversion,[3] sunken eye sockets, impotence

Fear causes qi to descend and the spirit to retreat. This results in symptoms such as incontinence. This is an emotion of longer duration than fright.

5. **Fright**: drooling, glazed eyes, mouth agape, dumbfounded and withdrawn,[4] sudden collapse, being unable to be roused

Fright causes the qi to become chaotic. This is due to the spirit having no place to gather, leading to symptoms such as difficulty thinking, palpitations, insomnia, heart irritability, shortness of breath, and, if severe, mental derangement.

6. **Mental exhaustion**: belching, hiccough, wheezing and rough breathing, coughing up blood, lower back pain, bone atrophy,[5] abnormal lung sounds, scanty sperm or no menses

Overwork causes qi to be consumed. Essentially, there is no qi being made and there is qi exhaustion. One feels very tired.

7. **Excessive thinking**: not eating, somnolence, confusion and dizziness, focal distention in the middle, blockage of the Triple Burner.

Excessive thinking causes qi to bind, which therefore causes a failure in qi circulation. Blockage of the Triple Burner refers to symptoms such as sensation of pressure in the head, heavy head, stifling sensation in the chest with blocked up breathing, reduced appetite, stifling sensation and distention in the gastric cavity, sagging distention in the lower abdomen, and dysfunctional bowel movements and urination.

---

2. Vessel atrophy (脉痿 *mài wěi*) is a type of atrophy pattern and may also be called Heart atrophy. In Ch. 44 of *Basic Questions*, "On Atrophy," it states: "The main channels are empty and deficient, which develops into muscle vessel painful obstruction, and then this spreads to vessel atrophy." Signs include joints of the limbs as if broken, inability to lift the limbs, and weakness in the lower leg preventing the patient from standing.

3. Atrophy inversion (痿厥 *wěi jué*) is a pattern of atrophy and weakness (usually of the legs) with simultaneous rebellious flow of qi and blood, manifesting in such symptoms as fire flow in the eyes, dizziness, and tinnitus.

4. Dumbfounded and withdrawn (痴癫 *chī diān*). This is a condition with a clouded sensorium, nonsensical talk, muscle twitches and rigidity, picking at bedclothes, and unconscious movements.

5. Bone atrophy (骨痿 *gǔ wěi*) is also called Kidney atrophy. It is due to internal overabundance of Kidney heat, pathogenic heat damaging the Kidneys, yin-essence depletion, or desiccated bone and marrow deficiency. This manifests as limp and weak lower back and/or spine and the inability to stretch or raise up, atrophy and weakness of the lower limbs making it impossible to walk about, very dark complexion, and desiccated teeth.

TREATMENT PRINCIPLES
Calm what is counterflowing.

Counterflow is essentially any flow that goes contrary to the normal direction. However, here it primarily refers to abnormal flow going upward. It is usually sudden or a short-term condition such as hiccough, belching, asthma attack, cough, or even emotional outbursts. In addition, an overabundance of qi will lead to fire, and an overabundance of fire leads to wind. Thus, fire and wind often accompany qi counterflow. Consequently, if these are present, one must also address them in treatment. Medicinals that calm counterflow are Bambusae Caulis in taeniam *(zhú rú)*, Pinelliae Rhizoma preparatum *(zhì bàn xià)*,Inulae Flos *(xuán fù huā)*, Aquilariae Lignum resinatum *(chén xiāng)*, and Haematitum *(dài zhě shí)*. There may also be Liver qi horizontal counterflow in which calming medicinals are used to correct the flow, such as Citri reticulatae viride Pericarpium *(qīng pí)*, Aurantii Fructus *(zhǐ ké)*, Toosendan Fructus *(chuān liàn zǐ)*, and Corydalis Rhizoma *(yán hú suǒ)*. Hence to calm means to redirect flow that is in counterflow. This does not have to be an acute situation.

Scatter what is clumped.

In the beginning, qi that stagnates leads to constraint (郁 *yù*) and requires the method of resolving constraint (解郁 *jiě yù*), using such medicinals as Bupleuri Radix *(chái hú)*, Cyperi Rhizoma *(xiāng fù)*, or a formula such as Rambling Powder *(xiāo yáo sǎn)*. Constraint can further lead to more serious clumping (结 *jié*) or qi nodules. This can come about from something as simple as receiving bad news during a meal. This can last for weeks, and requires slightly stronger medicinals such as Citri reticulatae viride Pericarpium *(qīng pí)* or Curcumae Rhizoma *(é zhú)*.

If there is even more severe stagnation, this can lead to blood stagnation (血滞 *xuè zhì*), where blood has some difficulty moving or there is slower flow in the vessels. Finally, if there is no movement at all or blockage, the stagnation can lead to blood stasis (血瘀 *xuè yū*).

Direct downward what is floating.

Conditions of qi floating often manifest as palpitations, fright, fear, and a spirit that is restless. In general, however, floating conditions are usually more chronic and ongoing, such as high blood pressure or chronic headaches and migraines, and thus often require stronger descending medicinals that anchor, such as Haliotidis Concha *(shí jué míng)*, Margaritiferae Concha usta *(zhēn zhū mǔ)*, or Ostreae Concha *(mǔ lì)*. Compared with 'counterflow' above, floating is not necessarily more serious, but the difference lies mostly in the duration of the condition.

Dredge what is constrained.

Regulating qi with medicinals such as Bupleuri Radix *(chái hú)* or Cyperi Rhizoma *(xiāng fù)* or formulas like Rambling Powder *(xiāo yáo sǎn)* is appropriate here.

> Gather in what is scattered.

This is essentially an astringent method using medicinals such as Mume Fructus *(wū méi)* or formulas such as Generate the Pulse Drink *(shēng mài yǐn)*.

> Pacify what is chaotic.

Pacifying is often used for conditions of Liver yang and Liver wind with medicinals such as Chrysanthemi Flos *(jú huā)*, Uncariae Ramulus cum Uncis *(gōu téng)*, Gastrodiae Rhizoma *(tiān má)*, Mori Folium *(sāng yè)*, Ostreae Concha *(mǔ lì)*, Margaritiferae Concha usta *(zhēn zhū mǔ)*, and Haliotidis Concha *(shí jué míng)*. Furthermore, if the mind is not calm, one can use medicinals such as Fossilia Dentis Mastodi *(lóng chǐ)*, Fossilia Ossis Mastodi *(lóng gǔ)*, Curcumae Radix *(yù jīn)*, and Polygalae Radix *(yuǎn zhì)*.

> **SUMMARY**
> Dredge, pacify, and ascend.

1. Dredge and Facilitate the Movement of Stagnant Qi
(疏利气滞 shū lì qì zhì)

[PRESENTATION] Anger, melancholy, and inhibited flow at the qi aspect; fullness and stifling sensation in the chest and flanks

Tribuli Fructus *(cì jí lí)*	9g
Processed Cyperi Rhizoma *(zhì xiāng fù)*	4.5g
Dry-fried Citri reticulatae viride Pericarpium *(chǎo qīng pí)*	4.5g
Alpiniae officinarum Rhizoma *(gāo liáng jiāng)*	9g
Aurantii Fructus *(zhǐ ké)*	4.5g
Curcumae Radix *(yù jīn)*	4.5g
Massa Fortunellae Fructus *(jīn jú bǐng)*	3p

COMMENTARY

ADDITIONAL SIGNS AND SYMPTOMS

- Frequent sighing or difficulty taking a deep breath
- Tight sensation in the trunk
- Lack of appetite
- Distention and pain in the epigastrium and abdomen
- Constipation, diarrhea, or alternating between the two
- Heaviness in the arms and legs
- Symptoms improve with warmth or passing of gas
- Mood swings

- The pulse is wiry, choppy, and stagnant
- The tongue is dark pale with no coating

PATHODYNAMIC AND LOCATION: There is usually an emotional aspect to this pattern, or some emotional experience that triggers its onset. This leads to mild qi and blood stagnation, primarily of the Liver. There may also be digestive complaints due to the Liver overacting on the Spleen and Stomach.

DURATION: This pattern is usually of a short-term nature but the method of treatment may be used for more chronic presentations. However, long-term qi stagnation is often complicated by dampness, phlegm, or heat from constraint, in which case this formula is inappropriate or must be modified.

TREATMENT PRINCIPLE: This condition requires a wide-ranging and comprehensive improvement of the qi dynamics utilizing such approaches as adjusting the qi (调气 *tiáo qì*), soothing qi (舒气 *shū qì*), regulating qi (理气 *lǐ qì*), facilitating the movement of qi (利气 *lì qì*), or promoting the movement of qi (行气 *xíng qì*).[ii]

MEDICINAL ANALYSIS

- Tribuli Fructus *(cì jí lí)* is acrid, bitter, and neutral. It soothes the Liver, regulates the qi, dispels wind, and opens the collaterals. It is excellent for soothing the Liver in emotionally sensitive people, especially when related to Liver qi constraint. It is said to circulate qi in the brain, chest, and throughout the entire body. It is especially useful when there is wind affecting the head with dizziness, facial tics, shaking, etc. However, these symptoms are not necessary for it to be used. It is very mild, neutral or slightly cold, and not overly acrid and bitter. It is used in place of the commonly used Bupleuri Radix *(chái hú)* (see below discussion). It is most effective if dry-fried and crushed.

- Alpiniae officinarum Rhizoma *(gāo liáng jiāng)* and Cyperi Rhizoma *(xiāng fù)* together benefit the Stomach, regulate the Liver qi, and are especially useful when there is both Liver and Stomach involvement resulting in pain. They also eliminate cold from the Liver's blood collaterals.

- The acrid and warm nature of Alpiniae officinarum Rhizoma *(gāo liáng jiāng)* moves qi stagnation in the chest, flanks, and epigastrium, as well as in the Spleen and Stomach, making it a good choice for pain. If there is no middle burner involvement, it can still be used at a lower dosage (2-3g) to help protect the Spleen and Stomach from the Liver. It should be noted that Alpiniae officinarum Rhizoma *(gāo liáng jiāng)* is milder than the true gingers, such as Zingiberis Rhizoma recens *(shēng jiāng)* or Zingiberis Rhizoma *(gān jiāng)*, and is not overly hot, especially when combined with the other medicinals in this formula (e.g. Curcumae Radix *(yù jīn)*).

- Cyperi Rhizoma *(xiāng fù)* is acrid, slightly sweet, and bitter. It dredges the Liver and promotes the movement of qi, and regulates the qi of the Triple Burner with a focus on the Liver and Stomach. It is especially appropriate for Liver qi in horizontal counterflow. It can also harmonize the blood aspect. It is fragrant and penetrating and should therefore be used with caution in blood deficient patients because it can scatter the qi and deplete the blood.

• Citri reticulatae viride Pericarpium *(qīng pí)* is acrid, bitter, and warm. It dredges the Liver while simultaneously regulating the Intestines and Stomach. This is an important herb for the treatment of Liver invading the Spleen or Stomach, especially with flank pain and abdominal distention.

• Aurantii Fructus *(zhǐ ké)* and Curcumae Radix *(yù jīn)* move qi in the epigastrium, costal regions, and chest. Aurantii Fructus *(zhǐ ké)* is acrid and regulates the Intestines, Stomach, and the qi of the Liver and Gallbladder. Curcumae Radix *(yù jīn)* is bitter, cool, and regulates the qi within the blood. It enters the Liver, Stomach, and Heart. It relaxes the mind, relieves depression, and treats various mental problems as well as distention, pain, and a stifling sensation in the chest and flanks.

• Massa Fortunellae Fructus *(jīn jú bǐng)* is kumquat that has been crushed and preserved with sugar. It is slightly sweet and slightly moist. It moves the Liver qi, tonifies the Spleen qi circulation, and is especially good if there is stagnant Spleen or Stomach qi with damage to the Stomach yin. If it is unavailable, one can substitute Akebiae Fructus *(bā yuè zhā)*, Aesculi Semen *(suō luó zǐ)*, or Citri sarcodactylis Flos *(fó shǒu huā)* (3-5g).[6] One may also use the fresh or candied kumquat, although the sugar should first be removed from the latter. It should only be boiled for 5-10 minutes.

• This formula is balanced and does not damage the yin if the patient's blood and yin are adequate. If the patient has a tendency toward blood or yin deficiency, this formula is inappropriate. All of these herbs are mild and are appropriate for sensitive or allergic people. When warranted, the formula may be used for a relatively long duration.

Dr. Qin's formula is based on Galangal and Cyperus Pill *(liáng fù wán)*.

Galangal and Cyperus Pill *(liáng fù wán)*
SOURCE: *Small Collection of Fine Formulas* (1842)

Alpiniae officinarum Rhizoma *(gāo liáng jiāng)*
Cyperi Rhizoma *(xiāng fù)*. . . . . (equal amounts)

MODIFICATIONS OF DR. QIN'S FORMULA

If this presentation occurs during menstruation or pre-menstrually:
    Dry-fried Angelicae sinensis radicis Cauda *(chǎo dāng guī wěi)* 4.5g
    Dry-fried Paeoniae Radix rubra *(chǎo chì sháo)* 9g

Stomach discomfort and belching:
    Citri sarcodactylis Fructus *(fó shǒu)* . . . . 4.5g[7]

---

6. These all have a similar ability to harmonize the Stomach and gently dredge the Liver, without damaging yin.

7. Although Citri sarcodactylis Fructus *(fó shǒu)* is milder than Citri reticulatae Pericarpium *(chén pí)*, it is still slightly drying. Therefore, if there is yin, blood, or fluid deficiency, or the patient is especially sensitive, one should use Citri sarcodactylis Flos *(fó shǒu huā)* 3g.

1. Dredge and Facilitate the Movement of Stagnant Qi

Burping or hiccough:

Inulae Flos *(xuán fù huā)* 4.5g

Citri sarcodactylis Flos *(fó shǒu huā)*
or Citri sarcodactylis Fructus *(fó shǒu)* 3g

Poor digestion:

Dry-fried Massa medicata fermentata *(chǎo shén qū)* 9g

Dry-fried Hordei Fructus germinatus *(chǎo mài yá)* 9g

Tight and painful flank:

Dry-fried Toosendan Fructus *(chǎo chuān liàn zǐ)* 4.5g

Tight and painful epigastrium:

Dry-fried Toosendan Fructus *(chǎo chuān liàn zǐ)* 4.5g

Corydalis Rhizoma *(yán hú suǒ)* 6g

Depression:

Rosae rugosae Flos *(méi guī huā)* 3g

Acori tatarinowii Rhizoma *(shí chāng pǔ)* 4.5g

Daidai Flos *(dài dài huā)*[8] 3g

Rosae chinensis Flos *(yuè jì huā)* 3g

Five-Flower Tea *(wǔ huā chá* — see below)

Insomnia:

Ziziphi spinosae Semen *(suān zǎo rén)* 9g

Poriae Sclerotium pararadicis *(fú shén)* 9g

Exhaustion, difficulty sleeping, and restlessness:

Tritici Fructus *(xiǎo mài)* 6-9g

Unquiet mind, can't stop thinking:

Polygalae Radix *(yuǎn zhì)* 4.5g

Acori tatarinowii Rhizoma *(shí chāng pǔ)* 4.5g

Yin deficiency:

Lilii Bulbus *(bǎi hé)* 6-9g

Tritici Fructus *(xiǎo mài)* 6-9g

▶ *Note:* Do not use cloying yin tonics such as Ophiopogonis Radix *(mài mén dōng)*, Glehniae/Adenophorae Radix *(shā shēn)*, or Rehmanniae Radix preparata *(shú dì huáng)*.[9] Remove Citri reticulatae viride Pericarpium *(qīng pí)* and add Rosae rugosae Flos *(méi guī huā)* 3-5g; or Rosae chinensis Flos *(yuè jì huā)* 3-5g.

---

8. Acrid, sweet, slightly bitter, and neutral. It regulates the qi, dredges the Liver, resolves constraint, unbinds the chest, and harmonizes the Stomach. It is important for focal distention and stifling sensation in the chest, distending pain in the stomach cavity, and can stop vomiting. Normal dosage is 1-2.5g a day.

9. These cloying medicinals can cause more stagnation by inhibiting the qi mechanism. If their use is necessary, dry-fry to ameliorate this side effect.

Yin deficiency with deficiency below and excess above:

Astragali complanati Semen *(shā yuàn zǐ)* 6-9g

▶ Remove Citri reticulatae viride Pericarpium *(qīng pí)* and add

Rosae rugosae Flos *(méi guī huā)* 3-5g

   or Rosae chinensis Flos *(yuè jì huā)* 3-5g

Blood deficiency:

Angelicae sinensis Radix *(dāng guī)* 6-9g

Paeoniae Radix alba *(bái sháo)* 6-9g

Remove Citri reticulatae viride Pericarpium *(qīng pí)* and add

Rosae rugosae Flos *(méi guī huā)* 3-5g

   or Rosae chinensis Flos *(yuè jì huā)* 3-5g

Blood stasis:

Angelicae sinensis Radix *(dāng guī)* 4.5g

   or dry-fried Angelicae sinensis radicis Cauda *(chǎo dāng guī wěi)* 3g

Chuanxiong Rhizoma *(chuān xiōng)* 3g

Five-Flower Tea *(wǔ huā chá)*

SOURCE: Wu Bo-Ping[10]

This formula can be used for mild cases of depression.
It is gentle and people can drink it throughout the day for years.

Rosae rugosae Flos *(méi guī huā)* 3g
Rosae chinensis Flos *(yuè jì huā)* 3g
Daidai Flos *(dài dài huā)* 3g
Citri sarcodactylis Flos *(fó shǒu huā)* 3g
Campsis Flos *(líng xiāo huā)*[11] 3g

Instructions: Using equal parts of the flowers, make 2g tea bags and steep.

Modifications:

Osmanthi Flos *(guì huā)*[12] improves the appetite.

Mume Flos *(méi huā)* very mildly calms the mind and moves qi.

Chrysanthemi Flos *(jú huā)* clears heat.

Chimonanthi Flos Immaturus *(là méi huā)*:[13] Use when stress causes the head
  to become red and feel hot.

Croci Stigma *(zàng hóng huā)*, 0.3g, moves blood.

  (Fresh flowers are best.)

---

10. This formula was drawn from the ideas of two of Dr. Wu's teachers, Qin Bo-Wei and Wei Chang-Chun. Other flowers may also be added, such as Magnoliae officinalis Flos *(hòu pò huā)* or Prunellae Flos *(xià kū huā)*, depending on the circumstances, creating Six-Flower Tea or Seven-Flower Tea.

11. Moves the blood and is especially good for premenstrual women with depression.

12. Acrid, warm, scatters cold, breaks up clumps, transforms phlegm, and stops coughing.

13. Acrid, sweet, slightly bitter, and cool. Enters the Lung and Stomach channels. Resolves toxicity, clears heat, regulates the qi, and opens up areas of constraint. It is slightly toxic.

1. Dredge and Facilitate the Movement of Stagnant Qi

QUESTIONS

1. *Why is Bupleuri Radix (chái hú) not used?*

There is a long history of debate surrounding the use of Bupleuri Radix *(chái hú)* in treating Liver constraint patterns. Although some believe it is invaluable in treating Liver disorders, others find it too harsh. For example, because of its ascending nature, Bupleuri Radix *(chái hú)* can cause insomnia and headaches, and can aggravate emotionally sensitive people, particularly those who easily get angry. This is especially true when one's nervous system is on edge or there is horizontal counterflow. It also can cause nausea in patients with preexisting stifling sensation in the chest (a common sign of qi constraint). Consequently, Dr. Qin follows the words of Ye Tian-Shi, "Bupleuri Radix *(chái hú)* plunders the yin," and Wang Meng-Ying, who said that it primarily "plunders the Liver yin." He therefore agrees that its dispersing nature makes it inappropriate, especially when this formula is taken over a long period of time. Thus, Bupleuri Radix *(chái hú)*, and even vinegar-fried Bupleuri Radix *(cù chái hú)*, poses too much of a risk for such a presentation.

2. *Why does Dr. Qin use Citri reticulatae viride Pericarpium (qīng pí) and not Citri reticulatae Pericarpium (chén pí)?*

Dr. Qin often uses Citri reticulatae viride Pericarpium *(qīng pí)* when there is Liver invading Spleen pathology. Citri reticulatae viride Pericarpium *(qīng pí)* dredges Liver qi constraint, whereas Citri reticulatae Pericarpium *(chén pí)* is best for regulating the qi in the Spleen, Stomach, and Lungs.

3. *Why is this formula warm? Doesn't Liver qi constraint usually have heat?*

Since this is a short-term problem, there is no buildup of heat. When there is stagnation, warm medicinals are the best for inducing movement. Cold medicinals can lead to further coagulation and more constraint. Thus it should be noted that it is incorrect that Liver qi constraint (or Liver qi stagnation) must have a heat component.

4. *Why does Dr. Qin choose Curcumae Radix (yù jīn) instead of dry-fried Toosendan Fructus (chǎo chuān liàn zǐ) or Corydalis Rhizoma (yán hú suǒ)?*

Both dry-fried Toosendan Fructus *(chǎo chuān liàn zǐ)* and Corydalis Rhizoma *(yán hú suǒ)* move the Liver qi and are suitable for this pattern, as noted in the modifications. However, both act more on the qi aspect, whereas Curcumae Radix *(yù jīn)* acts more on the blood aspect. Although this is not a blood stasis pattern per se, the use of Curcumae Radix *(yù jīn)* prevents the stagnation from going to a deeper level. Furthermore, Curcumae Radix *(yù jīn)* has a psychoemotional effect that the others do not.

5. *Why does this formula not look like other Liver-Spleen disharmony formulas, such as Important Formula for Painful Diarrhea (tòng xiè yào fāng) or Rambling Powder (xiāo yáo sǎn)?*

There are many variations to the way that Liver-Spleen disharmonies manifest and thus there are many other potentially appropriate formulas such as Resolve the Liver Decoction *(jiě gān jiān)*[14] and even Mume Pill *(wū méi wán)*. However, there are three key categories that are useful to understand.

   i. Wood overcontrols earth (木克土 *mù kè tǔ)*, also called horizontal counterflow, is caused by the condition called 'Liver qi'. This is Liver qi that is in excess where the Liver overwhelms the Spleen and/or attacks the Stomach. The treatment method centers on dredging the Liver (疏肝 *shū gān)* or calming the Liver, with a secondary approach of strengthening the Spleen or harmonizing the Stomach. Bupleurum Powder to Dredge the Liver *(chái hú shū gān sǎn)*[15] and Adjust the Qi Decoction *(tiáo qì tāng)*[16], as well as Dr. Qin's formula above, are appropriate.

   ii. Wood not controlling earth (木不克土 *mù bù kè tǔ),* also called wood not dredging earth, is caused by Liver constraint (肝郁 *gān yù)*. Constraint leads to a loss of free coursing of the Liver qi, causing the function of the Spleen and Stomach to slow. This is a deficient condition and the opposite of wood overcontrolling earth. Of note, because of the lack of movement of qi, if chronic, it is more apt to transform into heat, which becomes internally-constrained lurking heat.

     The appropriate strategy is to soothe the Liver (舒肝 *shū gān)* and build up the Spleen. The term 'soothe' is related to dredging with an element of tonification. Thus a soothing strategy, as the name implies, is a more gentle approach to eliminating stagnation. Rambling Powder *(xiāo yáo sǎn)* is a flagship formula for this method, which tonifies the Liver and Spleen. Merely dredging the Liver in such cases will cause further damage.

   iii. Earth conversely rebelling against wood (土反侮木 *tǔ fǎn wǔ mù)* occurs when the Spleen and Stomach are blocked and stagnant, influencing the orderly spreading out of Liver qi. The primary strategy is to improve the Spleen's transportation function and harmonize the Stomach so that the Liver recovers on its own. Formulas such as Resolve the Liver Decoction *(jiě gān jiān)* are appropriate.

Dredging qi is a core principle in all three patterns, although the first category—wood

---

14. Citri reticulatae Pericarpium *(chén pí)*, Pinelliae Rhizoma preparatum *(zhì bàn xià)*, Magnoliae officinalis Cortex *(hòu pò)*, and Poria *(fú líng)*, Paeoniae Radix alba *(bái sháo)*, Perillae Folium *(zǐ sū yè)*, Amomi Fructus *(shā rén)* and Zingiberis Rhizoma recens *(shēng jiāng)*.

15. Vinegar-fried Citri reticulatae Pericarpium *(cù chǎo chén pí)*, Bupleuri Radix *(chái hú)*, Chuanxiong Rhizoma *(chuān xiōng)*, dry-fried Aurantii Fructus *(chǎo zhǐ ké)*, Paeoniae Radix *(sháo yào)*, Glycyrrhizae Radix preparata *(zhì gān cǎo)*, and Cyperi Rhizoma *(xiāng fù)*.

16. Cyperi Rhizoma *(xiāng fù)*, Citri reticulatae viride Pericarpium *(qīng pí)*, Citri reticulatae Pericarpium *(chén pí)*, Linderae Radix *(wū yào)*, Aucklandiae Radix *(mù xiāng)*, Pogostemonis/Agastaches Herba *(huò xiāng)*?, Amomi Fructus *(shā rén)*, and Glycyrrhizae Radix *(gān cǎo)*.

overcontrols earth—will utilize it in its purest form. Understanding this method in its most basic form is important when addressing the combination patterns that often occur in wood earth disharmonies. In such situations, one can modify it with information found in other sections.

For example, if there is blood deficiency one can incorporates a strategy of tonifying blood by adding Angelicae sinensis Radix *(dāng guī)* and Paeoniae Radix alba *(bái sháo)* and removing Citri reticulatae viride Pericarpium *(qīng pí)*, as mentioned in the modification section above. This brings it one step closer to Rambling Powder *(xiāo yáo sǎn)*. However, as mentioned above, the key pathological process in Dr. Qin's method is that of excess, while in Rambling Powder *(xiāo yáo sǎn)* it is more one of deficiency.

Thus we end up with a spectrum of Liver Spleen disharmonies ranging from pure excess to mostly deficiency, with multiple secondary patterns such as the generation of heat, dampness, etc. Thus, even the categories above are a bit artificial and one must see this as a continuum of possibilities where one picks the appropriate treatment principles to match the specific person at a specific time.

2. Sedate Floating Qi (镇静浮气 *zhèn jìng fú qì*)

[PRESENTATION] Fear and panic from unanchored and unconserved qi; continuous palpitations and a disordered spirit

Fossilia Dentis Mastodi *(lóng chǐ)*	4.5g
Magnetitum *(cí shí)*	18g
Poriae Sclerotium pararadicis *(fú shén)*	9g
Ostreae Concha *(mǔ lì)*	9g
Ziziphi spinosae Semen *(suān zǎo rén)*	9g
Platycladi Semen *(bǎi zǐ rén)*	9g
Longan Arillus *(lóng yǎn ròu)*	5 pieces

COMMENTARY

ADDITIONAL SIGNS AND SYMPTOMS

- Palpitations may be accompanied by fear
- Insomnia with bad dreams in which the dreamer is in danger
- Headache
- Empty feeling in the head
- Difficulty thinking/disorientation
- Vertigo
- Shakiness
- Mood swings
- Extreme sadness[iii]
- Disorientation

- Complaint of having high 'stress'
- High blood pressure
- Possible history of stroke
- May have cardiac disease or be perimenopausal
- The pulse is thin and rapid; may have one of the irregular pulses
- The tongue has a red body (especially the tip) with no coating or a slightly yellow, thicker coating in the back (especially if there is a phlegm component)

DISCUSSION

LOCATION: Heart (secondarily the Liver and Kidneys)

PATHODYNAMIC AND ETIOLOGY: Heart (Liver and Kidneys) blood and yin deficiency leads to Heart/Liver yang rising and floating qi, which disturbs the spirit. This can occur due to an ongoing constitutional tendency or a more acute incident such as post-partum or post-surgical loss of blood. This is because blood and yin are needed to anchor the qi.

The Liver and Heart have a mother-child relationship, so when the Heart is not tranquil, the Liver yang ascends. When the Heart-spirit is not quiet and there is a lack of proper communication between the Heart and Kidneys, it is appropriate to direct the Heart fire downward (so that it can be received by the Kidneys), and raise and enrich the Kidney water. One should also pay attention to the Liver, because of the intimate connection between the Liver yin and blood and the Kidneys.

This method essentially relaxes and quiets the mind. If qi ascends, one easily becomes emotional (e.g., angry, restless, anxious, stressed) and cannot keep calm.

TREATMENT PRINCIPLE: Nourish the yin and blood, quiet the spirit, and direct the qi downward. Although the Heart is the primary focus of tonification in this case, one must not forget to also tonify the Liver and Kidneys.

MEDICINAL ANALYSIS

SUMMARY

Tonify, augment, and nourish the Heart blood and yin:

- Ziziphi spinosae Semen *(suān zǎo rén)*
- Platycladi Semen *(bǎi zǐ rén)*
- Longan Arillus *(lóng yǎn ròu)*
- Poriae Sclerotium pararadicis *(fú shén)*

Sedate and calm the spirit:

- Fossilia Dentis Mastodi *(lóng chǐ)* (enters the Heart and quiets floating qi from Heart yin deficiency)
- Ostreae Concha *(mǔ lì)* (enters the Liver, quiets yang rising from Liver yin deficiency)
- Magnetitum *(cí shí)* (enters the Kidney, quiets rising fire from Kidney yin deficiency)

INDIVIDUAL CHARACTERISTICS

- Fossilia Dentis Mastodi *(lóng chǐ)* enters the Heart and is a heavily sedating, anchoring, and descending medicinal. If unavailable, one can substitute Fossilia Ossis Mastodi *(lóng gǔ)* 9g. However, Fossilia Dentis Mastodi *(lóng chǐ)* is better for treating the Heart channel, while Fossilia Ossis Mastodi *(lóng gǔ)* is better for the Liver channel.

- Ostreae Concha *(mǔ lì)* enters the Liver and Heart, is astringent, and directs the Liver qi and yang downward.

- Magnetitum *(cí shí)* is heavy and enters the Kidneys and Liver. It reinforces the Kidneys' ability to receive. Dr. Wu has found that for this medicinal, a sufficient dose in the West is 9-12g.

- Poriae Sclerotium pararadicis *(fú shén)*, Longan Arillus *(lóng yǎn ròu)*, Platycladi Semen *(bǎi zǐ rén)*, and Ziziphi spinosae Semen *(suān zǎo rén)* all quiet the Heart/mind and allow one to sleep deeply. They all work in slightly different ways. Poriae Sclerotium pararadicis *(fú shén)* is able to sedate and calm the spirit as well as tonify and augment the Heart spirit. Longan Arillus *(lóng yǎn ròu)* is sweet and warm. It tonifies the Heart and Liver blood and Heart yang. Platycladi Semen *(bǎi zǐ rén)* nourishes the Heart blood and yin to calm the spirit, and also softens the Liver. Ziziphi spinosae Semen *(suān zǎo rén)* is sour, slightly bitter, and neutral. Its special characteristic is that it restrains the mind, allowing it to settle down in the face of excessive or overly busy thinking.

Dr. Qin's formula is based on Arborvitae Seed Pill to Nourish the Heart *(bái zǐ yǎng xīn wán)*.

Arborvitae Seed Pill to Nourish the Heart *(bái zǐ yǎng xīn wán)*

SOURCE: *Compilation of Materials of Benevolence for the Body* (1549)

Platycladi Semen *(bǎi zǐ rén)*	120g
Lycii Fructus *(gǒu qǐ zǐ)*	90g
Ophiopogonis Radix *(mài mén dōng)*	30g
Angelicae sinensis Radix *(dāng guī)*	30g
Acori tatarinowii Rhizoma *(shí chāng pǔ)*	30g
Poriae Sclerotium pararadicis *(fú shén)*	30g
Scrophulariae Radix *(xuán shēn)*	60g
Rehmanniae Radix preparata *(shú dì huáng)*	60g
Glycyrrhizae Radix *(gān cǎo)*	15g

MODIFICATIONS OF DR. QIN'S FORMULA

Palpitations, fear, inability to relax or stay quiet:

Schisandrae Fructus *(wǔ wèi zǐ)* 4.5g

WITH YIN DEFICIENCY:

Ophiopogonis Radix *(mài mén dōng)* 6g

Ginseng Radix *(rén shēn)* . . . . 4.5g[17]

---

17. These three make up Generate the Pulse Powder *(shēng mài sān)*, which, when added to this formula, tonifies

Irregular pulse:

Prepared Licorice Decoction *(zhì gān cǎo tāng)*[18]

High blood pressure, ascending fire (e.g., always feeling hot in the upper part of the body), severe insomnia:

Fluoritum *(zǐ shí yīng)* 6-9g

High blood pressure, fatigue, with rebellious Stomach qi (e.g., belching):

Haematitum *(dài zhě shí)* 6-9g

Briefly restless and loud, then fatigued and quiet, sensitive to stimulus (television or people's words), which easily produces palpitations or tachycardia:

Succinum *(hǔ pò)* 0.5g

> (with each dose, powder and do not cook)

Tinnitus:

Anemarrhenae Rhizoma *(zhī mǔ)* 6g

Phellodendri Cortex *(huáng bǎi)* 3g

Palpitations, poor memory, poor sleep (e.g., sleeps lightly and wakes up frequently), nightmares, foggy mind, and unclear thinking:

Polygalae Radix *(yuǎn zhì)* 4.5g

Acori tatarinowii Rhizoma *(shí chāng pǔ)* 4.5g

Polygoni multiflori Caulis *(yè jiāo téng)* 6g

Albiziae Cortex *(hé huān pí)* 4.5g

ADDITIONAL TIP: These patients usually benefit from some meditation or qi gong exercises that focus on guiding the qi downward.

QUESTIONS

1. If there is a component of blood deficiency, could one use Angelicae sinensis Radix (dāng guī) and Codonopsis Radix (dǎng shēn)?

Angelicae sinensis Radix *(dāng guī)* and Codonopsis Radix *(dǎng shēn)* are often used to tonify blood. However, in this case they are too warm and may aggravate the condition.

2. Why is there only a small dose of Fossilia Dentis Mastodi (lóng chǐ)?

Fossilia Dentis Mastodi *(lóng chǐ)* is used as a guiding herb to the Heart. One does not need to overly sedate the Heart, but merely change the directional flow of qi in this organ. Notice that the other 'heavy' herbs for the Kidneys and Liver have higher dosages.

---

the Heart yin and qi. It is an important combination for many cardiac patients, for example, irregular heart beats or coronary heart disease.

18. This is for Heart yin, yang, blood, and qi deficiency. Ingredients include Glycyrrhizae Radix preparata *(zhì gān cǎo)*, Ginseng Radix *(rén shēn)*, Cinnamomi Ramulus *(guì zhī)*, Rehmanniae Radix *(shēng dì huáng)*, Ophiopogonis Radix *(mài mén dōng)*, Asini Corii Colla *(ē jiāo)*, Cannabis Semen *(huǒ má rén)*, Zingiberis Rhizoma recens *(shēng jiāng)*, and Jujubae Fructus *(dà zǎo)*.

3. Lift Up Sunken Qi (升举气陷 *shēng jǔ qì xiàn*)

[PRESENTATION] Gathering qi has sunk and the clear yang is unable to ascend; exhaustion and encumbered fatigue

Dry-fried Codonopsis Radix *(chǎo dǎng shēn)* 4.5g

Dry-fried Citri reticulatae Pericarpium *(chǎo chén pí)* 4.5g

Atractylodis macrocephalae Rhizoma *(bái zhú)* 4.5g

Clear-Glycyrrhizae Radix preparata *(qīng zhì gān cǎo)* 1.5g

Prepared Cimicifugae Rhizoma *(zhì shēng má)* 2.4g

Honey-prepared Astragali Radix *(mì zhì huáng qí)* 4.5g

Bupleuri Radix *(chái hú)* 2.4g

COMMENTARY

ADDITIONAL SIGNS AND SYMPTOMS

SYMPTOMS RELATED TO QI DEFICIENCY

- Emotional fatigue
- Shortness of breath
- Easily catches colds
- Spontaneous sweating
- Tired limbs
- Weak knees[19]
- Unable to talk for long periods or at a loud volume (voice may be loud for about 10 minutes then becomes quiet)
- Poor digestion (may have a good appetite but have difficulty digesting the food)

SYMPTOMS RELATED TO THE CLEAR YANG UNABLE TO ASCEND

- Dizziness
- Poor memory
- Fuzzy thinking
- Pale, dark-yellow face

SYMPTOMS RELATED TO QI SINKING

- Sagging distention in the lower abdomen
- Frequent desire to defecate
- Chronic loose stools
- Organ prolapse
- Uterine bleeding
- Continuous white vaginal discharge

---

19. Although generally weak knees are associated with Kidney and Liver deficiency, this can result from any sort of normal qi deficiency.

Note: There is no mention of heat signs (yin fire symptoms). See question below.

- The pulse is soft, soggy, and weak
- The tongue is pale, swollen, wet, and tender with teeth marks

DISCUSSION

LOCATION: Middle burner

PATHODYNAMIC AND ETIOLOGY: Sinking of the middle qi with yang qi that is unable to ascend. Since the Spleen governs the middle qi, this pattern mostly relates to the Spleen and essentially arises from a qi deficiency. However, the fundamental issue is still one of an impaired qi dynamic and differs from a simple Spleen/middle qi deficiency pattern (see questions below). In today's clinic, this pattern arises from internal disharmonies.

It is important to gauge how much the qi dynamic has been impaired versus simple deficiency signs. This can help one tailor the treatment. Sinking qi and clear yang unable to ascend are essentially treated the same way. However, uncomplicated deficiency of the Spleen is treated differently (see the method "tonify, augment, and strengthen the middle" in Ch. 5, p. 120).

TREATMENT PRINCIPLE: Tonify, lift, and raise the middle qi

PRECAUTIONS: This formula is unsuitable for patterns of fire from either deficiency or excess with ascending counterflow. In these circumstances, it will cause even more fire to blaze upward.

MEDICINAL ANALYSIS

SUMMARY

- Honey-prepared Astragali Radix *(mì zhì huáng qí)* ascends and lifts the middle qi.
- Dry-fried Codonopsis Radix *(chǎo dǎng shēn)* tonifies the Spleen.
- Atractylodis macrocephalae Rhizoma *(bái zhú)* tonifies the middle qi and dries dampness.

INDIVIDUAL CHARACTERISTICS

- Honey-prepared Astragali Radix *(mì zhì huáng qí)* and dry-fried Codonopsis Radix *(chǎo dǎng shēn)* work together to augment the qi and tonify the middle qi. Honey-prepared Astragali Radix *(mì zhì huáng qí)* tonifies the gathering qi and lifts qi. It does not really tonify the Spleen qi circulation or aid in the Spleen's ability to digest. Thus, it can cause bloating if the Spleen's digestive function is too weak, and only a small dose should therefore be used. If there is deficiency fire ascending, do not use any form of Astragali Radix *(huáng qí)*. Dry-fried Codonopsis Radix *(chǎo dǎng shēn)* tonifies the middle burner qi and increases the Spleen circulation.
- Atractylodis macrocephalae Rhizoma *(bái zhú)* and clear-Glycyrrhizae Radix preparata *(qīng zhì gān cǎo)* augment the qi, build up the Spleen, and regulate dampness. Clear-Glycyrrhizae Radix preparata *(qīng zhì gān cǎo)* is used in a small dosage because it can be too sweet and lead to poor Spleen circulation.

- Dr. Wu prefers a dry-frying preparation for Bupleuri Radix *(chái hú)*. Prepared Cimicifugae Rhizoma *(zhì shēng má)* and dry-fried Bupleuri Radix *(chǎo chái hú)* are both mild, able to induce the qi to ascend, and are considered yang within yin. They guide the tonifying actions of Astragali Radix *(huáng qí)* and Codonopsis Radix *(dǎng shēn)* upward. One cannot ascend without tonifying, and tonifying without promoting movement will only further inhibit movement of the qi dynamic, leading to deficiency.

- Dry-fried Citri reticulatae Pericarpium *(chǎo chén pí)* is fragrant, awakens the Spleen, and promotes the circulation of qi. This is important because qi deficiency commonly leads to lack of movement (in the middle).

Question: There are many types of medicinal preparations for these herbs; what is their significance?

Paying attention to the above processing methods as well as changing them to fit the patient's individual presentation can greatly enhance the effect of this formula. Here are some key points to consider:

Dry-fried Codonopsis Radix *(chǎo dǎng shēn)*: This is not as cloying as Codonopsis Radix *(dǎng shēn)*. If there is focal distention and a stifling sensation in the chest and abdominal cavity, it is important that you not use the sweet and sticky Codonopsis Radix *(dǎng shēn)*.

Dry-fried Bupleuri Radix *(chǎo chái hú)*: Dry-frying Bupleuri Radix *(chái hú)* moderates its nature and enables it to work more on the Spleen to raise clear yang, as compared to Bupleuri Radix *(chái hú)*, which also ascends but is better for external conditions. Vinegar-fried Bupleuri Radix *(cù chái hú)* should not be used here because it has little ability to raise clear yang.

Prepared Cimicifugae Rhizoma *(zhì shēng má)*: This type of processing moderates its acrid, dispersing nature and emphasizes its ascending nature in the middle burner.

Dry-fried Citri reticulatae Pericarpium *(chǎo chén pí)*: Dry-frying Citri reticulatae Pericarpium *(chén pí)* moderates its drying and acrid, dispersing nature, which is then not as damaging to the Spleen yin. It also has a stronger effect on strengthening the middle burner.

Dr. Qin's formula is based on Tonify the Middle to Augment the Qi Decoction *(bǔ zhōng yì qì tāng)*.

Tonify the Middle to Augment the Qi Decoction *(bǔ zhōng yì qì tāng)*
SOURCE: *Discussion of the Spleen and Stomach* (13th century)

Astragali Radix *(huáng qí)* 1.5-3g
Ginseng Radix *(rén shēn)* 0.9g
Atractylodis macrocephalae Rhizoma *(bái zhú)* 0.9g
Glycyrrhizae Radix preparata *(zhì gān cǎo)* 1.5g
Angelicae sinensis Radix *(dāng guī)* 6g
Citri reticulatae Pericarpium *(chén pí)* 0.9g
Cimicifugae Rhizoma *(shēng má)* 0.9g
Bupleuri Radix *(chái hú)* 0.9g
   (this original dose is based on a powdered form)

MODIFICATIONS OF DR. QIN'S FORMULA

Blood deficiency (a common occurrence with qi-deficient patients):

Angelicae sinensis radicis Corpus *(dāng guī shēn)*.................... 2.5g

Severe bleeding:

Increase Astragali Radix *(huáng qí)* and add a small amount of
Angelicae sinensis Radix *(tǔ chǎo dāng guī)*

Kidney essence deficiency (commonly occurs with this pattern):

Prepared polygonatum *(zhì huáng jīng)* .... 9g[20]

Dioscoreae Rhizoma *(shān yào)* 9g

Reduced appetite and poor digestion:

Setariae (Oryzae)Fructus germinatus *(gǔ yá)* and
Hordei Fructus germinatus *(mài yá)*............................. 6-9g each

Achy and tight neck and back, easily fatigued, vertigo, and dizziness:[21]

Roasted Puerariae Radix *(wēi gé gēn)*[22] 6g
(especially if there are loose stools and frequent urination)

Extremely weak (e.g., after surgery, long-term diarrhea):

Korean Ginseng Radix *(gāo lí rén shēn)* 4.5g
(instead of Codonopsis Radix *(dǎng shēn)*)

Extremely weak (qi deficiency with yin deficiency):

Panacis quinquefolii Radix *(xī yáng shēn)*.......................... 4.5g
(instead of Codonopsis Radix *(dǎng shēn)*)

Extremely weak (long-term problem with easy contraction of colds and infection):

Ganoderma *(líng zhī)*... 1-5g[23]

Cordyceps *(dōng chóng xià cǎo)* 1-5g
(There are many types of preparations and qualities; hence, the dosage may vary
from less than a gram to 5g a day. One can therefore add the raw herb to the formula, make a soup or tea, or even take capsules.)

Dendrobii officinalis Caulis *(tiě pí shí hú)*[24]
(especially if yin is also damaged)

A combination of equal amounts Dendrobii officinalis Caulis, Ganoderma *(líng zhī)*, and
Panacis quinquefolii Radix *(xī yáng shēn)* can be ground and encapsulated. Take two capsules
(1 capsule =~ 0.33g) B.I.D. This is contraindicated if there is severe cold in the middle burner.

---

20. This is not as sticky as Rehmanniae Radix preparata *(shú dì huáng)* or Rehmanniae Radix *(shēng dì huáng)*.

21. Yang qi is unable to reach the head.

22. Lifts the qi and body fluids.

23. This not only 'boosts the immune system,' but also balances the immune system, thus making them suitable for many types of autoimmune disorders.

24. Dendrobii officinalis Caulis *(tiê pí shí hú)* is a special type of Dendrobii Herba *(shí hú)*. It is slightly cold, slightly sweet, and strongly supplements the blood, essence, and fluids, and regulates yin and yang balance. It tonifies the Heart, Liver, Spleen, Lung, and Kidney yin. It is especially effective in people who smoke, overwork, can't sleep, or overstrain their nerves.

QUESTIONS

1. *Does this formula treat the pattern of yin fire?*

    Tonify the Middle to Augment the Qi Decoction *(bǔ zhōng yì qì tāng)* was used by Li Dong-Yuan to treat a type of yin fire. This yin fire essentially refers to a qi deficiency (or qi sinking) pattern resulting in various heat signs, especially in the upper part of the body. However, there are no signs of heat or yin fire in the presentation above. This is because Drs. Qin and Wu want to emphasize the principal applications of the formula. Furthermore, in their clinical experience, a true yin fire presentation is seldom seen in modern times, only occurring in severe Spleen deficient patients. Consequently, one should be careful using this formula in the presence of heat, especially if the pathodynamic is unclear.

2. *Why does Dr. Qin use the term gathering qi (宗气 zōng qì) when middle qi (中气 zhōng qì) is usually used when describing Tonify the Middle to Augment the Qi Decoction (bǔ zhōng yì qì tāng)?*

    Dr. Qin uses the term 'gathering qi' to emphasize the systemic effect that the problem creates. Furthermore, due to the physiological relationship between the two aspects of qi, using gathering qi implies that middle qi is also involved and is sunken. For example, merely using the term middle qi primarily refers to problems centered on digestion (see method "tonify, augment, and strengthen the middle" in Ch. 5, p. 120); whereas gathering qi usually encompasses a wider range of symptoms and may or may not include specific digestive complaints.

3. *If one wants to have a more profound effect on raising qi should the dosage of Bupleuri Radix (chái hú) and Cimicifugae Rhizoma (shēng má) be increased?*

    The dosage of these two herbs is adequate as is, and should not be increased. They are merely guiding herbs, and in general, guiding herbs are best at relatively low dosages. Furthermore, Bupleuri Radix *(chái hú)* in a higher dosage can damage the yin and lead to more vertigo. One can increase Atractylodis macrocephalae Rhizoma *(bái zhú)*, Codonopsis Radix *(dǎng shēn)*, or even Astragali Radix *(huáng qí)* (if digestion is intact). For example, Atractylodis macrocephalae Rhizoma *(bái zhú)* and Codonopsis Radix *(dǎng shēn)* do not raise the qi in the same manner as Bupleuri Radix *(chái hú)*, but instead build the qi so that it can be raised.

4. *How does one differentiate this pattern from a basic pattern of Spleen qi deficiency and why does Dr. Qin say that fatigue is the key symptom for this pattern?*

    Fatigue is an important feature in this pattern as well as in simple middle burner deficiency, as found in Ch. 5. It is important to note that Dr. Qin does not mention any digestive complaint as the chief manifestation here, whereas in the section "tonify, augment, and strengthen the middle" he does. This pattern is less about digestive complaints and more about the qi dynamic. If there are digestive complaints, this formula must be modified or not used. Furthermore, one would also want to see some symptoms of qi sinking or clear yang failing to rise, such as vertigo, dizziness, or prolapse. In addition, in a basic pattern of middle burner deficiency, the right middle pulse will be deep and weak. In this pattern, the distal pulse will be weaker.

5. *Why does Dr. Qin not mention anything about prolapse as a key sign?*

Recognizing the full extent of the relationship of this pattern to internal organ prolapse is a relatively modern phenomenon. In the past, due to a lack of modern imaging tools, it was hard to definitively diagnose various internal organ prolapse. We now recognize the important relationship between prolapse and the sinking of Spleen qi.

6. *Why is Astragali Radix (huáng qí) used in its honey-prepared form?*

Honey-prepared Astragali Radix *(mì zhì huáng qí)* is better at tonifying than the un-prepared product. More specifically, its effects last longer and therefore both improves Spleen qi function for a longer period of time and also works on a deeper level. Consequently, the unprepared form works more on the surface, is more ascending, and quicker moving. Honey-prepared Astragali Radix *(mì zhì huáng qí)* is chosen because, to correct the root problem (qi sinking from deficiency), one must not only raise, but also substantially strengthen. Furthermore, Dr. Qin prefers milder versions of medicinals, to reduce the chance of side effects, enabling his formulas to be taken for longer periods of time.

7. *Why is Atractylodis macrocephalae Rhizoma (bái zhú) chosen instead of dry-fried Atractylodis macrocephalae Rhizoma (chǎo bái zhú)?*

The dry-fried version is better for digestive complaints, especially when there is dampness. Dry-fried Atractylodis macrocephalae Rhizoma *(chǎo bái zhú)* is better at strengthening the Spleen's circulation while Atractylodis macrocephalae Rhizoma *(bái zhú)* is better at strengthening the Spleen qi, enabling it to lift more. Normally this pattern has few associated digestive complaints. However, if these are present, one can choose dry-fried Atractylodis macrocephalae Rhizoma *(chǎo bái zhú)*.

CHAPTER SUMMARY

The treatment of qi disorders is relatively complex. It can be made relatively straightforward as long as one firmly grasps these key points:

• If there is constraint or clumping, one must regulate.

• If there is counterflow, floating, or scattering, one must sedate and preserve.

• If there is sinking, one must raise it.

• For treatment of the Liver, it is fundamental to dredge and regulate while simultaneously paying attention to the Spleen and Stomach.

- For treatment of the Heart, it is fundamental to pacify and preserve while simultaneously paying attention to the Liver and Kidney.
- For treatment of the Spleen, it is fundamental to raise up while simultaneously paying attention to the Lungs and Kidneys.

These methods all deal with an improper flow of qi. For qi deficiency, please consult Ch. 5 for specific principles of tonifying deficiency.

4

Treatment Guidelines for

Blood Disorders 血 *(xuè)*

SOURCE
- Blood comes about from the transformation of the essence of liquids and grains.

This essentially refers to blood production arising from a properly functioning Spleen and Stomach coupled with a good intake of nutrition. If either one is lacking, there can be blood deficiency.

PATHODYNAMICS
- Irregularity in daily life, excesses of the seven emotions, fatigue, excess sexual desire, and irregularities in diet all can stir up fire and damage the qi. When fire stirs, there is chaotic movement of hot blood. When the qi is damaged, the blood has nothing to attach to, resulting in chaotic movement outward (bleeding).

"Irregularity in daily life" primarily refers to sleep and eating habits.

Poor eating habits include eating meals at irregular times, eating late or missing meals, or eating too quickly. Poor sleep includes irregular sleep, going to bed too late, and/or not sleeping enough. In general, one needs 7-8 hours of sleep and should go to bed before 10:00 p.m.

The pathodynamics of fire and qi deficiency represent the core causes of bleeding. Other causes are blood stasis and cold in the blood. Blood stasis is not mentioned here because it only occurs secondarily to other causes such as qi stagnation, heat, cold, dampness, trauma, or qi and blood deficiency. Bleeding from cold in the blood is uncommon, although it is mentioned below.

SYMPTOMS

- If there is chaotic movement of blood in the upper body there will be vomiting of blood or nosebleeds.

This also includes other bleeding from the upper orifices such as bleeding from the ears or coughing up blood.

- If blood flows down into the lower part of the body there will be blood in the urine or stools.

There also can be vaginal bleeding.

- If blood clogs and stagnates in the channels and collaterals, there will be ulcers.

This also includes conditions such as carbuncles, toxic swellings (癰疽 *yōng jū*) and acne (when bright red and pus-filled), which are often a combination of blood heat and blood stasis. Thus when one sees pus, there is often blood stasis and not just fire/heat or cold toxin. These may also come about from underlying blood deficiency.

- If blood is constrained and clumped in the intestines and yin organs, there will be fixed abdominal masses.

For example, many times this manifests as endometriosis or uterine fibroids, which are caused when blood stasis forms nodules. However, it is not uncommon for there to be other complicating factors such as phlegm.

- If the blood is overwhelmed by wind and heat, there will be macules and papules.

This is essentially wind and heat in the blood aspect manifesting as many types of dermatological diseases such as urticaria, eczema, or allergic dermatitis.

- If the blood becomes stagnant from yin-cold, there will be pain and then painful obstruction.

This can occur in any number of locations such as the lower back, knees, joints, or muscles. This may also manifest as tingling and numbness in these areas. In addition to cold, there is usually an element of dampness. If severe, the extremities may turn white upon exposure to cold or black from gangrene, such as in the biomedical correlates, Raynaud's disease, rheumatoid arthritis, and Buerger's disease.

Accompanying symptoms may be lower abdominal pain and a sensation of cold, which is especially prevalent during menstruation. This often indicates a combination of blood stasis, cold, and dampness in the Womb.

Although many blood stasis formulas are warm in nature due to the likely occurrence of cold simultaneously occurring with blood stasis, it is more common to see heat (and dampness) stagnation with blood stasis in the modern clinic.[i]

Summary: Although there may be blood deficiency, blood heat, and blood stasis, it is not uncommon for these to be complicated by any number of other factors such as wind, dampness, phlegm, heat, or cold. This is especially true of blood stasis, which can be caused by many factors, and then, once present, can generate any number of secondary conditions.

PATTERN DIFFERENTIATION

- Accumulation of heat in the Lungs and Stomach: sensation of fullness in the chest with an excessive pulse

This is qi and blood aspect heat and is usually an acute situation. The chest is usually painful and there may be coughing of blood. The pulse is forceful and wiry. This may occur in conditions like pneumonia or from eating too much hot and spicy food.

- Great anger with qi counterflow: darkish green complexion and wiry pulse

This is a pattern of yang, fire, qi, and blood rising, which results in an overabundance of blood that becomes congested in the head. This is a serious pattern, not merely an issue of blood stasis. Two aspects are important to understand.

1. Although there is a component of heat/fire, the complexion is not red or purple. It is the color of the Liver, green-blue. This, as noted in the *Inner Classic*, is a true visceral color and indicates a severe pattern.

2. Although there is a heat/fire component in this pattern there will be cold hands and feet, cold nose, etc. This is because extreme yang transforms to yin, and extreme heat generates cold. This pattern could result in loss of consciousness. The treatment is to direct the counterflow downward and move and cool the blood, as opposed to directly treating the stasis and cold, which are secondary. One treatment approach is to use Flushing Away Roiling Phlegm Pill *(gǔn tán wán)* with the addition of blood cooling herbs such as Moutan Cortex *(mǔ dān pí)*, Paeoniae Radix rubra *(chì sháo)*, and Rehmanniae Radix *(shēng dì huáng)*.

- Yang deficiency and blood traveling outside the vessels: deficiency leading to cold with aversion to cold

This is a bleeding pattern with clear aversion to cold. Some examples are menstrual disorders, later stages of cancer, and bleeding in the elderly. This is much different from a simple qi deficiency pattern causing bleeding. Therefore, medicinals that tonify the Kidney yang, such as Aconiti Radix lateralis preparata *(zhì fù zǐ)* and Cinnamomi Cortex *(ròu guì)*, are essential, whereas merely using medicinals such as Astragali Radix *(huáng qí)* and Atractylodis macrocephalae Rhizoma *(bái zhú)* is insufficient.

The blood quality is thin, like water. Other signs include a puffy, swollen body or limbs, a pale tongue that is wet, possibly dark or even black, or white, greasy coating.

- Yin deficiency with ascending hyperactive fire: cough and wheezing with internal heat

The inclusion of this statement demonstrates Dr. Qin's understanding that blood deficiency often occurs simultaneously with yin deficiency. Thus, this presentation is fire from yin and blood deficiency. One should consider using medicinals such as Rehmanniae Radix *(shēng dì huáng)*, Scrophulariae Radix *(xuán shēn)*, Polygoni multiflori Radix *(hé shǒu wū)*, and Asini Corii Colla *(ē jiāo)* with this presentation.

Although yin and blood deficiency fire conditions can manifest in many ways, it is very common for serious patterns to include respiratory symptoms. In addition to the above-mentioned symptoms, others include difficulty taking a deep breath, shortness of breath, dry mouth, and dry throat. This is especially common in later stage lung cancer, chemotherapy patients, and tuberculosis. The extreme fire results in damage to both the yin and blood, and the resulting yin and blood deficiency further generates fire.

- Exhaustion of the Heart resulting in the inability to generate blood: irritability in the chest with restlessness and a stifling sensation

This is a blood deficiency pattern; for treatment, one should consult Ch. 5 on deficiency. This pattern may have bleeding, such as from the gums or nose, or visible blood vessels in the eyes, but such bleeding still requires tonification.

- Overworking resulting in an inability to contain the blood: spontaneous sweating and fatigue

First there is damage to the qi, which in turn damages the blood by essentially losing its ability to contain the blood. Thus there is bleeding, such as in the stool, from the vagina, coughing up blood, etc. The blood will be pale, thin, and continuously dribbling.

- Constraint and clumping damaging the Spleen: worry and reduced intake of food

This essentially has an underlying Liver blood deficiency component leading to Liver constraint, which over controls earth/Spleen. Diminished Spleen function leads to blood deficiency, creating a vicious cycle. Additional symptoms are deficiency types of insomnia, restlessness due to floating yang, dizziness marked by an empty feeling in the head, negative emotions (e.g., depression), and poor digestion.

- Consumption damaging the Lung qi: chronic cough without phlegm

This is damage to the Lung qi that leads to Lung yin and blood deficiency. Generally, this is not a bleeding pattern; however, there may be specks of blood or small clots mixed in with the dry phlegm. There may also be shortness of breath, palpitations, or just a frequent mild cough. It may come about from conditions such as general debilitation, tuberculosis, chronic fever, or following chemotherapy.

- Qi and blood failing to be governed: blood will certainly be scattered and diffuse

This is qi and blood deficiency that may occur anywhere, causing bleeding. "Scattered and diffuse" refers to the quality of the blood, which will be thin, watery, and have no smell. There is usually no sensation or pain.

- Accumulations and stasis collecting and building up: blood certainly will result in masses or lumps
- Constraint and clumping in the upper body: the blood will be purple

Purple signifies that the constraint and clumping is a chronic problem. This is older blood coming out of the upper part of the body, for example, through coughing or vomiting. This is in contrast to bleeding from the upper body that is bright red, which would be related to heat and is newly-occurring and would require a method of cooling the heat, such as with Rhinoceros Horn and Rehmannia Decoction *(xī jiǎo dì huáng tāng)*. If the blood is purple and dark, one cannot use a cooling method. Instead, one should use medicinals like Crinis carbonisatus *(xuè yú tàn)* or charred Nelumbinis Nodus rhizomatis *(ǒu jié tàn)*. Compare this with the following item.

- Blazing from deficiency or downward counterflow: blood will be bright colored (or fresh)

This is essentially bleeding due to yin (and blood) deficiency fire. The blood may also be thicker and sticky. The location/structure associated with the bleeding will feel hot (e.g., rectum/vagina). One should use medicinals that tonify the yin and are not too cloying, such as charred Paeoniae Radix alba *(bái sháo tàn)*, charred Rehmanniae Radix *(dì huáng tàn)*, and charred Nelumbinis Nodus rhizomatis *(ǒu jié tàn)*.

- Contraction of cold that mutually congeals with the blood - blood will be dark and black.
- Lungs generate abscess: blood will be accompanied by pus
- Phlegm first followed by bleeding: phlegm-fire accumulating heat

This is an excess presentation. An example is pneumonia in which one coughs up phlegm for a while and then starts to have blood mixed in with the phlegm.

- Bleeding first followed by phlegm: yin deficiency furious fire

This is a deficiency presentation where there is a chronic condition with weakness. One may first cough up blood and not be able to expel any phlegm. Thereafter, one may start to expel some phlegm. There may also be dry mouth, sore throat, insomnia, steaming bones, etc.

- Consuming food and drink to satiation with a stifling sensation and then spitting up blood: food damages the gastric cavity leading to impaired transportation

> • Excess consumption of liquor with intoxication and then spitting up blood: alcohol damages the clear pathways (blood vessels), resulting in chaotic movement of the blood
>
> **TREATMENT**
>
> • If there is spitting up of blood,[1] one should direct the qi downward but not give [cold and cooling medicinals] to direct the fire downward; one should promote the movement of blood but not directly stop the bleeding.

The cold and cooling medicinals referred to here are those like Gardeniae Fructus *(zhī zǐ)*, Gypsum fibrosum *(shí gāo)*, or Rhei Radix et Rhizoma *(dà huáng)*. While they may stop the bleeding, they can cause more stagnation and easily damage the normal qi. Quite often, patterns of spitting up or vomiting blood are from deficiency and one must be careful not to create further damage. For example, with coughing or vomiting blood not caused by fire, consider Mori Cortex *(sāng bái pí)*, Eriobotryae Folium *(pí pá yè)*, and honey-prepared Inulae Flos *(mì zhì xuán fù huā)*. Other medicinals that cause the qi to descend to stop bleeding are Nelumbinis Nodus rhizomatis *(ǒu jié)*, Rehmanniae Radix *(shēng dì huáng)*, Agrimoniae Herba *(xiān hè cǎo)*, charred Paeoniae Radix rubra *(chì sháo tàn)*, and charred Moutan Cortex *(mǔ dān pí tàn)*. Of note, bleeding from the nose and eyes is usually the exception to the rule and are more likely to be excess heat patterns. In these situations, one does not have to worry as much about damaging the normal qi.

It is also said that one should not directly stop the bleeding when there is bleeding. This refers to the inappropriate use of medicinals that directly stop bleeding, because these bind and can create stagnation. For example, medicinals like Crinis carbonisatus *(xuè yú tàn)*, charred Rehmanniae Radix preparata *(shú dì tàn)*, and Asini Corii Colla *(ē jiāo)* all have a tendency to create stagnation. Medicinals that promote movement, such as charred Moutan Cortex *(mǔ dān pí tàn)*, charred Nelumbinis Nodus rhizomatis *(ǒu jié tàn)*, and charred Paeoniae Radix rubra *(chì sháo tàn)*, can be used safely. This is especially true when one sees any hint of stagnation, such as clots. For example, with irregular uterine bleeding, many doctors will use medicinals that stop bleeding. Unless there is an emergency or the patient is very weak, this is incorrect. The bleeding may be reduced, but this treatment can create more stagnation, resulting in darker blood, increased lower abdominal pain, increased lower back pain, and insomnia; the condition thereupon becomes much more difficult to cure.

Although the first part of these treatment principles specifically refers to bleeding from the oral cavity, some believe that these principles are intended as general guidelines for all bleeding.

> **BLOOD DISORDERS ORIGINATING FROM THE:**
>
> LUNG: One should clear and direct downward and not raise and scatter.
> HEART: One should nourish the nutritive and not consume and dissipate.
> SPLEEN: One should warm the middle and not [use] sour and cold medicinals.

---

1. This refers to any bleeding that comes out of the oral cavity such as from coughing or vomiting.

> LIVER: One should dredge and promote the flow of qi with sweet and moderate medicinals and not make it more dense causing stagnation.
>
> KIDNEY: It is appropriate to fortify the water and enrich the yin and not to control and curtail.

"Control and curtail" refers to using a draining method with bitter cold or purging medicinals.

SUMMARY

- Promote movement and stop bleeding.

These are two separate but fundamental methods for the treatment of blood disorders. They will of course accompany other methods, such as cooling the blood.

> The methods in this chapter deal with manifestations of blood that are seen or felt, such as bleeding, pain, or masses. These are essentially blood stasis and bleeding patterns.

1. Clear and Cool the Blood (清凉血液 *qīng liáng xuè yè*)

[PRESENTATION] Build up of heat in the blood aspect; chaotic movement and overflowing of blood

Rehmanniae Radix *(shēng dì huáng)*[2]	9g
Moutan Cortex *(mǔ dān pí)*	4.5g
Paeoniae Radix alba *(bái sháo)*	4.5g
Black Gardeniae Fructus *(hēi zhī zǐ)*	4.5g
Lonicerae Flos *(jīn yín huā)*	4.5g
Scutellariae Radix *(huáng qín)*	4.5g
Nelumbinis Nodus Succus *(shēng ǒu zhī)*	1 cup

COMMENTARY

ADDITIONAL SIGNS AND SYMPTOMS

- There may be bleeding from any upper orifice (nose, ears, eyes, mouth, or skin) and the color of the blood will be bright red.
- Red face and red eyes
- Sensations of heat
- Tendency to sweat easily
- Headache or migraine
- Cough

---

2. Originally, Rehmanniae Radix recens *(xiān dì huáng)* 9g was used. It is more cooling and less tonifying than Rehmanniae Radix *(shēng dì huáng)*.

- Dry mouth and/or thirst with a strong desire to drink
- No appetite
- Insomnia with abundant dreams
- Irritability and restlessness at night (daytime is relatively peaceful)
- Ringing in ears like a train
- Constipation
- Dark yellow and burning urine with a strong odor
- Blood-streaked phlegm in the throat[ii]
- Menstrual diseases such as early or blocked menstruation[iii]
- Possible thrombocytopenia
- The pulse is jumpy or edgy and rapid, especially in the distal position; may also be thin and slippery
- The tongue is bright red, especially on the tip, with red prickles and a dry, yellow coating

DISCUSSION

LOCATION: This is a pattern of bleeding from the upper parts of the body due to heat in the blood. The phrase "heat in the blood aspect" is not the same as the blood level in a warm disease four-divisions model. In that model, this pattern is somewhere between the qi and nutritive levels.

ETIOLOGY AND PATHODYNAMIC: This pattern can arise from an invading external pathogen, internal damage from the seven emotions, dietary irregularities (e.g., spicy food), or hyperactivity of Liver fire, as all of these can lead to heat in this level. This results in damage to the yang collaterals, which leads to chaotic and upward movement of the blood.

DURATION: Although this is essentially for an acute stage, this method may be modified for chronic presentations.

TREATMENT STRATEGY:

ROOT: Nourish the yin and cool the blood
BRANCH: Clear heat, restrain and inhibit, and stop bleeding

Cooling (and quieting) the qi aspect is an important complement to addressing the blood aspect. Without it, the strategy is incorrect and the bleeding is difficult to stop.

MEDICINAL ANALYSIS

SUMMARY

- Cool the blood aspect: Rehmanniae Radix *(shēng dì huáng)*, Paeoniae Radix alba *(bái sháo)*, Moutan Cortex *(mǔ dān pí)*, Paeoniae Radix rubra *(chì sháo)*

- Cool the qi aspect: Lonicerae Flos *(jīn yín huā)* and Scutellariae Radix *(huáng qín)*

- Cool the qi and blood: black Gardeniae Fructus *(hēi zhī zǐ)*

- Tonify the blood: Paeoniae Radix alba *(bái sháo)* and Rehmanniae Radix *(shēng dì huáng)*

- All the medicinals are cool to cold.

INDIVIDUAL CHARACTERISTICS

- Rehmanniae Radix *(shēng dì huáng)* is slightly bitter, nourishes the yin, and cools the blood to stop bleeding.

- Paeoniae Radix alba *(bái sháo)* nourishes the yin and preserves the nutritive level. When used with Rehmanniae Radix *(shēng dì huáng)*, it cools and calms the blood.

- Moutan Cortex *(mǔ dān pí)* is considered the best choice for cooling the blood. It also stops bleeding and is able to transform stasis.

- Black Gardeniae Fructus *(hēi zhī zǐ)* is moist, cold, bitter, and clears heat from the three burners. This preparation is preferred because it enters the blood aspect whereas unprepared Gardeniae Fructus *(zhī zǐ)* enters the qi aspect.

- Lonicerae Flos *(jīn yín huā)*, Scutellariae Radix *(huáng qín)*, and Nelumbinis Nodus Succus *(shēng ǒu zhī)* all treat the branch by clearing heat, restraining, inhibiting, and stopping bleeding. The lotus root juice should not be cooked but should be consumed with the decoction. If unavailable, one may substitute Nelumbinis Nodus rhizomatis *(ǒu jié)* 9g.

Dr. Qin's formula is based on Rhinoceros Horn and Rehmannia Decoction *(xī jiǎo dì huáng tāng)*.[iv]

Rhinoceros Horn and Rehmannia Decoction *(xī jiǎo dì huáng tāng)*
SOURCE: *Important Formulas Worth a Thousand Gold Pieces [for any Emergency]* (7th century)

Rhinocerotis Cornu *(xī jiǎo)* 3g
Rehmanniae Radix *(shēng dì huáng)* 24g
Paeoniae Radix *(sháo yào)* 9g
Moutan Cortex *(mǔ dān pí)* 6g

MODIFICATIONS OF DR. QIN'S FORMULA

Difficult to stop bleeding or heavy bleeding:

Charred Rehmanniae Radix *(dì huáng tàn)*, charred Paeoniae Radix alba *(bái sháo tàn)*, charred Moutan Cortex *(mǔ dān pí tàn)*, charred Lonicerae Flos *(jīn yín huā tàn)*, or charred Nelumbinis Nodus rhizomatis *(ǒu jié tàn)* (instead of lotus root liquid). However, one should not use too many charred medicinals (see question below).

Bubali Cornu *(shuǐ niú jiǎo)* 15g

Chronic nosebleeds:

Cirsii japonici Herba sive Radix *(dà jì)*
and Cirsii Herba *(xiǎo jì)* . . . . 6g each[3]

If there is concurrent blood stasis (e.g., purplish lips,
stasis spots on the tip of the tongue, or red-streaked eyes):

---

3. These two can be used alone to stop nosebleeds in children. One can boil the two medicinals for 7-10 minutes and add some flavoring (e.g., vanilla, but not chocolate because it can exacerbate the bleeding).

Paeoniae Radix rubra *(chì shǎo)* instead of Paeoniae Radix alba *(bái shǎo)* or a combination of both

Emotional, restless, with a red face:

Junci Medulla *(dēng xīn cǎo)* 2-3g
Lophatheri Herba *(dàn zhú yè)* 3-5g
Acori tatarinowii Rhizoma *(shí chāng pǔ)*[v] 3-5g

Yin deficiency (e.g., steaming bones or night sweating):

Scrophulariae Radix *(xuán shēn)* 9g

Hot sensation in the chest and Stomach with constipation:

Forsythiae Fructus *(lián qiáo)* 4.5g
Steamed Rhei Radix et Rhizoma *(shú dà huáng)* 4.5g

Bleeding based on location:

• NOSEBLEEDS:

Imperatae Rhizoma *(bái máo gēn)* 6g
Cirsii japonici Herba sive Radix *(dà jì)* and
Cirsii Herba *(xiǎo jì)* . . . . 6g each

• EYES (VERY RED OR BLEEDING):

Celosiae Semen *(qīng xiāng zǐ)* 4.5g
Dry-fried Cassiae Semen *(chǎo jué míng zǐ)* 4.5g

• COUGHING OF BLOOD:

Platycladi Cacumen *(cè bǎi yè)* 4-6g
Rubiae Radix *(qiàn cǎo gēn)* 6-9g
Phragmitis Rhizoma *(lú gēn)* . . . . 9g (dry)
or 1 foot (fresh)

• COUGHING OF BLOOD AND YELLOW PHLEGM:

Trichosanthis Pericarpium *(guā lóu pí)* 4.5g

• BLEEDING FROM EARS:

Anemarrhenae Rhizoma *(zhī mǔ)* 9g
Gentianae Radix *(lóng dǎn cǎo)* 4.5g

If there is chronic lurking heat, consider clearing and draining with Cool the Bones Powder *(qīng gǔ sǎn)*.[4]

QUESTIONS

1. When there is noticeable blood loss, is it appropriate to also include blood tonics like Polygoni multiflori Radix (hé shǒu wū), Angelicae sinensis Radix (dāng guī), or Rehmanniae Radix preparata (shú dì huáng)?

Even though a fundamental treatment strategy here is to nourish the yin, and yin is closely related to blood, one's approach must be clear, soft, quick, and light. Therefore,

---

4. Artemisiae annuae Herba *(qīng hāo)*, Trionycis Carapax *(biē jiǎ)*, Stellariae Radix *(yín chái hú)*, Picrorhizae Rhizoma *(hú huáng lián)*, Anemarrhenae Rhizoma *(zhī mǔ)*, Lycii Cortex *(dì gǔ pí)*, Gentianae macrophyllae Radix *(qín jiāo)*, and Glycyrrhizae Radix *(gān cǎo)*.

one should not use the above medicinals because they are rich and greasy and are too warm for this situation and can actually lead to an increase in bleeding.

2. *Why is Lonicerae Flos (jīn yín huā) in this prescription? Is there some toxin or exterior involvement?*

Lonicerae Flos *(jīn yín huā)* mainly clears the qi level. However, it also has the ability to vent heat outward, especially from the qi and nutritive levels as well as in between the two. By contrast, an herb like Menthae haplocalycis Herba *(bò hé)* has the ability to expel, but works too much on the surface. Gardeniae Fructus *(zhī zǐ)* can clear heat from the qi and blood aspects, but has little ability to thrust the pathogen outward. Lonicerae Flos *(jīn yín huā)* is light and has an affinity for the upper part of the body. It also has a slight ability to moisten the fluids, although in this situation this is not that relevant. The main thrust of the formula is to eliminate the heat. There is no toxin or exterior involvement in this pattern, and Lonicerae Flos *(jīn yín huā)* is accordingly chosen to guide heat to the surface and simultaneously cool internal heat.

3. *If there is bleeding, why doesn't Dr. Qin use the common preparation method of charring the medicinals (e.g., charred Rehmanniae Radix (dì huáng tàn) or charred Paeoniae Radix alba (bái sháo tàn)) to further enhance the formula's ability to stop bleeding?*

One will notice that in the modifications section, charred preparations are suggested if the bleeding is severe. However, charred medicinals, especially when coupled with cold medicinals, will create stagnation, causing further complications. If one follows the above treatment strategy and the problem is not severe, charred medicinals should not be needed. Thus one should use normally-processed Rehmanniae Radix *(shēng dì huáng)* or Paeoniae Radix alba *(bái sháo)* because these are better at cooling the blood.

4. *If this formula is based on Rhinoceros Horn and Rehmannia Decoction (xī jiǎo dì huáng tāng), why does Dr. Qin take out Rhinocerotis Cornu (xī jiǎo) or a suitable substitute such as Bubali Cornu (shuǐ niú jiǎo)?*

In general, Dr. Qin likes to use formulas that are on the milder side. Rhinocerotis Cornu *(xī jiǎo)* is a very strong medicinal and he only uses it when absolutely necessary (see the method "calm and quiet the sovereign fire" in Ch. 11, p. 245). Furthermore, removing Rhinocerotis Cornu *(xī jiǎo)* creates a more flexible formula (making it suitable for acute and chronic presentations) and is also a generally safer approach. If the presentation is serious, one may of course add Bubali Cornu *(shuǐ niú jiǎo)*. This formula substitutes Lonicerae Flos *(jīn yín huā)*, Nelumbinis Nodus rhizomatis *(ǒu jié)*, black Gardeniae Fructus *(hēi zhī zǐ)*, and Scutellariae Radix *(huáng qín)* for Rhinocerotis Cornu *(xī jiǎo)*. These are milder, are not animal products, and are less expensive.

5. *If there is no bleeding, should one remove Nelumbinis Nodus Succus (ǒu zhī) / Nelumbinis Nodus rhizomatis (ǒu jié)?*

Actually, one should keep Nelumbinis Nodus Succus *(ǒu zhī)* / Nelumbinis Nodus rhizomatis *(ǒu jié)* in the prescription. They are excellent mild medicinals for cooling the blood and moving blood stasis.

6. *If this is a pattern of heat in the upper burner, why are there symptoms of menstrual disorders, constipation, and dark urination mentioned?*

Although this is primarily an upper burner pattern (e.g., dry mouth, sore throat, dry cough, chest pain, high fever, or headache) there will likely be some lower burner symptoms, given the systemic involvement of the heat. Of course, once heat is located in one region of the body, it can be transferred to other locations with the many inherent physiological relationships that exist (e.g., constipation resulting from the pairing of the Lungs and Large Intestine, where Lung heat is unable to be removed via the bowels).

2. Warm and Harmonize the Blood (温和血液 *wēn hé xuè yè*)

[PRESENTATION] Cold in the blood aspect; blood stasis binds, congeals, and stagnates

Cinnamomi Cortex *(ròu guì)*[5]	1.2g
Dry-fried Angelicae sinensis Radix *(chǎo dāng guī)*	4.5g
Artemisiae argyi Folium *(ài yè)*	4.5g
Wine-fried Paeoniae Radix alba *(jiǔ chǎo bái sháo)*	4.5g
Charred Zingiberis Rhizoma preparata *(páo jiāng tàn)*	2.4g
Chuanxiong Rhizoma *(chuān xiōng)*	2.4g
Dalbergiae odoriferae Lignum *(jiàng xiāng)*	1.5g

COMMENTARY

ADDITIONAL SIGNS AND SYMPTOMS

- Lower abdomen that is subjectively and/or objectively cool; symptoms may improve with local application of heat
- Painful lower abdomen, especially with the menses or pressure on CV-3 *(zhōng jí)* or CV-4 *(guān yuán)*
- Menses:
    Delayed menses (e.g., 40-50 days)
    Dark or brown menstrual blood that contains clots
    Bleeding that starts with just spotting, which may continue for a day or two before the flow actually starts
    Cramps or cold pain with menstruation
    If severe, there may be amenorrhea

- The stools may contain blood (muddy-looking stools/dark color)
- Infrequent bowel movements that can be either loose or soft
- Watery diarrhea

---

5. The original text prescribed cinnamon heart *(ròu guì xīn)* 1.2g.

- Lower back pain and fatigue that is more severe during menses
- Infertility
- The pulse is deep and choppy
- The tongue is swollen, dark pale, with a greasy, sticky, white or grey coating

This is common in women's diseases.

DISCUSSION

LOCATION: Cold in the blood aspect (Womb)

ETIOLOGY AND PATHODYNAMIC: This is usually caused by cold and dampness in the blood which can come about for two reasons:

1. Internally-generated cold. This is very commonly a deficiency of the *chōng* and *rèn* that leads to congealing and binding of the blood.

2. External cold. This may include exposure to cold weather or consumption of cold foods, which leads to delayed or difficult menses or cramping. Such an external exposure, if unresolved, can lead to internal cold and affect subsequent periods.

TREATMENT PRINCIPLE: When the blood obtains warmth, movement is promoted. Thus one should give warm and harmonizing medicinals that promote the movement of qi and invigorate the blood.

MEDICINAL ANALYSIS

- Artemisiae argyi Folium *(ài yè)* warms the Womb, warms and opens the blood vessels, and relieves pain. This is an important herb for many women's disease caused by cold and dampness.
- Dry-fried Angelicae sinensis Radix *(chǎo dāng guī)* and Chuanxiong Rhizoma *(chuān xiōng)* are yang medicinals that act on the blood. Together they warm and nourish the blood, promote the movement of qi and blood, and stop pain. Dry-frying Angelicae sinensis Radix *(dāng guī)* increases its warmth and decreases the oils that can damage the Spleen circulation.
- Wine-fried Paeoniae Radix alba *(jiǔ chǎo bái sháo)* is a yin medicinal that acts on the blood. It tonifies the yin and blood. Wine processing changes its nature from cool to warm and moderates its sour nature, enabling it to mildly regulate the blood, relax increased tension, and stop pain.
- Charred Zingiberis Rhizoma preparata *(páo jiāng tàn)* enters and warms the blood to warm and dry cold-dampness (see question no. 3 below).
- Cinnamomi Cortex *(ròu guì)* is warm and enters and nourishes the blood aspect of the Heart and Liver. It has the ability to move stagnation at this level. It also warms and nourishes the Kidneys.
- Dalbergiae odoriferae Lignum *(jiàng xiāng)* is very aromatic and acrid. It warms the qi dynamic, primarily promoting the movement of qi and secondarily dispersing stasis (especially of blood, cold, and dampness). It enables the menstrual period to arrive with less effort.

Note: Both Dalbergiae odoriferae Lignum *(jiàng xiāng)* and Cinnamomi Cortex *(ròu guì)* should be taken directly as a powder, capsule, or added to the strained decoction.

Suggestion: Take this prescription one week prior to menstruation and discontinue once menstruation begins.

This formula is roughly based on Ass-Hide Gelatin and Mugwort Decoction *(jiāo ài tāng)* and Drive Out Stasis from the Lower Abdomen Decoction *(shào fù zhú yū tāng).*

Ass-Hide Gelatin and Mugwort Decoction *(jiāo ài tāng)*

SOURCE: *Essentials from the Golden Cabinet* (c. 220)

Chuanxiong Rhizoma *(chuān xiōng)* 6g
Asini Corii Colla *(ē jiāo)* 6g
Glycyrrhizae Radix *(gān cǎo)* 6g
Artemisiae argyi Folium *(ài yè)* 9g
Angelicae sinensis Radix *(dāng guī)* 9g
Paeoniae Radix alba *(bái sháo)* . . . . 12 g
Rehmanniae Radix *(shēng dì huáng)* . . . . 12 g

---

Drive Out Stasis from the Lower Abdomen Decoction *(shào fù zhú yū tāng)*

SOURCE: *Corrections of Errors among Physicians* (1830)

Dry-fried Foeniculi Fructus *(chǎo xiǎo huí xiāng)* 1.5g
Dry-fried Zingiberis Rhizoma *(chǎo gān jiāng)* 0.6g
Corydalis Rhizoma *(yán hú suǒ)* 3g
Angelicae sinensis Radix *(dāng guī)* 9g
Chuanxiong Rhizoma *(chuān xiōng)* 3g
Myrrha *(mò yào)* 3g
Cinnamomi Cortex *(ròu guì)* 3g
Paeoniae Radix rubra *(chì sháo)* 6g
Typhae Pollen *(pú huáng)* 9g
dry-fried Trogopterori Faeces *(chǎo wǔ líng zhī)* 6g

---

MODIFICATIONS OF DR. QIN'S FORMULA

Deficient *chōng* and *rèn*:

Fluoritum *(zǐ shí yīng)* 9g

(can also use Quartz album *[bái shí yīng]*[vi] or Gingko Semen *[bái guǒ]*)

• KEY SIGNS OF A DEFICIENT *chōng* AND *rèn* ARE:

Frequent lower back soreness

Low sexual desire

Infertility or miscarriage

Pulse: weak in the proximal position

Irregular menses:

Spatholobi Caulis *(jī xuè téng)* 4-6g

Leonuri Fructus *(chōng wèi zǐ)* 6-9g

(if there is a headache)

Leonuri Herba *(yì mǔ cǎo)*

(use cautiously where there is significant cold)

Premenstrual syndrome marked by distention in the breasts and chest along with shallow breathing:

Dry-fried Toosendan Fructus *(chuān liàn zǐ)* 4-6g

Corydalis Rhizoma *(yán hú suǒ)* 4-6g

Emotionally restless with insomnia:

Polygoni multiflori Caulis *(yè jiāo téng)* 6g

Polygalae Radix *(yuǎn zhì)* 4.5g

Cramping, pain, internal nodules or lumps, and blood clots:

Sudden Smile Powder *(shī xiào sǎn)*

Trogopterori Faeces *(wǔ líng zhī)* 4.5g

Typhae Pollen *(pú huáng)* 3g

Low sexual desire, lower back pain, cold hands and feet, and frequent urination:

Epimedii Herba *(yín yáng huò)* 4.5g

Kidney deficiency (feeling very cold):

Dry-fried Rehmanniae Radix preparata *(chǎo shú dì huáng)* 9g,

with Asari Radix et Rhizoma *(xì xīn)* . . . . 1g[vii]

In general, for this pattern one can also consider adding Campsis Flos *(líng xiāo huā)*, Rosae rugosae Flos *(méi guī huā)*, and Phaseoli Semen *(chì xiǎo dòu)*, all of which are mild but can move the blood.

QUESTIONS

1. *If this formula is based on Four-Substance Decoction (sì wù tāng), why is Rehmanniae Radix preparata (shú dì huáng) or Rehmanniae Radix (shēng dì huáng) absent?*

   Rehmanniae Radix *(shēng dì huáng)* is bitter and cold, Rehmanniae Radix preparata *(shú dì huáng)* is rich and greasy, and for these reasons they are not included.

2. *Since Cinnamomi Cortex (ròu guì) and Zingiberis Rhizoma preparata (páo jiāng) are used, could one also use Aconiti Radix lateralis preparata (zhì fù zǐ) or Zingiberis Rhizoma (gān jiāng) for this pattern?*

   Aconiti Radix lateralis preparata *(zhì fù zǐ)* and Zingiberis Rhizoma *(gān jiāng)* should not be used because they are too drying and harsh and are unsuitable for the blood aspect. Furthermore, Zingiberis Rhizoma recens *(shēng jiāng)* is also inappropriate; it is best for upper burner problems.

Three types of ginger:

Zingiberis Rhizoma recens *(shēng jiāng)* is best for the upper burner (e.g., wind-cold); it is the most moving and expelling.

Zingiberis Rhizoma (*gān jiāng*) in best for the middle burner; it warms the Spleen and Stomach.

Zingiberis Rhizoma preparata (*páo jiāng*) is best for the lower burner; it is especially good for the Womb.

---

3. Why does Dr. Qin use charred Zingiberis Rhizoma preparata (páo jiāng tàn) instead of Zingiberis Rhizoma preparata (páo jiāng)?

This pattern usually has a deep level of damp and cold stagnation. The charring enables Zingiberis Rhizoma preparata *(páo jiāng tàn)* to enter the deep collaterals and deep blood vessels, separating out the dampness and cold. By contrast, Zingiberis Rhizoma preparata *(páo jiāng)* does not go as deeply and mainly enters the organ level, not the blood aspect.

In addition, charred Zingiberis Rhizoma preparata *(páo jiāng tàn)* is milder and may be needed because many of these patients have some underlying deficiency and a tendency toward sensitive stomachs. Zingiberis Rhizoma preparata *(páo jiāng)* can irritate the stomach, resulting in abdominal pain, and is considered more acrid and dispersing than charred Zingiberis Rhizoma preparata *(páo jiāng tàn)*. However, if there is a large amount of dampness, one can make use of this additional acrid quality and use Zingiberis Rhizoma preparata *(páo jiāng)*.

3. Unblock the Menses and Dispel Stasis (通经去瘀 *tōng jīng qù yū*)

[PRESENTATION] Static blood in the lower burner; menstruation is blocked and stagnant

Angelicae sinensis Radix *(dāng guī)*	4.5g
Chuanxiong Rhizoma *(chuān xiōng)*	2.4g
Dry-fried Paeoniae Radix rubra *(chì sháo)*	4.5g
Spatholobi Caulis *(jī xuè téng)*	4.5g
Achyranthis bidentatae Radix *(niú xī)*	4.5g
Leonuri Fructus *(chōng wèi zǐ)*	4.5g
Rosae chinensis Flos *(yuè jì huā)*	3 flowers

COMMENTARY

ADDITIONAL SIGNS AND SYMPTOMS

MENSTRUAL PERIOD:

- Black or dark blood
- Many clots
- Amenorrhea with abdominal pain
- An often transient sensation of small masses in the lower abdomen
- Premenstrual lower back, abdominal, or breast pain
- Premenstrual constipation
- Premenstrual red spots, patches, or changes in pigment on the face (which disappear after menses)

- Endometriosis (mild)

OTHER:

- Sensations of hot and cold do not usually occur in this pattern.
- All the symptoms tend to be worse in the afternoon and evening.
- The pulse is deep and choppy
- The tongue has a dark purple body, thin white coating, and thick and dark sublingual veins

DISCUSSION

This is a pattern of congealing in the blood aspect, and the stasis is more severe than in the previous method. It is pathogen with form. There is no predominant temperature associated with this presentation. This method only applies to women and revolves around menstruation. It is relatively common.

TREATMENT PRINCIPLE: Promote the movement of qi and blood. This treatment method is stronger than the previous ones.

MEDICINAL ANALYSIS

- Dry-fried Paeoniae Radix rubra *(chǎo chì sháo)* promotes the movement of stasis in the channels and collaterals. Dry-frying reduces the cooling nature of Paeoniae Radix rubra *(chì sháo)* and enhances its moving properties. Unprepared Paeoniae Radix rubra *(chì sháo)* is more binding.
- Spatholobi Caulis *(jī xuè téng)* is able to unblock the collaterals, unblock menstruation, nourish blood without congealing, and eliminate stasis without damaging the normal. One can use a relatively large dosage.
- Leonuri Fructus *(chōng wèi zǐ)* enters the blood aspect, regulates the Liver channel, and unblocks the *chōng* and *rèn* so as to eliminate stasis. It is an excellent medicinal for freeing up menstruation. It has the special ability of being able to direct qi downward as well as direct water qi down and out of the body. For example, it can benefit conditions such as migraines during menstruation.
- Achyranthis bidentatae Radix *(niú xī)* is sour and neutral. It moves and tonifies the blood while guiding the blood downward.
- Rosae chinensis Flos *(yuè jì huā)* is sweet and warm and moves the qi and blood, especially in the Liver. It is commonly used for menstrual disorders and is especially effective for intense emotions (e.g., intense sadness) that occur during or prior to menstruation, or insomnia with many bad dreams. If this is unavailable, one can substitute Rosae rugosae Flos *(méi guī huā)* 2-3g, Campsis Flos *(líng xiāo huā)* 2-3g, or Croci Stigma (*zàng hóng huā)* 0.5g.

———————————————————

While it is stronger than the previous methods, this is still a relatively mild formula that can be taken one week prior to menses. If there are irregular or late menses, it can be taken for a longer period of time.

As with the previous formula, there is no single base formula. One may view it as a modification of Four-Substance Decoction *(sì wù tāng)*, where dry-fried Paeoniae Radix rubra *(chǎo chì sháo)* replaces Paeoniae Radix alba *(bái sháo)*, which increases the blood-invigorating and stasis-transforming functions of Four-Substance Decoction *(sì wù tāng)*.

Four-Substance Decoction *(sì wù tāng)*

SOURCE: *Formulary of the Bureau of Medicines of the Taiping Era* (1078)

Rehmanniae Radix preparata *(shú dì huáng)*. 9-12g
Paeoniae Radix alba *(bái sháo)* 9-12g
Angelicae sinensis Radix *(dāng guī)*. 9-12g
Chuanxiong Rhizoma *(chuān xiōng)* 3-6g

---

MODIFICATIONS OF DR. QIN'S FORMULA

Abdominal or breast tenderness with pressure:

Processed Cyperi Rhizoma *(zhì xiāng fù)* 4.5g

Dry-fried Aurantii Fructus *(chǎo zhǐ ké)* 4.5g

Severe pain:

Corydalis Rhizoma *(yán hú suǒ)*. 4.5g

Dry-fried Toosendan Fructus *(chuān liàn zǐ)*. 6g

Menstrual period that is difficult to expel along with inhibited urination:

Leonuri Herba *(yì mǔ cǎo)*. 9g

Discharge (water/mucus) with menses:

Lycopi Herba *(zé lán)*[6]. 4.5g

Emotional problems (e.g., restlessness, insomnia, or profuse dreams):

Rosae rugosae Flos *(méi guī huā)*. 3g

Campsis Flos *(líng xiāo huā)* 3g

Constipation during or preceding menses:[viii]

Persicae Semen *(táo rén)*. 9g

Carthami Flos *(hóng huā)*. 3g

QUESTIONS

1. *If this formula is based on Four-Substance Decoction (sì wù tāng), why does Dr. Qin remove Rehmanniae Radix preparata (shú dì huáng)?*

   Rehmanniae Radix preparata *(shú dì huáng)* is too cloying, which can create more stagnation.

2. *Why does Dr. Qin choose Leonuri Fructus (chōng wèi zǐ) instead of Leonuri Herba (yì mǔ cǎo)?*

---

6. Lycopi Herba *(zé lán)* can enter the collaterals and somewhat the channels. It has a light diuretic function as well as the ability to dry dampness, similar to Eupatorii Herba *(pèi lán)*.

Leonuri Fructus *(chōng wèi zǐ)* are the seeds of Leonuri Herba *(yì mǔ cǎo)*. Both medicinals are similar and able to unblock the menses and invigorate and promote the movement of blood. However, Leonuri Fructus *(chōng wèi zǐ)* is stronger and enters the deep collaterals and thus moves blood at a deeper level than Leonuri Herba *(yì mǔ cǎo)*, which only moves stagnation in the blood vessels. One of the key indications for its use is that the patient's head has been affected, for example, they have a deep headache that may be difficult to pinpoint. This shows that the deep collaterals have been affected, rather than just lower burner stagnation.

In this pattern, if there are no head symptoms, one may choose to use Leonuri Herba *(yì mǔ cǎo)*. However, if there is also backache and/or chest pain, one can use both. This additional pain shows there is a greater degree of blood stagnation, and more force is required. Leonuri Fructus *(chōng wèi zǐ)* and Leonuri Herba *(yì mǔ cǎo)* have a synergistic relationship and can be used together to enhance each others' function of moving blood, especially in the lower burner.

3. *Why does Dr. Qin choose Achyranthis bidentatae Radix (niú xī) instead of Cyathulae Radix (chuān niú xī)?*

Although Cyathulae Radix *(chuān niú xī)* has a stronger ability to move the blood, Achyranthis bidentatae Radix *(niú xī)* is chosen because of its additional ability to tonify, which is required here due to the loss of blood that occurs during menstruation. Achyranthis bidentatae Radix *(niú xī)* has about a 50:50 ratio of tonification and moving, whereas Cyathulae Radix *(chuān niú xī)* is more around 80:20. One may choose Cyathulae Radix *(chuān niú xī)* if the menses are very stagnant and there is difficulty urinating.

4. Attack and Break Up Blood Accumulation (攻破血积 *gōng pò xuè jī*)

[PRESENTATION] Static blood accumulations and clusters; fixed lumps or stone-like mobile abdominal masses

Angelicae sinensis radicis Cauda *(dāng guī wěi)*	6g
Sparganii Rhizoma *(sān léng)*	4.5g
Carthami Flos *(hóng huā)*	2.4g
Curcumae Rhizoma *(é zhú)*	4.5g
Salviae miltiorrhizae Radix *(dān shēn)*	4.5g
Persicae Semen *(táo rén)*	4.5g
Lycopi Herba *(zé lán)*	4.5g

COMMENTARY

ADDITIONAL SIGNS AND SYMPTOMS

• Abdominal masses, accumulations and clusters such as nodules, neuromas, myomas, fibromas, or any palpable mass in the abdomen. Although the masses may come and go with the menses, they are usually distinct, large, and palpable. Even if impalpable, modern biomedical diagnostic tests will show masses deep in the body or endometriosis.

- Severe pain
- Difficulty falling asleep
- Menstrual flow may have difficulty getting started or may start and stop.
- Patients may have biomedical diagnoses such as endometriosis, pelvic infection, cancers, or infertility.
- The pulse is deep and choppy. Sometimes the pulse is so deep that it is difficult to find. This does not show deficiency, but rather that the stagnation is serious and at a very deep level.
- The tongue is purple, dark, with many blood stasis spots

DISCUSSION

DURATION AND TREATMENT COURSE: This presentation is one that advances slowly over time and therefore takes a long time to cure, at least six months.

The formula can be given 7-10 days prior to menstruation to expel blood stasis. One may also choose to give it during menses to further aid in expelling the blood stasis. If many clots are expelled, this is a positive sign. One may end up giving the formula 15 days out of the cycle for many months. This formula is safe for long-term use; however, if the patient is deficient, it is best to follow-up with a tonifying formula after menstruation.

TREATMENT PRINCIPLE: Promote the movement of blood and drive out stasis while still keeping a foundation of nourishing the blood. This method is stronger than the previous ones, and should be appropriately differentiated.

MEDICINAL ANALYSIS

- Angelicae sinensis radicis Cauda *(dāng guī wěi)* nourishes the blood, enters the channels and deep collaterals (at the blood aspect), and breaks up blood stasis.

- Salviae miltiorrhizae Radix *(dān shēn)* is bitter and slightly cold. It enters the organ level, invigorates the blood, and also mildly nourishes the blood. In addition, it is chosen because it is a mild herb.

- Persicae Semen *(táo rén)* and Carthami Flos *(hóng huā)* work together to invigorate the blood and eliminate stasis. Persicae Semen *(táo rén)* is bitter, neutral, and slightly sweet. It enters the organs and is specific for the treatment of hard obstructions and the buildup of blood and menstrual obstruction. It should be crushed. Carthami Flos *(hóng huā)* is acrid and warm and enters the channels and vessels.

- Sparganii Rhizoma *(sān léng)* and Curcumae Rhizoma *(é zhú)* are similar and work together to break up accumulation and drive out blood stasis, as well as move qi stagnation. However, Curcumae Rhizoma *(é zhú)* is bitter, neutral to warm, and functions more on the qi aspect, while Sparganii Rhizoma *(sān léng)* is acrid, bitter, slightly cool, and functions more on the blood aspect.

- Lycopi Herba *(zé lán)* is bitter, acrid, slightly warm, and very mild. It invigorates the blood, moves water and eliminates swelling, and frees the menses. It enters the Liver, making it suitable for many gynecological diseases, especially when there is some element of blood stasis mixed with water issues (e.g., body swelling or an abdomen that is painful and tight from edema). Note that when there is chronic blood stasis, there is often accompanying pathogenic water and phlegm.

Dr. Qin's formula is based on Four-Substance Decoction with Safflower and Peach Pit *(táo hóng sì wù tāng)*.

Four-Substance Decoction with Safflower and Peach Pit *(táo hóng sì wù tāng)*

SOURCE: *Golden Mirror of the Medical Tradition* (1742)

Chuanxiong Rhizoma *(chuān xiōng)* 3g
Angelicae sinensis Radix *(dāng guī)* 6g
dry-fried Paeoniae Radix alba *(chǎo bái sháo)* 6g
Rehmanniae Radix preparata *(shú dì huáng)* 6g
Persicae Semen *(táo rén)* 6g
Carthami Flos *(hóng huā)* 3g

MODIFICATIONS OF DR. QIN'S FORMULA

Chronic disease that is difficult to cure (e.g., neuromas). **Use animal products:**

Wine-fried Pheretima *(jiǔ chǎo dì lóng)* 6g

Eupolyphaga/Stelophaga *(tǔ biē chóng)* (wine fried) 4.5g

Trogopterori Faeces *(wǔ líng zhī)* 4.5g

Consider other bugs and insects (e.g. Tabanus *[méng chóng]* or black ant — Formica fusca *[mǎ yǐ]*)[7]

Chronic disease with simultaneous deficiency:

Notoginseng Radix *(sān qī)* . . . . 3g (powder)

Menses that are difficult to get started:

Leonuri Herba *(yì mǔ cǎo)* 9g

Also consider adding Gigeriae galli Endothelium corneum *(jī nèi jīn)*, which dissolves nodules.

CONCURRENT PATTERNS

With congealing cold:

Cinnamomi Cortex *(ròu guì)* 1-2g
   (powdered and added to the strained decoction)
Zingiberis Rhizoma preparata *(páo jiāng)* /
   charred Zingiberis Rhizoma preparata *(páo jiāng tàn)* 3-5g

---

7. Formica fusca *(mǎ yǐ)* enters the Liver and Kidneys, is salty, sour, and balanced. It tonifies the Kidneys, augments the essence, frees the channels, invigorates the collaterals, resolves toxicity, and disperses swelling.

Artemisiae argyi Folium *(ài yè)*.....................................4-6g

With qi stagnation:

Cyperi Rhizoma *(xiāng fù)*.....................................4-6g

Citri reticulatae Pericarpium *(chén pí)*.............................4-6g

With dampness and/or phlegm:

Gleditsiae Spina *(zào jiǎo cì)*.....................................4.5g

ADDITIONAL CONSIDERATIONS

1. Patent medicine for blood stasis nodules: Rhubarb and Ground Beetle Pill *(dà huáng zhè chóng wán)* (see below)

2. If the patient is tired after menstruation (as in blood deficiency), and one has already given a blood-moving formula before menstruation, one should then tonify after the period stops with a formula like Four-Substance Decoction with Safflower and Peach Pit *(táo hóng sì wù tāng)*. If there is more severe weakness, fatigue, and/or insomnia following the period, one may consider a formula like Restore the Spleen Decoction *(guī pí tāng)*,[8] Black Restore the Spleen Decoction *(hēi guī pí tāng)*,[9] or Ginseng Decoction to Nourish Luxuriance *(rén shēn yǎng róng tāng)*.[10]

3. **Food therapy:** If the patient is not overtly deficient, it is enough to use food therapy (instead of herbs) after menstruation. For example, consider Phaseoli Semen *(chì xiǎo dòu)* [adzuki beans] 30g (soaked overnight) plus Croci Stigma *(zàng hóng huā)* [saffron] 0.25g, and one teaspoon of brown sugar cooked into a soup. This will move and tonify the blood.

4. **External treatment:** Four-Substance Decoction with Safflower and Peach Pit *(táo hóng sì wù tāng)* plus Caryophylli Flos *(dīng xiāng)*, Foeniculi Fructus *(xiǎo huí xiāng)*, Aconiti Radix lateralis preparata *(zhì fù zǐ)*, and Ephedrae Herba *(má huáng)* (6-9 each). Grind into a coarse powder. Mix with 250g of rock salt. Place in cloth bag, warm it, and place on any location that is stagnant. Treatment course is 7-10 days.

5. **Enema:** Add Caryophylli Flos *(dīng xiāng)* 6g and Foeniculi Fructus *(xiǎo huí xiāng)* 6g to Dr. Qin's formula above. Boil to a very concentrated 100cc and use as an enema. This is a slow drip enema, over one hour. One should heat the liquid to just above body temperature

---

8. Ginseng Radix *(rén shēn)*, dry-fried Astragali Radix *(chǎo huáng qí)* , Atractylodis macrocephalae Rhizoma *(bái zhú)*, Poria *(fú líng)*, dry-fried Ziziphi spinosae Semen *(chǎo suān zǎo rén)*, Longan Arillus *(lóng yǎn ròu)*, Aucklandiae Radix *(mù xiāng)*, Glycyrrhizae Radix preparata *(zhì gān cǎo)*, Angelicae sinensis Radix *(dāng guī)*, processed Polygalae Radix *(zhì yuǎn zhì)*, Zingiberis Rhizoma recens *(shēng jiāng)*, and Jujubae Fructus *(dà zǎo)*.

9. This is Restore the Spleen Decoction *(guī pí tāng)* plus dry-fried Rehmanniae Radix preparata *(chǎo shú dì huáng)*.

10. Paeoniae Radix alba *(bái sháo)*, Angelicae sinensis Radix *(dāng guī)*, Citri reticulatae Pericarpium *(chén pí)*, Astragali Radix *(huáng qí)*, Cinnamomi Cortex *(ròu guì)*, Ginseng Radix *(rén shēn)*, Atractylodis macrocephalae Rhizoma *(bái zhú)*, Glycyrrhizae Radix preparata *(zhì gān cǎo)*, Rehmanniae Radix preparata *(shú dì huáng)*, Schisandrae Fructus *(wǔ wèi zǐ)*, Poria *(fú líng)*, and Polygalae Radix *(yuǎn zhì)*.

and slowly allow the enema to drip into the bowels. If it enters too quickly (or the body just cannot absorb the medicinals), it can cause diarrhea and will be ineffective.

6. **Moxa cake:** Add Caryophylli Flos *(dīng xiāng)* 6g to Dr. Qin's formula above. Instead of cooking, grind it into a powder and then make into a paste, using water or ginger liquid plus flour. One can then place the cakes on points such as CV-3 *(zhōng jí)*, CV-4 *(guān yuán)*, CV-8 *(shén què)*, ST-28 *(shuǐ dào)*, and ST-29*(guī lái)*, then burn moxa on top of the cake. This will move stagnation in the abdomen. Do this one week prior to menstruation or any time there is abdominal cramping. This has been successful for such problems as endometriosis and uterine fibroids.

QUESTIONS

1. *If this formula is based on Four-Substance Decoction with Safflower and Peach Pit (táo hóng sì wù tāng), why are three of the six ingredients absent?*

   Paeoniae Radix alba *(bái sháo)* and Rehmanniae Radix preparata *(shú dì huáng)* are too cloying. Chuanxiong Rhizoma *(chuān xiōng)* is also counterproductive because it is ascending and the formula needs to descend.

2. *What is Rhubarb and Ground Beetle Pill (dà huáng zhè chóng wán) and how can it be used?*

   Rhubarb and Ground Beetle Pill *(dà huáng zhè chóng wán)* is derived from Ch. 6 of the *Essentials from the Golden Cabinet.* Although it may be difficult to find outside of China, it is a very effective formula for accumulations, especially with menstrual periods that contain dark clots, and for conditions like endometriosis. Therefore, if there is no result with above methods, consider giving 4.5g boiled with other herbs, taken over a long period of time (e.g., 4-6 months). This can greatly reduce the impact of endometriosis, and help to eliminate infertility[11] that commonly occurs with such patterns. However, even after the patient becomes pregnant, she should continue some type of herbal or food therapy for 1-2 months to continue to eliminate stasis. Following the pregnancy, it is also very important to limit exposure to cold (e.g., avoid getting chilled as well as foods such as ice cream) while continuing to nourish and move the blood. If all these steps are followed, it is possible to cure the endometriosis or other blood stasis patterns.

3. *Why are Sparganii Rhizoma (sān léng) and Curcumae Rhizoma (é zhú) chosen?*

   They are chosen because abdominal masses have already formed, and one must use these somewhat harsh herbs to break the blood stasis and promote the movement of qi. Consequently, one must pay attention to dosage, the stage of the disease, and the patient's constitution so as not to damage the patient. These are the strongest herbs in the formula.

---

11. If infertility is a concern, one may consider adding medicinals to strengthen the eight extraordinary vessels, such as Fluoritum *(zǐ shí yīng)*, Quartz album *(bái shí yīng)*, and Gingko Semen *(bái guǒ)*.

5. Facilitate the Movement of Qi and Disperse Blood Stasis
(利气散瘀 *lì qì sàn yū*)

[PRESENTATION] Qi gathers in the upper burner, leading to a stoppage and stasis of blood; expectoration of blood and pain in the collaterals

Platycladi Cacumen *(cè bǎi yè)* 4.5g
dry-fried Paeoniae Radix rubra *(chǎo chì sháo)* 4.5g
vinegar-prepared Olibanum *(cù zhì rǔ xiāng)* 3g
Curcumae Radix *(yù jīn)* 4.5g
Dalbergiae odoriferae Lignum *(jiàng xiāng)* 2.4g
Aurantii Fructus *(zhǐ ké)* 4.5g
Luffae Fructus Retinervus *(sī guā luò)* 9g

COMMENTARY

ADDITIONAL SIGNS AND SYMPTOMS:

- Chest, back, and/or flank pain. The pain is usually sharp, stabbing, moving, and will suddenly come and go. It has a quality similar to a fast pricking needle and usually occurs on the surface of the body. The exact location may be unclear. This pain is not serious, in that if one is working hard, he will not feel it. It may also manifest as ongoing pressure or tightness where the patient may feel the need to pound on their chest. The pain usually occurs more in the daytime.[ix]
- Chest oppression
- Dry mouth and throat
- Intense emotions (e.g., depression)
- Insomnia
- Restlessness
- Dry cough, possibly with blood
- The pulse is choppy and wiry
- The tongue is dark red

DISCUSSION

This pattern is mainly for pain in the chest and flanks. It is principally a pattern of qi stagnation, which leads to a secondary, somewhat minor, pattern of blood stasis in the superficial collaterals. Although there may be heat present (see question no. 4 below), bleeding in this case is caused by stasis and not heat. There should not be a lot of bleeding, but there may be slight clots. One can also use this formula if there is no bleeding.

ETIOLOGY: This pattern may occur after an accident where there is residual blood stasis in the chest. It may also occur from internal imbalances such as emotional influences (e.g., anger or depression) leading to Liver qi stagnation, which in turn affects the chest.

MEDICINAL ANALYSIS

SUMMARY

This formula essentially moves qi and blood stasis in the chest and is most appropriate when there are some heat signs.

INDIVIDUAL CHARACTERISTICS

* Dry-fried Paeoniae Radix rubra *(chǎo chì sháo)* promotes the movement of stasis in the channels and collaterals. Dry-frying reduces its cooling nature and enhances its moving properties. Regular Paeoniae Radix rubra *(chì sháo)* is more binding and cooler.
* Olibanum *(rǔ xiāng)* is acrid, aromatic, and warm. It is a blood-within-the-qi medicinal and strongly promotes the movement of qi, invigorates the blood, and stops pain.
* Curcumae Radix *(yù jīn)* is acrid, bitter, and cold. It is a qi-within-the-blood medicinal, allowing it to regulate the qi and disperse stasis, which makes it quite effective at relieving pain.
* Dalbergiae odoriferae Lignum *(jiàng xiāng)* is aromatic, acrid, and warm. It alleviates pain by moving qi stagnation in the blood, especially in the upper burner.
* Platycladi Cacumen *(cè bǎi yè)* cools the blood and stops bleeding and should only be used if there is bleeding.
* Aurantii Fructus *(zhǐ ké)* is slightly warm. It regulates the Liver and disperses qi, especially in the flanks.
* Luffae Fructus Retinervus *(sī guā luò)* is neutral, cool, and light. It enters the qi aspect, guiding the other medicinals to enter the collaterals.

MODIFICATIONS OF DR. QIN'S FORMULA

Constipation with dry stool:
Persicae Semen *(táo rén)* 9g

Recent accident or trauma (use with caution if there are significant heat signs):
Notoginseng Radix *(sān qī)* 3g
Yunnan Baiyao (prepared medicine)

Accident with neck involvement (e.g., whiplash):
Puerariae Radix *(gé gēn)* 9g
Notopterygii Rhizoma seu Radix *(qiāng huó)* 4.5g

Joint and muscle pain:
Spatholobi Caulis *(jī xuè téng)* 4.5g
Salviae miltiorrhizae Radix *(dān shēn)* 4.5g

Generalized pain:
Vaccariae Semen *(wáng bù liú xíng)* 4-6g
Liquidambaris Fructus *(lù lù tōng)* 4-6g

More severe pain:
Myrrha *(mò yào)* 4-6g
Corydalis Rhizoma *(yán hú suǒ)* 4.5g

Chest pressure with difficulty taking a deep breath:

Liquidambaris Fructus *(lù lù tōng)* 4-6g

Emotional upset accompanied by pain that is not severe:

Rosae rugosae Flos *(méi guī huā)*, Rosae chinensis Flos *(yuè jì huā)*,
and Campsis Flos *(líng xiāo huā)* . . . . 3g each

Poor digestion with a blocked sensation in the epigastrium:

Scorched Crataegi Fructus *(jiāo shān zhā)* 9g

Fried Massa medicata fermentata *(chǎo shén qū)* 9g

Headache:

Viticis Fructus *(màn jīng zǐ)* 4-6g

Leonuri Fructus *(chōng wèi zǐ)* 6-9g

Cough:

Platycodi Radix *(jié gěng)* 3g

To further circulate qi in the collaterals:

Citri reticulatae Vascular *(jú luò)* 2-3g

To further stop bleeding by eliminating blood stasis in the collaterals:

Rubiae Radix *(qiàn cǎo gēn)* 6-9g

More obvious blood stasis, including dark spots on tongue, a taste of blood in the throat, purple blood coming up when clearing the throat, or even dark black stools with constipation:

Persicae Semen *(táo rén)* 4.5g

Carthami Flos *(hóng huā)* 4.5g

QUESTIONS

1. Since there is a qi stagnation component, is it suitable to use Bupleuri Radix (chái hú)?

Yes, one can use Bupleuri Radix *(chái hú)* unless there is a tendency for headaches, high blood pressure (due to yang rising), or any sensation of heat rising. The dosage should be 4.5g.

2. Why does Dr. Qin use Olibanum (rǔ xiāng) instead of Myrrha (mò yào)?

Both of these medicinals regulate the blood. However, Olibanum *(rǔ xiāng)* primarily goes to the qi aspect and channels, whereas Myrrha *(mò yào)* mainly goes to the blood aspect. Since this is essentially a qi aspect problem, Dr. Qin chose Olibanum *(rǔ xiāng)*. However, both can be used together if there is severe pain.

3. Are there any considerations if the etiology is more from an emotional cause?

Consider adding Tribuli Fructus *(cì jí lí) and* Campsis Flos *(líng xiāo huā)*. If more serious, one can add Inulae Flos *(xuán fù huā)* 4-6g, Croci Stigma *(zàng hóng huā)* 0.5g, and Allii fistulosi Bulbus *(cōng bái)* 3-4 pieces.

4. Is there a heat component in this pattern?

One may notice the symptoms of dry mouth, dry throat, dry cough (with blood), insomnia, and restlessness. These are not from heat per se. The dry symptoms are linked to the blood stasis, which interferes with the circulation of fluids, leading to dryness. As noted above, the bleeding itself is from stasis. In addition, blood stasis can lead to some production of heat, which can lead to insomnia and restlessness. The formula is fairly balanced thermally and the objective is to remove the root cause, stagnation. Consequently, one should not cool the blood or add heavy moistening medicinals, which would lead to more stagnation. In addition, a formula that is too acrid and warm could easily exacerbate this situation.

---

6. Restrain and Inhibit the Blood Vessels (收敛血管 *shōu liàn xuè guǎn*)

[PRESENTATION] Chaotic movement of blood; spitting of blood or continuous uterine bleeding

Clear-prepared Astragali Radix (*qīng zhì huáng qí*)	4.5g
Calcined Fossilia Ossis Mastodi (*duàn lóng gǔ*)	9g
Dry-fried Codonopsis Radix (*chǎo dǎng shēn*)	4.5g
Calcined Ostreae Concha (*duàn mǔ lì*)	15g
Atractylodis macrocephalae Rhizoma (*bái zhú*)	4.5g
Pearls of Asini Corii Colla (*ē jiāo zhū*)	9g
Terra flava usta (*zào xīn tǔ*)	15g

COMMENTARY

ADDITIONAL SIGNS AND SYMPTOMS:

- Lack of appetite
- Pale face
- Fatigue
- Shortness of breath
- Lack of desire to open one's eyes
- Visual floaters
- Reduced auditory acuity
- Insomnia
- Restlessness
- If severe, there may be labored breathing, sweating from the head, continuous palpitations, profuse uterine bleeding, lightheadedness, dizziness, or vertigo. This is severe qi abandonment and requires urgent treatment by securing the qi.
- The pulse is deficient, deep, and thin; if severe, hollow, rapid, and floating
- The tongue is pale, swollen, and dry, with cracks

DISCUSSION

This is a pattern of Spleen/middle qi deficiency where the qi is unable to contain and govern the blood. The main issue is bleeding, which usually occurs from the lower orifices (bowels, urine, or vagina), although there may also be coughing or vomiting of blood. The flow is usually not heavy and may be pink or slightly dark colored, watery, thin, runs gently, and does not clot quickly. Overwork or fatigue are the most common causes of this condition.

DURATION: This is often an acute situation, where the bleeding must be stopped quickly. However, one may also use this strategy for chronic or moderate situations.

Note: If there is continuous bleeding, even light, that persists for 2-3 weeks with treatment, refer to a biomedical practitioner. If there is severe, profuse bleeding, one should not wait for more than a couple days.

TREATMENT PRINCIPLE: Stop the bleeding and tonify the blood and qi.

MEDICINAL ANALYSIS

- Clear prepared Astragali Radix *(qīng zhì huáng qí)*, dry-fried Codonopsis Radix *(chǎo dǎng shēn)*, and Atractylodis macrocephalae Rhizoma *(bái zhú)* augment the qi and build up the Spleen in order to contain the blood. If there is deficiency abandonment,[12] use Ginseng Radix *(rén shēn)*.

- Calcined Fossilia Ossis Mastodi *(duàn lóng gǔ)* and calcined Ostreae Concha *(duàn mǔ lì)* secure, contain, and stop the bleeding.

- Pearls of Asini Corii Colla *(ē jiāo zhū)* tonify the blood and stop the bleeding. They should be crushed and dissolved into the strained decoction.

- Terra flava usta *(zào xīn tǔ)* is sweet and warm and builds up the middle in order to stop the bleeding. It should be cooked first for 30 minutes.

- One may also consider using charred Rehmanniae Radix preparata *(shú dì tàn)*.

MODIFICATIONS OF DR. QIN'S FORMULA

Weakness, palpitations, and sweating, with a pulse that is deficient, weak, or hollow:
Ginseng Radix *(rén shēn)* 4.5g
Ophiopogonis Radix *(mài mén dōng)* 6g
Schisandrae Fructus *(wǔ wèi zǐ)* 3g

Bleeding that is difficult to stop (heavy or light):
Ten Partially-charred Substances Powder *(shí huī sǎn)*ˣ
   (stop bleeding in emergencies)
Charred Trachycarpi Petiolus *(zōng lǘ tàn)* 6g

---

12. Deficiency abandonment (虚脱 *xū tuō*) is a sudden change in the patient's condition where yin and yang separate from each other. If severe, there may be critical life symptoms. In general, there is extreme fatigue, fear, pain, hunger, bleeding, pale face, deficiency sweating, dizziness, blurred vision, nausea, vomiting, throbbing of the heart, low blood pressure, loss of control of the urine and bowels, or fainting.

Charred Nelumbinis Receptaculum *(lián fáng tàn)* 4.5g

Charred Saposhnikoviae Radix *(fáng fēng tàn)* 4.5g

Charred Schizonepetae Herba *(jīng jiè tàn)* 4.5g

Heavy bleeding from sinking of middle qi:

Charred Cimicifugae Rhizoma *(shēng má tàn)* 3-5g

Incessant uterine bleeding:

Charred aged Trachycarpi Petiolus *(chén zōng tàn)* 4-6g

Expectoration of blood or spitting up of blood:

Charred Rehmanniae Radix *(dì huáng tàn)* 4-6g

Expectoration of blood (later stages where the yin and blood have become exhausted):

Charred Rehmanniae Radix preparata *(shú dì tàn)* 6-9g

Bletillae Rhizoma *(bái jí)* 4-6g

Nosebleeds:

Charred Cirsii Herba *(xiǎo jì tàn)* 4.5g

Charred Imperatae Rhizoma *(máo gēn tàn)* 4.5g

Cough with blood:

Charred Nelumbinis Nodus rhizomatis *(ǒu jié tàn)* 4.5g

Agrimoniae Herba *(xiān hè cǎo)* 6g

For any type of upper body bleeding:

Omit Astragali Radix *(huáng qi)*

Blood in the urine:

Charred Platycladi Cacumen *(cè bǎi tàn)*[13] 4.5g

Charred Imperatae Rhizoma *(máo gēn tàn)* 4.5g

Uterine bleeding:

Charred aged Trachycarpi Petiolus *(chén zōng tàn)* 4.5g

Charred Nelumbinis Receptaculum *(lián fáng tàn)* 4.5g

After or during bleeding there are additional yin deficiency symptoms:

Testudinis Plastri Colla *(guī bǎn jiāo)* 9g

Charred Rehmanniae Radix *(dì huáng tàn)* . . . . 4-6g, or

Charred Rehmanniae Radix preparata *(shú dì tàn)* 6g

Blood deficiency (e.g., pale face, pale tongue, anemia, etc.):

Charred Rehmanniae Radix preparata *(shú dì tàn)* 9g

(cold presentation)

---

13. One should not use unprocessed Platycladi Cacumen *(cè bǎi yè)*. Not only can it be difficult to digest, it is inappropriate for deficient patients. The charring aids the digestion, is less cool, and is better at stopping bleeding.

Charred Rehmanniae Radix preparata *(shú dì tàn)* 6-9g
+ charred Rehmanniae
Radix *(dì huáng tàn)* 4-6g
(if on the warm side, e.g., with red face, dry mouth, heat, or a mixed pattern)

Concurrent blood stasis (e.g., dark blood, clots, purple or black spots
on the tongue, more serious in the evening):
Crinis carbonisatus *(xuè yú tàn)* 4-6g

QUESTIONS

1. *Since the basic principle is tonify the blood and qi to stop the bleeding, why is Angelicae sinensis Radix (dāng guī) not used?*

   This question is in reference to the formula Tangkuei Decoction to Tonify the Blood *(dāng guī bǔ xuè tāng)*,[14] which is the flagship formula for blood loss with qi and blood deficiency. Although the same treatment principle applies to the above method, Angelicae sinensis Radix *(dāng guī)* should not be used because it is too warm and can cause more bleeding. Asini Corii Colla *(ē jiāo)* is a better choice because it is cool. This also applies to the basic formula of Four-Substance Decoction *(sì wù tāng)*; it is inappropriate in this situation, even with extensive blood loss.

2. *What is the significance of the various processing of the medicinals?*

   The calcined Ostreae Concha *(mǔ lì)* and Fossilia Ossis Mastodi *(lóng gǔ)* increases the astringent properties of these herbs and increases their ability to stop the bleeding. Pearls of Asini Corii Colla *(ē jiāo zhū)* are much easier to digest than regular Asini Corii Colla *(ē jiāo)*, which is important because of the middle burner deficiency in this case. Furthermore, pearls of Asini Corii Colla *(ē jiāo zhū)* are more effective here in stopping bleeding. Dry-fried Codonopsis Radix *(chǎo dǎng shēn)* is less cloying and more tonifying to the Spleen's circulation than Codonopsis Radix *(dǎng shēn)*.

3. *If there is serious bleeding, can one use the patent medicine Yunnan Baiyao?*

   This ready-made prepared formula is inappropriate because it is too moving and too drying for this pattern of deficiency. However, without any better options, one may use it for at most 2-3 days to control bleeding, if the bleeding is severe.

---

14. Astragali Radix *(huáng qí)* 30g and Angelicae sinensis Radix *(dāng guī)* 6g.

5

Treatment Guidelines for

Deficiency 虛 *(xū)*

ETIOLOGY

External damage from excessive drinking and sex, internal damage from the seven emotions, dietary irregularities, overwork and fatigue, and immoderate desires

Included with the above etiologies are various types of substance abuse, excessive exercise, greed, as well as some genetic factors. Substance abuse here includes inappropriate use of pharmaceuticals (such as steroids, birth control pills, or other hormones) as well as illicit drugs and smoking, as all of these can lead to the presence of toxins in the body. This can also occur, to a much lesser extent, by eating too much hot and spicy foods.

PATHODYNAMIC

Alcohol damages the Lungs; once damp-heat fumes and steams, the Lung yin melts.

Excessive sex damages the Kidneys; once the essence chamber becomes empty, ministerial fire becomes unrestrained.

This will manifest with symptoms such as lower back pain, dizziness, frequent urination, steaming bones, night sweats, and tinnitus.

Excessive thought and deliberation damages the Heart; once the blood is consumed, fire easily ascends.

Excessive thought and deliberation can also damage the Spleen, Liver, Kidneys, and Lungs, but typically it will first affect the Heart. This manifests as an unclear or tired mind, insomnia or poor sleep, anxiety, and a poor memory. Restore the Spleen Decoction *(guī pí tāng)* is an appropriate treatment. There is usually a progression of insomnia leading to poor memory leading to generalized weakness.

Secondarily, excessive thought and deliberation can lead to qi constraint, which leads to poor circulation of Spleen qi, which damages the Spleen. This will manifest as poor digestion and reduced appetite.

> Overwork and fatigue damage the Spleen; once heat is internally generated, it harms the true yin.

This pattern is not very common and is yin fire, as conceptualized by Li Dong-Yuan. This process can also damage the Kidneys, leading to qi, blood, and essence deficiency. At first, one may just feel tired, and then this may develop into full blown chronic fatigue and depression. At this point, all the organs are somewhat deficient, and this is difficult to cure. It should be kept in mind that sleep deprivation can easily contribute to fatigue.

> Anger damages the Liver; once Liver fire internally blazes, it ascends and scorches the blood, leading to spitting of blood.

This may also manifest as headaches, migraines, hypertension, red face and ears, mood swings, and irregular menses.

> **PATTERN DIFFERENTIATION**
> * Crimson cheeks and red lips: yin deficiency below forcing the yang upwards

This commonly occurs in the afternoon; there may also be red eyes.

> * The mouth is usually dry and thirsty: Kidney yin insufficiency and patients will take in fluids to save themselves.

This is Kidney water deficiency, which commonly occurs at night, and is often a pattern of Heart fire and Kidney water failing to connect. This will manifest as insomnia, palpitations that may be easily triggered by even the slightest sound, a thin and rapid pulse, and a purple red, dry, cracked tongue. Sample formulas are Emperor of Heaven's Special Pill to Tonify the Heart *(tiān wáng bǔ xīn dān)*,[1] Anemarrhena, Phellodendron, and Rehmannia Pill *(zhī bǎi dì huáng wán)*,[2] and Coptis and Ass-Hide Gelatin Decoction *(huáng lián ē jiāo tāng)*.[3]

---

1. Rehmanniae Radix *(shēng dì huáng)*, Ginseng Radix *(rén shēn)*, Asparagi Radix *(tiān mén dōng)*, Ophiopogonis Radix *(mài mén dōng)*, Scrophulariae Radix *(xuán shēn)*, Salviae miltiorrhizae Radix *(dān shēn)*, Poria *(fú líng)*, Polygalae Radix *(yuǎn zhì)*, wine-washed Angelicae sinensis Radix *(jiǔ xî dāng guī)*, Schisandrae Fructus *(wǔ wèi zǐ)*, Platycladi Semen *(bâi zî rén)*, dry-fried Ziziphi spinosae Semen *(châo suān zâo rén)*, Platycodi Radix *(jié gêng)*, and Cinnabaris *(zhū shā)*.

2. Rehmanniae Radix preparata *(shú dì huáng)*, Corni Fructus *(shān zhū yú)*, Dioscoreae Rhizoma *(shān yào)*, Poria *(fú líng)*, Moutan Cortex *(mǔ dān pí)*, Alismatis Rhizoma *(zé xiè)*, salt-fried Anemarrhenae Rhizoma *(yán châo zhī mǔ)*, and salt-fried Phellodendri Cortex *(yán châo huáng bâi)*.

3. Coptidis Rhizoma *(huáng lián)*, Scutellariae Radix *(huáng qín)*, Asini Corii Colla *(ē jiāo)*, Paeoniae Radix *(sháo yào)*,

Also common is Kidney and Lung yin deficiency with yang rising (e.g., dry cough), for which one should consider Seven-Ingredient Metropolis Qi Pill *(qī wèi dū qì wán)*[4] or Eight-Immortal Pill for Longevity *(bā xiān cháng shōu wán)*.[5]

The phrase "take in fluids to save themselves" refers to patients self-treating their thirst and dryness with "known" remedies such as Dendrobii Herba *(shí hú)* or Panacis quin-quefolii Radix *(xī yáng shēn)* in soups, or purposely eating moist, nourishing foods. This should be differentiated from the dry mouth and thirst that occur in *yáng míng* or qi level diseases, for which White Tiger Decoction *(bái hǔ tāng)*[6] is appropriate; these are usually acute presentations.

> • Hoarse voice with little sound coming out: Kidney qi expended

This is Kidney qi deficiency damaging the Lungs. However, apart from expended qi, there may also be a component of Kidney yin and essence deficiency contributing to the damage of Lung yin. The throat will be purple, dark, and dry. The main point here is that one cannot just treat the Lung/voice, but must also consider the Kidneys. Medicinals such as Testudinis Plastrum *(guī bǎn)*, Anemarrhenae Rhizoma *(zhī mǔ)*, Corni Fructus *(shān zhū yú)*, and Asparagi Radix *(tiān mén dōng)* should be considered. A sample formula is Great Tonify the Yin Pill *(dà bǔ yīn wán)* (see p. 134) plus Lung medicinals such as Glehniae/Adenophorae Radix *(shā shēn)*, Herba Dendrobii Officinalis *(tiě pí shí hú)*, Trichosanthis Radix *(tiān huā fěn)*, Asparagi Radix *(tiān mén dōng)*, and Ophiopogonis Radix *(mài mén dōng)*; plus medicinals that aid in rebuilding the voice/vocal chords such as Sterculiae lych-nophorae Semen *(pàng dà hǎi)*, Oroxyli Semen *(mù hú dié)*, Physalis Calyx seu Fructus *(guà jīn dēng)*, and Galli Membrana Ovi *(fēng huáng yī)*.[7]

This pattern comes about from overwork, talking too much, singing too much, not sleeping enough, or from very serious conditions such as lung cancer. If hoarseness continues, the voice will eventually be lost.

> • Rough breathing and wheezing: yin deficiency withers the Lungs; qi is without a place to return

This is chronic wheezing or asthma; often there will be shortness of breath after light exertion or even shaking of the hands. This is Lung yin deficiency with Kidney yin deficiency. The yin must be strong for the qi to reside and for the yin to connect. If the yin is weak, the qi floats and separates, leading to difficulty in breathing. This also can be viewed as Kidneys unable to grasp the qi, which can lead to Lung deficiency. Apart from treating the

---

and Egg yolk *(jī zi huáng)*.

4. This is Six-Ingredient Pill with Rehmannia *(liù wèi dì huáng wán)* plus Schisandrae Fructus *(wǔ wèi zǐ)*.

5. This is Six-Ingredient Pill with Rehmannia *(liù wèi dì huáng wán)* plus Ophiopogonis Radix *(mài mén dōng)* and Schisandrae Fructus *(wǔ wèi zǐ)*.

6. Gypsum fibrosum *(shí gāo)*, Anemarrhenae Rhizoma *(zhī mǔ)*, Glycyrrhizae Radix preparata *(zhì gān cǎo)*, and Nonglutinous rice *(jīng mǐ)*.

7. All of these should be very small dosages.

Lung yin, consideration should also be given to the Kidney yin and essence as well as the Lung and Heart qi. For treatment, consider capsules of Cordyceps *(dōng chóng xià cǎo)* or Ginseng Radix *(rén shēn)* plus Gecko *(gé jiè)*[8] as well as formulas such as Galenite Elixir *(hēi xī dān)*[9] or Ginseng and Gecko Powder *(rén shēn gé jiè sǎn)*,[10] etc.

> • Sore and dry throat: when true water is exhausted below, deficiency fire floats upward.

This is usually a chronic and frequently occurring sore throat that comes about from over-work and fatigue and may be accompanied by floating fire symptoms such as toothache. This is Kidney water unable to hold onto fire. One should include the idea of Great Tonify the Yin Pill *(dà bǔ yīn wán)* into the treatment plan. For symptomatic relief, one can make a tea out of Momordicae Fructus *(luó hàn guǒ)*, Pyri Exocarpium *(lí pí)* [pear skin], or Mume Fructus *(wū méi)* to ease the dry throat. However, there are times where chronic sore throat is just from Lung yin deficiency, in which case Glehnia and Ophiopogonis Decoction *(shā shēn mài mén dōng tāng)*[11] is an appropriate base formula (see method no. 1 below).

> • Insomnia with disorientation: the blood fails to nourish the Heart, so the spirit cannot be stored.

This is essentially a pattern of Heart blood deficiency with manifestations such as restlessness, inability to concentrate, poor memory, profuse dreaming, frequent waking, dizziness, and tinnitus. There may also be a component of Liver blood and Kidney essence deficiency that leads to a lack of tranquility in the Heart. This is common in menopause. Consider Arborvitae Seed Pill to Nourish the Heart *(bǎi zǐ yǎng xīn wán)*,[12] Restore the Spleen Decoction *(guī pí tāng)*, or Coptis and Ass-Hide Gelatin Decoction *(huáng lián ē jiāo tāng)*.

> • Frequent irritability and restlessness: lack of yin within yang, softness failing to aid the hard

Because of yin deficiency, there is an inability to moisten and accept yang. This is no different than 'yin unable to preserve yang,' 'non-interaction of yin and yang,' 'frail yin floating

---

8. Two capsules three times per day. Each capsule should have around 0.3g of herbs in equal parts. This is good for long-term deficiency with easy shortness of breath.

9. Aquilariae Lignum resinatum *(chén xiāng)*, Aconiti Radix lateralis preparata *(zhì fù zǐ)*, Trigonelle Semen *(hú lú bā)*, Actinolitum *(yáng qǐ shí)*, Foeniculi Fructus *(xiǎo huí xiāng)*, Psoraleae Fructus *(bǔ gǔ zhī)*, Myristicae Semen *(ròu dòu kòu)*, Toosendan Fructus *(chuān liàn zǐ)*, Aucklandiae Radix *(mù xiāng)*, Cinnamomi Cortex *(ròu guì)*, Galenite *(hēi xī)*, and Sulfur *(liú huáng)*.

10. Gecko *(gé jiè)*, Ginseng Radix *(rén shēn)*, Poria *(fú líng)*, Mori Cortex *(sāng bái pí)*, Armeniacae Semen *(xìng rén)*, Fritillariae cirrhosae Bulbus *(chuān bèi mǔ)*, Anemarrhenae Rhizoma *(zhī mǔ)*, and Glycyrrhizae Radix preparata *(zhì gān cǎo)*.

11. Glehniae/Adenophorae Radix *(shā shēn)*, Ophiopogonis Radix *(mài mén dōng)*, Polygonati odorati Rhizoma *(yù zhú)*, Mori Folium *(sāng yè)*, Trichosanthis Radix *(tiān huā fěn)*, Lablab Semen album *(bái biǎn dòu)*, and Glycyrrhizae Radix *(gān cǎo)*.

12. Platycladi Semen *(bǎi zǐ rén)*, Lycii Fructus *(gǒu qǐ zǐ)*, Ophiopogonis Radix *(mài mén dōng)*, Angelicae sinensis Radix *(dāng guī)*, Acori tatarinowii Rhizoma *(shí chāng pú)*, Poriae Sclerotium pararadicis *(fú shén)*, Scrophulariae Radix *(xuán shēn)*, Rehmanniae Radix preparata *(shú dì huáng)*, and Glycyrrhizae Radix *(gān cǎo)*.

yang,' or 'yin deficiency with hyperactive yang.'

There also may be a sensation of heat or emotions that change easily, as often seen in menopause. This is a pattern of yin deficiency leading to an inability of yin to connect with yang, or a separation of yin and yang. One can consider a formula such as Grand Communication Pill *(jiāo tài wán)*.[13]

> • Easily angered, tense sinews with aches and pains: with exhausted water and parched wood, the Liver is deprived of nourishment.

The sinews may also feel tight upon palpation. This commonly manifests in the neck, upper back, and shoulders. The yin is unable to nourish the sinews. There may also be tinnitus, insomnia, hypertension, migraines, and lower back pain. This is Liver and Kidney yin deficiency that may also have a component of Liver yang rising. Two key points in diagnosis are a thin and rapid pulse (especially in the proximal position) and a dry, cracked, and tender tongue that may be pink, red, or purple; there will either not be any coating or only a patchy (geographic) coating. In these cases, consider the formula Lycium Fruit, Chrysanthemum, and Rehmannia Pill *(qǐ jú dì huáng wán)*[14] with added medicinals such as Puerariae Radix *(gé gēn)*, Lycopodii Herba *(shēn jīn cǎo)*, Trachelospermi Caulis *(luò shí téng)*, Spatholobi Caulis *(jī xuè téng)*, or Gentianae macrophyllae Radix *(qín jiāo)*.

> • No pleasure in food, flesh is gradually diminished: the Spleen base is not conserved so the dynamic of transformation worsens daily.

There may also be dry skin, diarrhea/loose bowels (2-3 per day), or no bowel movement for 2-3 days, and loss of body weight. The tongue is swollen with teeth marks, pale, and dry. This is Spleen qi and yin deficiency. Consider the formulas Ginseng, Poria, and White Atractylodes Powder *(shēn líng bái zhú sǎn)* and/or Aid Life Pill *(zī shēng wán)*.

> • Throbbing below the Heart with continuous palpitations: qi unable to return to the essence

This is essence and qi deficiency affecting the spirit. Qi deficiency leads to essence deficiency and vice versa. Other symptoms related to the spirit, such as insomnia and restlessness, may also be present.

> • Continuous night sweating: with fire, the yin is unable to be conserved; without fire, the yang is unable to be secured.

This describes the patterns of yin and/or yang deficiency leading to night sweats. First, if there is pathological fire, it will push out the body liquids. Second, if there is deficiency in the fire at the gate of vitality, the protective yang will be unable to keep the fluids secure. In

---

13. Coptidis Rhizoma *(huáng lián)* and Cinnamomi Cortex *(ròu guì)*.

14. Six-Ingredient Pill with Rehmannia *(liù wèi dì huáng wán)* plus Chrysanthemi Flos *(jú huā)* and Lycii Fructus *(gôu qî zî)*.

practice, these often occur together, although one may be more dominant than the other. However, both patterns can, in and of themselves, result in sweating. Understanding this helps clarify why merely clearing the heat or tonifying the yin does not always work for night sweats. Consequently, one must often tonify the fire at the gate of vitality or yang qi to stop night sweats. However, it should be noted that formulas like Kidney Qi Pill from the *Golden Cabinet (jīn guì shèn qì wán)*[15] that contain Cinnamomi Cortex *(ròu guì)* and Aconiti Radix lateralis preparata *(zhì fù zǐ)* are inappropriate because there is already heat.[16] One may consider a formula such as Tangkuei and Six-Yellow Decoction *(dāng guī liù huáng tāng)*[17] or Two-Immortal Decoction *(èr xiān tāng)*[18] plus medicinals that stop sweating.

> • Profuse amounts of phlegm like clear water with lots of foam: as overflowing fluids become phlegm, the Spleen is deficient and unable to control water.

This is primarily a Spleen (yang) deficiency with dampness leading to phlegm and thin mucus. This may occur in conditions such as asthma and bronchitis. There may also be copious amounts of frothy saliva. Consider the formula Poria, Licorice, Schisandra, and Ginger Decoction *(líng gān wǔ wèi jiāng tāng)*.[19]

> • The bones are as painful as if they've been broken: true yin is defeated and expended.

One must use medicinals with an affinity to flesh and blood, such as Testudinis Plastrum *(sū guī bǎn)*, Testudinis Plastri Colla *(guī bǎn jiāo)*, Trionycis Carapax *(biē jiǎ)*, Trionycis Carapacis Colla *(biē jiǎ jiāo)*, and Hominis Placenta *(zǐ hé chē)*. These are usually combined with medicinals such as Rehmanniae Radix preparata *(shú dì huáng)*, Corni Fructus *(shān zhū yú)*, and Ligustri lucidi Fructus *(nǚ zhēn zǐ)*.

> • Lower back and flank pain: Liver and Kidney deficiency

There may also be a sense of heaviness in the lower back, hips, or down to the knees. Regardless of the biomedical diagnosis (e.g., sciatica), one must consider Kidney deficiency, which usually includes both yin and yang. Consider the formula Pubescent Angelica and Taxillus Decoction *(dú huó jì shēng tāng)*.[20]

---

15. Rehmanniae Radix *(shēng dì huáng)*, Corni Fructus *(shān zhū yú)*, Dioscoreae Rhizoma *(shān yào)*, baked Aconiti Radix lateralis *(bāo fù zǐ)*, Cinnamomi Ramulus *(guì zhī)*, Alismatis Rhizoma *(zé xiè)*, Poria *(fú líng)*, and Moutan Cortex *(mǔ dān pí)*.

16. There are times, albeit infrequently, that pure yang deficiency will cause night sweats. In such cases, one would choose a formula such as True Warrior Decoction *(zhēn wǔ tāng)*, Aconite Accessory Root Decoction *(fù zǐ tāng)*, or Cinnamon Twig and Aconite Accessory Root Decoction *(guì zhī fù zǐ tāng)* plus medicinals that stop sweating.

17. Dry-fried Angelicae sinensis Radix *(chǎo dāng guī)* 6g, Rehmanniae Radix *(shēng dì huáng)* 9g, Rehmanniae Radix preparata *(shú dì huáng)* 9g, dry-fried Coptidis Rhizoma *(chǎo huáng lián)* 3g, dry-fried Scutellariae Radix *(chǎo huáng qín)* 3g, salt-fried Phellodendri Cortex *(yán chǎo zhī mǔ)*, 3g, and Astragali Radix *(huáng qí)* 9g.

18. Curculiginis Rhizoma *(xiān máo)*, Epimedii Herba *(yín yáng huò)*, Morindae officinalis Radix *(bā jǐ tiān)*, Phellodendri Cortex *(huáng bǎi)*, Anemarrhenae Rhizoma *(zhī mǔ)*, and Angelicae sinensis Radix *(dāng guī)*.

19. Poria *(fú líng)*, Glycyrrhizae Radix preparata *(zhì gān cǎo)*, Schisandrae Fructus *(wǔ wèi zǐ)*, and Zingiberis Rhizoma *(gān jiāng)*.

20. Angelicae pubescentis Radix *(dú huó)*, Asari Radix et Rhizoma *(xì xīn)*, Saposhnikoviae Radix *(fáng fēng)*, Genti-

- Ice-cold sensation below the knees: the fire at the gate of vitality is debilitated and expended and is unable to return to its source.

This may also manifest merely as cold hands and feet.

- Urination is yellow, rough, and dribbling: the true yin is exhausted, and the qi is unable to transform water.

This is Kidney yin deficiency with damp-heat and symptoms that occur when people are tired. Urine may also be difficult to pass, burn, and have an odor. This may correspond to prostatitis.

Although there are apparent heat signs, the solution is more about tonification (80%) than clearing heat (20%). The root problem is qi unable to process the fluids, so the urine becomes stagnant in the Bladder, which then produces heat. There is not an excess of heat or fire in the body. If one increases the body's natural ability to process fluids, the problem will be resolved.

- Hearts of the soles of the feet are as if burning: deficiency fire is parching the yin, and the root of the Kidneys is desiccated and expended.

This also includes pain or heat on the heel or pain on the sole of the foot. If a patient has these symptoms they must have Kidney yin/essence depletion. The pain can be from something like a bone spur, which is still considered due to deficiency.[i] One must therefore tonify with a formula such as Restore the Left [Kidney] Pill *(zuǒ guī wán)*[21] or Great Tonify the Yin Pill *(dà bǔ yīn wán)*.

- Cold and shivering at the level of the skin interstices, and spitting up of foamy oral mucus: protective level deficiency

There may also be aversion to wind, goose bumps, and a tendency to sweat easily.

- Cough with internal heat, and spitting up of fishy-smelling mucus: nutritive level deficiency

The internal heat may manifest as only a slight fever or high fever, dry mouth, and dry and burning throat, or with a taste of blood in the throat. The cough is usually dry and all the symptoms worsen at night. The tongue is purple-red with no coating and the pulse is thin and rapid.

---

anae macrophyllae Radix *(qín jiāo)*, Taxilli Herba *(sāng jì shēng)*, Eucommiae Cortex *(dù zhòng)*, Achyranthis bidentatae Radix *(niú xī)*, Cinnamomi Cortex *(ròu guì)*, Angelicae sinensis Radix *(dāng guī)*, Chuanxiong Rhizoma *(chuān xiōng)*, Rehmanniae Radix *(shēng dì huáng)*, Paeoniae Radix alba *(bái sháo)*, Ginseng Radix *(rén shēn)*, Poria *(fú líng)*, and Glycyrrhizae Radix preparata *(zhì gān cǎo)*.

21. Rehmanniae Radix preparata *(shú dì huáng)*, dry-fried Dioscoreae Rhizoma *(chǎo shān yào)*, Lycii Fructus *(gǒu qǐ zǐ)*, Corni Fructus *(shān zhū yú)*, wine-prepared Cyathulae Radix *(jiǔ chuān niú xī)*, Cuscutae Semen *(tù sī zǐ)*, Cervi Cornus Colla *(lù jiǎo jiāo)*, and Testudinis Plastri Colla *(guī bǎn jiāo)*.

- Great loss of blood and loss of semen: damage to the Liver and Kidneys
- Clumping of blood with a dry cough: constraint and clumping leading to blazing fire

Clumping of blood is a deficiency pattern, where there is exhaustion of yin fluids with blood stasis that generates heat. It is not the same as 'clumping of the blood' in the *Discussion of Cold Damage.*

- Reduced intake of food and drink, wheezing, cough, and diarrhea: medicinals damaging the Spleen and Stomach

1. Tonify the Lungs and Nourish the Yin (补肺养阴 *bǔ fèi yǎng yīn*)

[PRESENTATION] Heat damages the Lung qi and yang fluids; Lung atrophy and dry cough

Panacis quinquefolii Radix *(xī yáng shēn)*	2.4g
Aristolochiae Fructus *(mǎ dōu líng)*[22]	4.5g
Glehniae Radix *(běi shā shēn)*	4.5g
Armeniacae Semen dulce *(tián xìng rén)*	9g
Ophiopogonis Radix *(mài mén dōng)*	4.5g
Fritillariae cirrhosae Bulbus *(chuān bèi mǔ)*	4.5g
Imperatae Rhizoma *(bái máo gēn)*	4.5g

COMMENTARY

ADDITIONAL SIGNS AND SYMPTOMS

- Shortness of breath
- Sore throat
- Dry throat, mouth, skin, and hair
- Loss of voice or low, tentative voice
- Fatigue
- Dry cough without phlegm, scanty phlegm, or, if severe, scanty phlegm with blood
- Copious sweat and aversion to wind
- Constipation
- The tongue is red or dark red and dry body with cracks and no coating
- The pulse is thin, rapid, and dry, especially in the distal position

DISCUSSION

PATTERN: This is dual deficiency of Lung yin and qi.

PHYSIOLOGY, ETIOLOGY, AND PATHODYNAMIC: The Lungs' root is in yin and their function is yang. They are in charge of breathing and respiration, master the skin and hair,

---

22. See discussion below for possible substitutions.

promote the movement of fluids, and irrigate the hundred vessels. In chronic disease, where the Lungs are damaged and the lobes of the Lungs are scorched and withered, there is impairment of distribution and transformation. Thus the Lungs are unable to transform qi and promote the movement of yang fluids.

DURATION: This is usually a chronic presentation.

MEDICINAL ANALYSIS

- Panacis quinquefolii Radix *(xī yáng shēn)* is cool, sweet, moist, tonifies yin (70-80%) and qi (20-30%), and clears heat. If unavailable, one may substitute Pseudostellariae Radix *(tài zǐ shēn)*, but this is not as effective.

- Aristolochiae Fructus *(mǎ dōu líng)* clears and clarifies the Lungs, moistens Lung yin, stops coughing, and calms wheezing. However it is *toxic* and one should therefore substitute one of the following:

    1. honey-prepared Mori Cortex *(mì zhì sāng bái pí)* 4.5-6g, honey-prepared Asteris Radix *(mì zhì zǐ wǎn)* 6g, or Tremella *(yín ěr)* 9g if there is mainly a dry cough
    2. honey-prepared Eriobotryae Folium *(mì zhì pí pá yè)* 6g if there is an incessant cough
    3. honey-prepared Farfarae Flos *(mì zhì kuǎn dōng huā)* 6g if there is a cough with phlegm that is difficult to expel and comes out in small pieces.

- Glehniae Radix *(bĕi shā shēn)* and Ophiopogonis Radix *(mài mén dōng)* clear and nourish the Lung and Stomach yin, moisten dryness, and generate fluids. Glehniae Radix *(bĕi shā shēn)* is more moist and better at tonifying the fluids than Adenophorae Radix *(nán shā shēn)*, which is better at promoting circulation of the Spleen. Glehniae Radix *(bĕi shā shēn)* better addresses the Stomach yin, while Ophiopogonis Radix *(mài mén dōng)* is better for the Lungs.

- Armeniacae Semen dulce *(tián xìng rén)* moistens the Lungs, stops coughing, and is suitable for deficiency consumption panting and coughing. If unavailable, one can substitute Pruni Amygdali Semen *(bā dàn xìng rén)* [almonds] 9g, which is more moistening then Armeniacae Semen dulce *(tián xìng rén)*.

- Fritillariae cirrhosae Bulbus *(chuān bèi mǔ)* is sweet and cool. It stops coughing and is strongly enriching and moistening, enabling it to moisten dryness and tonify Lung yin. One may choose to dissolve half the dose of powdered Fritillariae cirrhosae Bulbus *(chuān bèi mǔ)* into each dose of the strained decoction.

- Imperatae Rhizoma *(bái máo gēn)* clears heat. It travels to the blood aspect, cooling the blood, and is especially appropriate if there is bleeding (e.g., blood in the phlegm, dry and bloody nose). Phragmitis Rhizoma *(lú gēn)* can be substituted, especially if there is no bleeding. Both are cool and moist; however, Imperatae Rhizoma *(bái máo gēn)* is better at clearing heat and Phragmitis Rhizoma *(lú gēn)* is better at moistening. The suggested dosage is 6g each.

117

Dr. Qin's formula is based on Glehnia and Ophiopogonis Decoction *(shā shēn mài mén dōng tāng).*

Glehnia and Ophiopogonis Decoction *(shā shēn mài mén dōng tāng)*

SOURCE: *Systematic Differentiation of Warm Pathogen Diseases* (1798)

Glehniae/Adenophorae Radix *(shā shēn)* 9g
Ophiopogonis Radix *(mài mén dōng)* 9g
Polygonati odorati Rhizoma *(yù zhú)* 6g
Mori Folium *(sāng yè)* 4.5g
Trichosanthis Radix *(tiān huā fěn)* 4.5g
Lablab Semen album *(bái biǎn dòu)* 4.5g
Glycyrrhizae Radix *(gān cǎo)* 3g

MODIFICATIONS OF DR. QIN'S FORMULA

Dry cough with wheezing:

Gingko Semen *(bái guǒ)* 5g

Farfarae Flos *(kuǎn dōng huā)* 6g

Severe dry cough:

Asteris Radix *(zǐ wǎn)* 4.5g

Honey-prepared Eriobotryae Folium *(mì zhì pí pá yè)* 6g

Trichosanthis Radix *(tiān huā fěn)* 6g

Dry cough with blood:

Nelumbinis Nodus rhizomatis *(ǒu jié)* or Nodus rhizomatis *(ǒu jié tàn)* . . 6g

Charred Imperatae Rhizoma *(máo gēn tàn)* 4.5g

Pearls of Asini Corii Colla *(ē jiāo zhū)* 4.5g
(if there is blood deficiency)

Dry cough with deep ear pain:

Anemarrhenae Rhizoma *(zhī mǔ)* 6g

Trichosanthis Radix *(tiān huā fěn)* 6g

Dry cough due to a lingering pathogen from a common cold:

Snake Gallbladder and Fritillariae Liquid *(shé dǎn chuān bèi yè)*
[prepared medicine]

Cough with yellow, sticky phlegm:

Powdered Indigo naturalis *(qīng dài)* 1g

Meretricis/Cyclinae Concha *(gé qiào)* 9g

▶ These two ingredients are stirred into the decoction for the last 3-5 minutes of cooking. Note that this combination is known as Indigo and Clam Shell Powder *(dài gé sǎn).*

Mori Cortex *(sāng bái pí)* 6g
(especially if there is a sensation of heat)

Chest pain following coughing:

Paeoniae Radix alba *(bái sháo)* 6g

Luffae Fructus Retinervus *(sī guā luò)* 4.5g

Dry mouth, scanty urine, tinnitus, and lower back pain:

Asparagi Radix *(tiān mén dōng)* 4.5g

Scrophulariae Radix *(xuán shēn)* 6g

Dry throat and hoarseness:

Sterculiae lychnophorae Semen *(pàng dà hǎi)* 2-3p

Dendrobii Herba *(shí hú)* 4.5g

Dry mouth with thirst:

Polygonati odorati Rhizoma *(yù zhú)* 6g

Dry lips and mouth, more severe dryness:

Dendrobii Herba *(shí hú)*[23] 4.5g

Dryness accompanied by emotional problems (e.g., restless, easy angered):

Lilii Bulbus *(bǎi hé)* 6g

Rehmanniae Radix *(shēng dì huáng)* 6g

Steaming bones:

Lycii Cortex *(dì gǔ pí)* 6g

Moutan Cortex *(mǔ dān pí)* 4.5g

Constipation:

Cannabis Semen *(huǒ má rén)* 6g

Platycladi Semen *(bǎi zǐ rén)* 6g

FOOD THERAPY

Fritillariae and Pear *(chuān bèi lí)*: Remove the top of an Asian pear, core it, and add 3g of Fritillariae cirrhosae Bulbus *(chuān bèi mǔ)* powder and 3 pieces of rock sugar or 1 tablespoon of honey. Replace the top and steam or double boil for 20-30 minutes until the pear is soft. Remove the top and bottom and mash, and then eat as a dessert after meals. This is especially good for chronic dry cough with a bit of phlegm.

Pear malt-sugar candy *(lí gāo tāng)*: This is a pear candy that is very effective at alleviating yin deficiency cough. It can be purchased at many Asian food stores.

QUESTIONS

1. *When there is Lung yin deficiency, what other patterns should one pay attention to?*

There is always some component of Lung qi deficiency when there is a Lung yin deficiency pattern. The yin may be damaged first or the qi may be damaged first. There is also usually Stomach yin deficiency whenever there is Lung yin deficiency. Paying

---

23. For this purpose, Dendrobii officinalis Caulis *(tiê pí shí hú)* is preferred.

attention to these aspects is therefore important for treatment, as we can see from the inclusion of Panacis quinquefolii Radix *(xī yáng shēn)* and Glehniae/Adenophorae Radix *(shā shēn)* in the formula above.

2. *Can one use Armeniacae Semen amarum (kǔ xìng rén) instead of Armeniacae Semen dulce (tián xìng rén)?*

If one simply writes a prescription with *xìng rén,* a pharmacy will usually dispense Armeniacae Semen amarum *(kǔ xìng rén),* which is said to be slightly bitter, slightly sweet, warm, diffusing, scattering, and directs Lung qi downward, and is also somewhat toxic in nature. However, it is not really appropriate in this situation. Armeniacae Semen dulce *(tián xìng rén)* is superior because it has no scattering or diffusing nature. However, in reality, due to modern cultivation practices, Armeniacae Semen amarum *(kǔ xìng rén)* has lost most of its bitter nature and is more similar to Armeniacae Semen dulce *(tián xìng rén)* than in the past and can thus also be used here.

3. *Why does Qin sometimes mention yang fluids and sometimes yin fluids?*

Generally speaking, a yang fluid issue is more superficial compared to that of a yin fluid. Yang fluids are thin, clear, and watery, and spread to the more superficial parts of the body, nourishing the muscles, flesh, and orifices. Yin fluids are thick and viscous and flow in the deeper regions of the body where they nourish the bones, joints, brain, and marrow.

For example, in this section, Dr. Qin mentions damage to the yang fluids of the Lungs. Above this section in the introduction to this chapter, Dr. Qin mentions the damage to the yin fluids of the Lungs. The latter situation is from 'clumping of blood' and corresponds to a deeper problem involving blood stasis. In addition, notice the fourth method described later in this chapter, "generate yang fluids and enrich the yin fluids," which addresses a wasting and thirsting disorder. This certainly is a deeper or chronic problem where just generating yang fluids is not sufficient. One must include the deeper strategy of enriching the yin fluids. Thus, deeper-acting medicinals are chosen, such as Rehmanniae Radix *(shēng dì huáng)*.

2. Tonify, Augment, and Strengthen the Middle (补益建中 *bǔ yì jiàn zhōng*)

[PRESENTATION] Spleen and Stomach qi deficiency; urgent morning diarrhea

Dry-fried Codonopsis Radix *(chǎo dǎng shēn)*	4.5g
Clear-Glycyrrhizae Radix preparata *(qīng zhì gān cǎo)*	1.5g
Atractylodis macrocephalae Rhizoma *(bái zhú)*	4.5g
Poria *(fú líng)*	9g
Dioscoreae Rhizoma *(shān yào)*	9g
Dry-fried Lablab Semen album *(chǎo biǎn dòu)*	9g
Dry-fried Setariae (Oryzae) Fructus germinatus *(chǎo gǔ yá)*	9g

COMMENTARY

ADDITIONAL SIGNS AND SYMPTOMS

- The diarrhea is loose rather than watery, usually occurring 2-3 times in the morning or after eating.

- Bowel movements are irregular (e.g., constipation then loose stools), but there is often incomplete voiding.

- Poor digestion (abdominal fullness and focal distention after eating; stuck feeling at CV-12 *[zhōng wǎn]*)

- Bland taste in the mouth

- Reduced or little appetite or will have an appetite and then feel a blockage or fullness after eating

- Fatigue and lack of strength in the limbs

- Shortness of breath

- No strength to speak

- Dark pale or withered-yellow facial complexion

- The pulse is soft and soggy, especially deep and weak in the right middle position

- The tongue is pale, tender, and cracked (if more on yin deficiency side) or swollen and pale with teeth marks and a wet body with a white or grey, slightly greasy coating (if more on damp side; see question no. 1 below). The formula must be modified if significant dampness is present.

DISCUSSION

DURATION: this is usually a chronic problem.

ETIOLOGY: this presentation is often due to dietary irregularities, overwork, fatigue, internal damage, or congenital insufficiency.

MEDICINAL ANALYSIS

- Dry-fried Codonopsis Radix *(chǎo dǎng shēn)*, Poria *(fú líng)*, Atractylodis macrocephalae Rhizoma *(bái zhú)*, and clear-Glycyrrhizae Radix preparata *(qīng zhì gān cǎo)* augment the qi, tonify the center, build up the Spleen, and nourish the Stomach. Dry-fried Codonopsis Radix *(chǎo dǎng shēn)* also increases the Spleen's circulation. Dry-fried Codonopsis Radix *(chǎo dǎng shēn)* is not as cloying as Codonopsis Radix *(dǎng shēn)*. Thus, if there is focal distention and a stifling sensation in the chest and gastric cavity, it is important that one not use the sweet and sticky Codonopsis Radix *(dǎng shēn)*.

- Poria *(fú líng)* is sweet and neutral. It tonifies the Spleen circulation, moves dampness, and promotes urination. Atractylodis macrocephalae Rhizoma *(bái zhú)* strengthens digestion and also dries dampness (20-30%) along with its ability to tonify (70-80%).

- Dioscoreae Rhizoma *(shān yào)* and dry-fried Lablab Semen album *(chǎo biǎn dòu)* are both sweet, neutral, and tonify both the Spleen qi and yin. Dioscoreae Rhizoma *(shān yào)* also has a binding nature and is used to stop diarrhea.

- The tonifying and augmenting function of dry-fried Lablab Semen album *(chǎo biǎn dòu)* is not as strong as Atractylodis macrocephalae Rhizoma *(bái zhú)* and Dioscoreae Rhizoma *(shān yào)*, but it is neither drying nor cloying. It is an excellent medicinal to tonify the Spleen to eliminate dampness.

- Dry-fried (Oryzae) Fructus germinatus *(chǎo gǔ yá)* increases the circulation of Spleen qi, helping to eliminate dampness and aiding digestion.

Dr. Qin's formula is based on Ginseng, Poria, and White Atractylodes Powder *(shēn líng bái zhú sǎn)*

Ginseng, Poria, and White Atractylodes Powder *(shēn líng bái zhú sǎn)*

SOURCE: *Formulary of the Pharmacy Service for Benefiting the People in the Taiping Era* (1107)

Ginseng Radix *(rén shēn)* 1000g
Atractylodis macrocephalae Rhizoma *(bái zhú)* 1000g
Glycyrrhizae Radix preparata *(zhì gān cǎo)* 1000g
Dioscoreae Rhizoma *(shān yào)* 1000g
Lablab Semen album *(bái biǎn dòu)* 750g
Nelumbinis Semen *(lián zǐ)* 500g
Coicis Semen *(yì yǐ rén)* 500g
Amomi Fructus *(shā rén)* 500g
Platycodi Radix *(jié gěng)* 500g

MODIFICATIONS OF DR. QIN'S FORMULA

Frequent loose stools or easily-stimulated diarrhea (e.g., after eating a small amount of cold foods):

Nelumbinis Semen *(lián zǐ)* 9g
Euryales Semen *(qiàn shí)* 9g

Serious diarrhea (e.g., immediate watery diarrhea that is difficult to control with such precipitants as a slight change in the weather or eating a small amount of cold food):

Dry-fried Chebulae Fructus *(chǎo hē zǐ)* 6g
Roasted Puerariae Radix *(wēi gé gēn)* 9g

Poor appetite with easy food stagnation (e.g., difficult digestion, fullness, and an uncomfortable sensation at center of the epigastrium):

Dry-fried Gigeriae galli Endothelium corneum *(chǎo jī nèi jīn)* 4.5g
Dry-fried Massa medicata fermentata *(chǎo shén qū)* 9g

Bland taste or sticky sensation in the mouth (dampness):

Amomi Fructus *(shā rén)* 3g
Amomi Fructus rotundus *(bái dòu kòu)* 3g

Nausea:

Pogostemonis/Agastaches Herba *(huò xiāng)* 4.5g

Perillae Caulis *(zǐ sū gěng)* 4.5g

Easy fullness and distention after eating a small amount of food:

Hordei Fructus germinatus *(mài yá)* 9g

QUESTIONS

1. Is there dampness or yin deficiency in this pattern?

This formula fundamentally addresses Spleen qi deficiency. However, Spleen qi deficiency can also be accompanied by either dampness or yin deficiency. This formula addresses a pattern that is approximately 70% qi deficiency and 30% yin deficiency. Thus, it does not really address dampness.

However, patterns of Spleen qi deficiency with digestive problems almost always include some dampness, especially when one sees symptoms such as loose stools, bloating, gas, etc. But in this pattern, the dampness is secondary and will not be seen on the tongue and so forth, as in the patterns in Ch. 9 on dampness. Consequently, Dr. Qin uses medicinals such as Atractylodis macrocephalae Rhizoma *(bái zhú)* and Dioscoreae Rhizoma *(shān yào)* to improve the Spleen's function, which will eliminate the small amount of dampness that may exist in this pattern. If there are more signs and symptoms of dampness (e.g., wet and slightly greasy tongue), one should make the appropriate modifications, for example, by using dry-fried Atractylodis macrocephalae Rhizoma *(chǎo bái zhú)* or dry-fried Dioscoreae Rhizoma *(chǎo shān yào)*, or adding medicinals such as Amomi Fructus *(shā rén)* and Amomi Fructus rotundus *(bái dòu kòu)*. In general, however, these medicinals should be avoided for this pattern because they can further aggravate the yin deficiency that is most likely present.

2. Can you have Spleen qi deficiency without dampness?

Yes. For example, in a Tonify the Middle to Augment the Qi Decoction *(bǔ zhōng yì qì tāng)* pattern there is no dampness.

3. Why does Dr. Qin take out Nelumbinis Semen (lián zǐ) from the original formula when there is diarrhea?

The current formula already contains enough astringent medicinals for the basic presentation. For example, Dioscoreae Rhizoma *(shān yào)*, Lablab Semen album *(bái biǎn dòu)*, and Atractylodis macrocephalae Rhizoma *(bái zhú)* are sufficient to control the diarrhea. Of course, if there is more diarrhea, one can add Euryales Semen *(qiàn shí)*, Nelumbinis Semen *(lián zǐ)*, roasted Puerariae Radix *(wēi gé gēn)*, and/or Chebulae Fructus *(hē zǐ)*.

4. Why is Pinelliae Rhizoma preparatum (zhì bàn xià) not chosen as a modification for nausea, while Pogostemonis/Agastaches Herba (huò xiāng) and Perillae Caulis (zǐ sū gěng) are?

Since this pattern is usually a Spleen qi and yin deficiency presentation, Pinelliae Rhizoma preparatum *(zhì bàn xià)* is inappropriate. If there are clear signs of dampness, such as a thick tongue coating, then it can be used. Perillae Caulis *(zǐ sū gěng)* and Pogostemonis/ Agastaches Herba *(huò xiāng)* are better for this type of presentation. These two circulate the qi to gently eliminate the stagnation that is leading to the nausea. Perillae Caulis *(zǐ sū gěng)* is especially appropriate when there is Spleen qi and yin deficiency. One can also add Bambusae Caulis in taeniam *(zhú rú)* as a symptomatic herb to control the nausea.

5. *Why does Dr. Qin use some dry-fried and some unprocessed medicinals?*

The simple answer to the question is balance. For example, although unprocessed Setariae (Oryzae) Fructus germinatus *(gǔ yá)* can raise Spleen qi and is best for patterns of Spleen qi deficiency, Dr. Qin chooses the dry-fried form because it is better at eliminating the small amount of dampness that most likely is present in this pattern. This is because the formula already includes enough other medicinals that raise and tonify the Spleen qi. Dr. Qin avoids a lopsided formula by carefully selecting and not dry-frying every ingredient. For example, Atractylodis macrocephalae Rhizoma *(bái zhú)* and Dioscoreae Rhizoma *(shān yào)* are left unprocessed to address the Spleen yin (e.g., scanty tongue coating and poor appetite).

3. Tonify the Protective Level and Secure the Exterior
(补卫固表 *bǔ wèi gù biǎo*)

[PRESENTATION] Protective qi insecurity; spontaneous sweating with aversion to cold

Astragali Cortex *(huáng qí pí)* 9g
Ginseng Radix capillaris *(rén shēn xū)* 2.4g
Dry-fried Atractylodis macrocephalae Rhizoma *(chǎo bái zhú)* 4.5g
Oryzae glutinosae Radix *(nuò dào gēn xū)* 6g
Aconiti Radix lateralis preparata *(zhì fù zǐ)* 2.4g
Tritici Fructus levis *(fú xiǎo mài)* 9g
Jujubae Fructus *(dà zǎo)* 3p

COMMENTARY

ADDITIONAL SIGNS AND SYMPTOMS

- Easily sweats, such as after drinking hot water or mild exertion
- Frequently catches colds
- Aversion to wind or easily feels cold
- Fatigue and lack of strength
- Faint low voice
- Dizziness and vertigo
- Bright white facial complexion

- The pulse is weak in the distal position.
- The tongue is swollen, puffy, and tooth-marked, with a wet coating that is not thick

Note: Securing the exterior has a strong component of stopping sweating.

MEDICINAL ANALYSIS

- Ginseng Radix capillaris *(rén shēn xū)*, Astragali Cortex *(huáng qí pí)*, and Atractylodis macrocephalae Rhizoma *(bái zhú)* all are very similar and are considered the chiefs of the formula. However, there are some minor differences.

  Astragali Cortex *(huáng qí pí)* is a 'skin' (cortex) that travels to the skin and is excellent at securing the exterior and stopping sweating. If unavailable, one can substitute Astragali Radix *(huáng qí)*. However, Astragali Cortex *(huáng qí pí)* is better at tonifying the protective level.

  Ginseng Radix capillaris *(rén shēn xū)* and Atractylodis macrocephalae Rhizoma *(bái zhú)* work more on strengthening the central qi and aiding digestion.

  Ginseng Radix capillaris *(rén shēn xū)* is the tail of the ginseng root and has the additional ability to enter the surface's collaterals, preventing sweating by aiding in closing the pores. If unavailable, one can use Ginseng Radix *(rén shēn)* or Codonopsis Radix *(dǎng shēn)*. One may also choose red Ginseng *(hóng shēn)* if there is more yang and qi deficiency, or Panacis quinquefolii Radix *(xī yáng shēn)* if there is more yin deficiency.

- Aconiti Radix lateralis preparata *(zhì fù zǐ)* is very acrid and very warm and intensely tonifies the original yang of the lower burner.

- The combination of Oryzae glutinosae Radix *(nuò dào gēn xū)* and Tritici Fructus levis *(fú xiǎo mài)* is excellent at stopping sweating. Tritici Fructus levis *(fú xiǎo mài)* is neutral (to slightly cool). It enters the Heart, stops sweating, and has the secondary function of strengthening the Spleen's circulation. It is best when slightly crushed. Oryzae glutinosae Radix *(nuò dào gēn xū)* is neutral (to slightly warm). It secures and binds in order to keep the sweat in.

- Jujubae Fructus *(dà zǎo)* is sweet and moderate. It harmonizes the middle and protects it from any possible harm from the other medicinals.

Dr. Qin's formula is based on Tonify the Middle to Augment the Qi Decoction *(bǔ zhōng yì qì tāng)* and Ginseng and Aconite Accessory Root Decoction *(shēn fù tāng)*.

Tonify the Middle to Augment the Qi Decoction *(bǔ zhōng yì qì tāng)*

SOURCE: *Clarifying Doubts about Damage from Internal and External Causes* (1247)

Astragali Radix *(huáng qí)* 12-24g
Ginseng Radix *(rén shēn)* 9-12g
Atractylodis macrocephalae Rhizoma *(bái zhú)* 9-12g
Glycyrrhizae Radix preparata *(zhì gān cǎo)* 3-6g
Wine-washed Angelicae sinensis Radix *(jiǔ xǐ dāng guī)* 6-12g

Citri reticulatae Pericarpium *(chén pí)* 6-9g
Cimicifugae Rhizoma *(shēng má)* 3-6g
Bupleuri Radix *(chái hú)* 3-9g

Ginseng and Aconite Accessory Root Decoction *(shēn fù tāng)*

SOURCE: *Classified Compilation of Medical Prescriptions* (1445)

Ginseng Radix *(rén shēn)* 12g
Aconiti Radix lateralis preparata *(zhì fù zǐ)* 9g

---

MODIFICATIONS OF DR. QIN'S FORMULA

Palpitations, flusteredness, or insomnia (with sweating):

Calcined Fossilia Ossis Mastodi *(duàn lóng gǔ)* 9g

Calcined Ostreae Concha *(duàn mǔ lì)* 9g

(If there is no sweating, consider unprocessed versions.)

Poor digestion:

Alpiniae officinarum Rhizoma *(gāo liáng jiāng)* 4.5g

Cyperi Rhizoma *(xiāng fù)* 6g

Daybreak diarrhea:

Psoraleae Fructus *(bǔ gǔ zhī)* 4.5g

Alpiniae oxyphyllae Fructus *(yì zhì rén)* 4.5g

QUESTIONS

1. *Why does Dr. Qin use Ginseng Radix (rén shēn) and Aconiti Radix lateralis preparata (zhì fù zǐ)?*

   In Ch. 18 of the *Divine Pivot* it states that the protective qi stems from the lower burner (Kidney and Bladder). With long-term deficiency, one cannot simply tonify the protective qi with medicinals such as Astragali Radix *(huáng qí)* or formulas like Jade Windscreen Powder *(yù píng fēng sǎn)*. One must take into account the lower burner, which many times relates to an underlying root problem. For example, this strategy can be important for some chronic sinus problems with frequent sneezing. The formula addresses all three of the major organs that produce protective qi: the Kidneys, Spleen, and Lungs.

2. *Why is dry-fried Atractylodis macrocephalae Rhizoma (chǎo bái zhú) chosen here, where Atractylodis macrocephalae Rhizoma (bái zhú) was used in the previous method?*

   Dry-fried Atractylodis macrocephalae Rhizoma *(chǎo bái zhú)* is better at strengthening the Spleen's yang, which is an important component of building protective qi. It also circulates more. In the previous method there was more Spleen qi and yin deficiency, for which Atractylodis macrocephalae Rhizoma *(bái zhú)*, which is moister, is more appropriate.

4. Generate Yang Fluids and Enrich the Yin Fluids (生津滋液 *shēng jīn zī yè*)

[PRESENTATION] Intestines and Stomach are dry; wasting and thirsting disorder and
constipation

Rehmanniae Radix *(shēng dì huáng)*[24]	9g
Cannabis Semen *(huǒ má rén)*	9g
Dendrobii Herba *(shí hú)*[25]	9g
Phragmitis Rhizoma *(lú gēn)*	30g
Paeoniae Radix alba *(bái sháo)*	4.5g
Anemarrhenae Rhizoma *(zhī mǔ)*	4.5g
Trichosanthis Radix *(tiān huā fěn)*	9g

COMMENTARY

ADDITIONAL SIGNS AND SYMPTOMS

- Dry mouth and thirst with a desire to drink
- Dry skin and hair with hair loss
- Food is difficult to swallow or there is dysphagia-occlusion
- Food is difficult to digest, and if severe, there may be reduced intake (due to lack of fluids/saliva)
- Constant hunger
- The stools are dry and hard or even goat-like, and are difficult to expel
- Profuse urination
- Frequent sensation of heat
- Muscle atrophy (from the muscles becoming dry)
- The pulse is thin and rapid
- The tongue is red, dry, and cracked

DISCUSSION

PATTERN: This method is suitable for a pattern of internal damage dryness with insufficient fluids.

ETIOLOGY AND PATHODYNAMIC: This pattern most often arises from constitutional yin deficiency and fluid exhaustion, general weakness (often in the elderly), postnatal depletion with damage to the yang fluids and blood, or later stages of warm diseases where the fluids are depleted and injured. All of these can lead to dry and exhausted Stomach yang fluids and a dysfunction of the intestinal tract.

DURATION: Chronic or acute. For example, an acute situation might occur after a high fever, where the heat dries out the fluids.

---

24. Originally 9g of the fresh herb was used.

25. Originally 9g of the fresh herb was used.

MEDICINAL ANALYSIS

- Rehmanniae Radix *(shēng dì huáng)* is sweet and cold. It enriches and moistens to treat insufficiency of the yin and fluids.

- Cannabis Semen *(huǒ má rén)* is sweet, balanced, oily, and moist. It can moisten dryness and lubricate the Intestines, and tonifies deficiency.

- Dendrobii Herba *(shí hú)* nourishes the Stomach and generates fluids, alleviates thirst and moistens dryness. If unavailable, one can substitute Glehniae Radix *(běi shā shēn)*.

- Phragmitis Rhizoma *(lú gēn)* is mild and not cloying. It generates fluids and has the advantage of not constraining the pathogen.

- Paeoniae Radix alba *(bái sháo)* tonifies the blood and preserves the yin.

- Anemarrhenae Rhizoma *(zhī mǔ)* enriches the yin, causes fire to descend, moistens dryness, and lubricates the Intestines. It is usually used when there is more severe heat.

- Trichosanthis Radix *(tiān huā fěn)* is bitter, cool, and moist. It clears heat and generates fluids (especially yang fluids).

Dr. Qin's formula is based on Hemp Seed Pill *(má zǐ rén wán)*.

Hemp Seed Pill *(má zǐ rén wán)*
SOURCE: *Discussion of Cold Damage* (c. 220)

Cannabis Semen *(huǒ má rén)*	500-600g
Armeniacae Semen *(xìng rén)*	150-250g
Paeoniae Radix *(sháo yào)*	150-250g
Aurantii Fructus immaturus *(zhǐ shí)*	150-250g
Magnoliae officinalis Cortex *(hòu pò)*	150-250g
Rhei Radix et Rhizoma *(dà huáng)*	300-500g

---

MODIFICATIONS OF DR. QIN'S FORMULA

When there is increased dryness, one can consider the following medicinals to increase the moistening capacity of the formula:

- Glehniae Radix *(běi shā shēn)* 6-9g
  (oral or generalized dryness)

- Trichosanthis Pericarpium *(guā lóu pí)* 4-6g
  (oral or generalized dryness)

- Nelumbinis Nodus rhizomatis *(ǒu jié)* 4-6g
  (dry skin and hair)

- Mume Fructus *(wū méi)* . . . . 1-2 pieces
  (dry mouth)

5. Nourish the Nutritive and Tonify the Blood (养营补血 *yáng yíng bǔ xuè*)

[PRESENTATION] Desiccation of blood; anemia and amenorrhea

Polygoni multiflori Radix preparata (*zhì hé shǒu wū*)	9g
Pearls of Asini Corii Colla (*ē jiāo zhū*)	4.5g
Angelicae sinensis radicis Corpus (*dāng guī shēn*)	4.5g
Cuscutae Semen (*tù sī zǐ*)	4.5g
Dry-fried Paeoniae Radix alba (*chǎo bái sháo*)	4.5g
Astragali complanati Semen (*shā yuàn zǐ*)	9g
Longan Arillus (*lóng yǎn ròu*)	6p

COMMENTARY

ADDITIONAL SIGNS AND SYMPTOMS

- Frequent vertigo or dizziness
- Unclear mind, especially when tired
- Heart palpitations and rapid heart rate with light exertion or work
- Pale face
- Easily chilled, especially hands and feet
- May or may not correspond to Western diagnosis of anemia
- The pulse is thin, weak, and soft
- The tongue is pale

DISCUSSION

While the blood is dependent on the Spleen, Heart, and Liver, when tonifying the blood one should pay special attention to the Liver blood, unless of course there are compelling symptoms suggesting that other organs need more attention. For example, light-colored bleeding indicates a need to focus on the Spleen, and if there is poor circulation in the blood vessels, pay more attention to the Heart.

PATTERN: This is Liver blood deficiency with Kidney yin, yang, and essence deficiency. The Kidney aspect must be present to use this formula. Blood deficiency can be divided into blood yin (more heat signs) or blood yang (more cold signs) deficiency. This presentation is blood yang deficiency. Therefore, tonification is more on the warm side. Compare this with the following method, which emphasizes Kidney yin deficiency.

ETIOLOGY AND PATHODYNAMIC: This method is suitable when there is source of transformation insufficiency (inadequate blood and qi production), loss of nourishment from the Liver blood, chronic disease that damages and consumes essence blood, or excessive loss of blood.

MEDICINAL ANALYSIS

SUMMARY

All of these medicinals are warm except for dry-fried Paeoniae Radix alba *(chǎo bái sháo)* and Pearls of Asini Corii Colla *(ē jiāo zhū)*.

INDIVIDUAL CHARACTERISTICS

- Polygoni multiflori Radix preparata *(zhì shǒu wū)* is slightly warm, bitter, and astringent, but harmonious and moderate in nature, hence not cloying, hot, or dry. Although it tonifies the Kidneys, Liver, yin, yang, blood, and essence, it is an important medicinal for the regulation and nourishment of Liver blood, and is particularly able to tonify the yin. Unprepared Polygoni multiflori Radix *(hé shǒu wū)* tonifies the blood but is cool and can cause diarrhea. Therefore, it can be used if there is constipation. Most of the Polygoni multiflori Radix *(hé shǒu wū)* available in the West is the processed form.

- Pearls of Asini Corii Colla *(ē jiāo zhū)* are sweet, sour, and cooling. This is an essential medicinal for enriching the yin and tonifying the blood, especially of the Liver. It can also stop bleeding. It performs this last function by repairing the blood vessels. It is most suitable when there is blood deficiency with dizziness, palpations, and insomnia. From a biomedical perspective, it can increase red blood cells. Pearls of Asini Corii Colla *(ē jiāo zhū)* are easier to digest than Asini Corii Colla *(ē jiāo)*, which is sticky and has a tendency to damage the Spleen circulation.

- Angelicae sinensis radicis Corpus *(dāng guī shēn)* and dry-fried Paeoniae Radix alba *(chǎo bái sháo)* both tonify the blood and nourish the nutritive. Angelicae sinensis radicis Corpus *(dāng guī shēn)* is the body of Angelicae sinensis Radix *(dāng guī)* and is an important medicinal for tonifying the Liver blood. Dry-fried Paeoniae Radix alba *(chǎo bái sháo)* is neutral to cool and is an important medicinal for nourishing the Liver yin.

- Cuscutae Semen *(tù sī zǐ)* and Astragali complanati Semen *(shā yuàn zǐ)* are neither dry nor greasy; they enrich and nourish the Liver and Kidney yin, essence, and yang. Astragali complanati Semen *(shā yuàn zǐ)* is more tonifying for the Liver, whereas Cuscutae Semen *(tù sī zǐ)* is more tonifying for the Kidneys. Cuscutae Semen *(tù sī zǐ)* is unique in that, for Kidney yang insufficiency, it can assist the yang medicinals to form yin, and in Kidney yin insufficiency, it can assist the yin medicinals to form yang.

- Longan Arillus *(lóng yǎn ròu)* tonifies the blood, augments the qi, and specifically the Heart yang and blood.

Dr. Qin's formula is based on Fleeceflower Special Pill to Extend Life *(shǒu wū yán shòu dān)* and Restore the Spleen Decoction *(guī pí tāng)*.[26]

---

26. One of Dr. Qin's formal formulas, based on this method, is Major Cuscutae Seed Drink *(dà tù sī zǐ yǐn)*: Cuscutae Semen *(tù sī zǐ)*, Astragali complanati Semen *(shā yuàn zǐ)*, Polygoni multiflori Radix preparata *(zhì hé shǒu wū)*, Rehmanniae Radix preparata *(shú dì huáng)*, Pearls of Asini Corii Colla *(ē jiāo zhū)*,Testudinis Plastri Colla *(guī bǎn jiāo)*, Hominis Placenta *(zǐ hé chē)*, Psoraleae Fructus *(bǔ gǔ zhī)*, and Corni Fructus *(shān zhū yú)*. Dosages unknown.

Fleeceflower Special Pill to Extend Life (*shǒu wū yán shòu dān*)

SOURCE: *Small Collection of Fine Formulas* (1842)

Polygoni multiflori Radix (*hé shǒu wū*)
Cuscutae Semen (*tù sī zǐ*)
Siegesbeckiae Herba (*xī xiān cǎo*)
Mori Folium (*sāng yè*)
Ligustri lucidi Fructus (*nǚ zhēn zǐ*)
Lonicerae Flos (*jīn yín huā*)
Eucommiae Cortex (*dù zhòng*)
Achyranthis bidentatae Radix (*niú xī*)
Rehmanniae Radix (*shēng dì huáng*)[27]

Restore the Spleen Decoction (*guī pí tāng*)

SOURCE: *Categorized Essentials for Normalizing the Structure* (1529)

Ginseng Radix (*rén shēn*) 3-6g
Astragali Radix (*huáng qí*). 9-12g
Atractylodis macrocephalae Rhizoma (*bái zhú*) 9-12g
Poria (*fú líng*). 9-12g
Ziziphi spinosae Semen (*suān zǎo rén*) 9-12g
Longan Arillus (*lóng yǎn ròu*) 6-9g
Aucklandiae Radix (*mù xiāng*). 3-6g
Glycyrrhizae Radix preparata (*zhì gān cǎo*). 3-6g
Angelicae sinensis Radix (*dāng guī*). 6-9g
processed Polygalae Radix (*zhì yuǎn zhì*) 3-6g

MODIFICATIONS OF DR. QIN'S FORMULA

Spirit failing to keep to its abode (e.g., loss of normal clarity of mind and composure):

Platycladi Semen (*bǎi zǐ rén*) 4-6g

Ziziphi spinosae Semen (*suān zǎo rén*). 4-6g

In general, also consider adding to the formula:

Mori Fructus (*sāng shèn*) 6-9g

   (gently tonifies the Liver blood and yin, which is a useful strategy in chronic blood deficiency. It is especially useful when there is unclear vision and hearing.)

Ligustri lucidi Fructus (*nǚ zhēn zǐ*). 4-6g

   (tonifies the Liver yin and relaxes and quiets the mind. It is especially useful when there is difficulty falling asleep as well as overactive emotions and thoughts.)

QUESTIONS

1. *Why does Dr. Qin choose herbs that are known to be Kidney yang tonics?*

   Both Cuscutae Semen (*tù sī zǐ*) and Astragali complanati Semen (*shā yuàn zǐ*) are considered to be yang tonics, however it should be noted that this is not a yang deficiency pattern per se. Because the Liver and Kidneys share the same source, if one desires to tonify the Liver blood then one must also augment the Kidneys, particularly the essence.

---

27. Dosages unknown.

Because the condition is on the colder side, warming herbs are best. However, both of these medicinals tonify Kidney yin, essence, and yang, as well as the Liver. Cuscutae Semen *(tù sī zǐ)* is additionally said to tonify the *rèn* and *chōng* vessels, qi, and blood. It is also especially appropriate for problems such as low hemoglobin.

2. *Why does Dr. Qin choose to use dry-fried Paeoniae Radix alba (chǎo bái sháo) in this method and the unprepared form in the previous method?*

In general, unprocessed Paeoniae Radix alba *(bái sháo)* is best in cases where yin deficiency predominates. If there are more digestive problems or the patient is more on the cold side, then dry-fried Paeoniae Radix alba *(chǎo bái sháo)* is more appropriate. Furthermore, dry-fried Paeoniae Radix alba *(chǎo bái sháo)* better circulates the qi, while unprocessed Paeoniae Radix alba *(bái sháo)* has too much of a binding effect to be appropriate for this pattern.

3. *Why does Dr. qin not use Rehmanniae Radix preparata (shú dì huáng)?*

This pattern is more about the Liver blood than Kidney deficiency. Dr. Qin considers Polygoni multiflori Radix *(hé shǒu wū)* the primary herb for tonifying the Liver, the second being Angelicae sinensis Radix *(dāng guī)*. Rehmanniae Radix preparata *(shú dì huáng)*, while it does tonify the Liver, is best for the Kidneys, as demonstrated in the next method's formula. However, if the appropriate result is not achieved with the formula above, one can add Rehmanniae Radix preparata *(shú dì huáng)*.

4. *Since the blood is made by the Spleen, should the Spleen be considered in this case?*

It is not uncommon to have blood deficiency without Spleen deficiency; thus there is no need to address the Spleen. The idea that just because one has blood deficiency one must tonify the Spleen with Atractylodis macrocephalae Rhizoma *(bái zhú)*, Codonopsis Radix *(dǎng shēn)*, or Astragali Radix *(huáng qí)* is incorrect. Furthermore, because this pattern has no Spleen deficiency, there is no dampness and one can safely use Longan Arillus *(lóng yǎn ròu)* and Polygoni multiflori Radix *(hé shǒu wū)*.

6. Enrich the Yin and Replenish the Water (滋阴填坎 *zī yīn tián kǎn*)

[PRESENTATION] Kidney water exhausted and consumed; sore lower back, blurry and unclear vision, and deafness

Vinegar-fried Testudinis Plastrum *(cù chǎo guī bǎn)*	9g
Corni Fructus *(shān zhū yú)*	9g
Rehmanniae Radix preparata *(shú dì huáng)*	6g
Ligustri lucidi Fructus *(nǚ zhēn zǐ)*	9g
Eucommiae Cortex *(dù zhòng)*	9g
Lycii Fructus *(gǒu qǐ zǐ)*	9g
Sesami Semen nigrum *(hēi zhī má)*	9g

COMMENTARY

ADDITIONAL SIGNS AND SYMPTOMS

KEY SYMPTOMS

- Lower or mid-back pain (often more severe at night)
- Foot, sole, or heel pain

OTHER KIDNEY SYMPTOMS

- Sore and weak knees
- Lack of strength in legs
- Tinnitus, deafness, sensation of pain inside the ear, or sounds that seem further away than they actually are
- Vertigo and dizziness
- Headache (deep in the head), which is worse after fatigue or sex
- Seminal emissions
- Loose teeth, unhealthy gums, or sore jaw

YIN DEFICIENT SYMPTOMS MAY ALSO BE PRESENT, SUCH AS

- Heat in the five centers
- Night sweating
- Dry throat
- Insomnia

- The pulse is thin, rapid, and the proximal position is difficult to find
- The tongue is thin, red, dry, cracked, geographic, and larger dark red or purple bumps at the root of the tongue

DISCUSSION

PATTERN: Kidney yin and essence exhaustion and desiccation

ETIOLOGY: This pattern arises from internal damage due to excessive sex, long-term diseases that reach the Kidneys, or later stages of warm diseases where extreme heat damages the yin.

MEDICINAL ANALYSIS

- Rehmanniae Radix preparata *(shú dì huáng)* is slightly warm to neutral and is an essential medicinal to tonify and augment the Kidneys and Liver. Not only does it enrich the yin and nourish the blood, it also generates essence and tonifies the marrow. It is suitable to use in all patterns of yin deficiency, blood deficiency, and essence depletion. This is a cloying medicinal that should be used with caution when there are digestive issues.
- Corni Fructus *(shān zhū yú)* is sour, neutral (Wu) to warm (Qin), and is able to bind the essence as well as tonify the Liver and Kidneys. It also enriches and nourishes the essence and yin. It is especially good for symptoms such as fatigue, dizziness, insomnia, and a scattered mind. With Rehmanniae Radix preparata *(shú dì huáng)* it makes a strong

herbal pair that tonifes the blood and nourishes the yin. Neither Dr. Qin nor Dr. Wu consider Corni Fructus *(shān zhū yú)* a medicinal that tonifies the yang.

• Ligustri lucidi Fructus *(nǔ zhēn zǐ)* and Lycii Fructus *(gǒu qǐ zǐ)* simultaneously tonify the yin and yang. Ligustri lucidi Fructus *(nǔ zhēn zǐ)* is slightly bitter, neutral to slightly cool, and is balanced in nature, very mild and not cloying, and fortifies the yin of the Kidneys and Liver. The nature of Lycii Fructus *(gǒu qǐ zǐ)* is balanced and able to fortify the yin, yang, and essence of the Kidneys as well as the Liver yin.

• Sesami Semen nigrum *(hēi zhī má)* tonifies the Liver and Kidneys and tonifies and augments the yin, essence, and blood. It is especially good for cloudy eyes.

• Vinegar-fried Testudinis Plastrum *(cù chǎo guī bǎn)* nourishes the yin and clears heat from yin deficiency. It is preferred over the unprepared medicinal because it is more tonifying and has a much better absorption rate.

• Eucommiae Cortex *(dù zhòng)* tonifies and augments the Liver and Kidneys, strengthens and fortifies the sinews and bones, and is especially useful for Kidney deficiency lower back pain and soreness.

Dr. Qin's formula is based on Six-Ingredient Pill with Rehmannia *(liù wèi dì huáng wán)* and Great Tonify the Yin Pill *(dà bǔ yīn wán).*

Six-Ingredient Pill with Rehmannia *(liù wèi dì huáng wán)*
SOURCE: *Craft of Medicines and Patterns for Children* (1119)

Rehmanniae Radix preparata *(shú dì huáng)* 240g
Corni Fructus *(shān zhū yú)* 120g
Dioscoreae Rhizoma *(shān yào)* 120g
Poria *(fú líng)* 90g
Moutan Cortex *(mǔ dān pí)* 90g
Alismatis Rhizoma *(zé xiè)* 90g

Great Tonify the Yin Pill *(dà bǔ yīn wán)*
SOURCE: *Essential Teachings of [Zhu] Dan-Xi* (1481)

Rehmanniae Radix preparata *(shú dì huáng)* 180g
Crisp Testudinis Plastrum *(sū guī bǎn)* 180g
Dry-fried Phellodendri Cortex *(chǎo huáng bǎi)* 120g
Wine-fried Anemarrhenae Rhizoma *(jiǔ chǎo zhī mǔ)* 120g

---

MODIFICATIONS OF DR. QIN'S FORMULA

Tinnitus:

Magnetitum *(cí shí)* 12g

Anemarrhenae Rhizoma *(zhī mǔ)* 6g

Dizziness:

Tribuli Fructus *(cì jí lí)* 6g

Astragali complanati Semen *(shā yuàn zǐ)* 9g

More severe lower back pain:

Cibotii Rhizoma *(gǒu jǐ)* 9g

Dipsaci Radix *(xù duàn)* 9g

FOOD THERAPY

Consider soft-shelled turtle *(jiǎ yú)*, bird's nest *(yàn wō)*, and sea cucumber *(hǎi shēn)*.

QUESTIONS

1. *One often hears the term 'cloying' used to describe herbs. When should one use or not use a cloying medicinal?*

   Cloying herbs not only can be difficult to digest but may also contribute to all sorts of problems related to stagnation. For example, anything that clogs the qi dynamic can exacerbate anything that is contributing to or resulting from stagnation. Thus, medicinals that are too cloying are usually avoided when there is a greasy tongue coating and/or signs of impaired digestion, dampness, phlegm, stasis, or heat.

   However, when there is a deep deficiency, such as essence deficiency, thick flavored 'cloying' herbs are indicated. One will notice that the treatment principles outlined in this chapter treat progressively deeper and deeper deficiencies, and consequently utilize progressively more and more cloying medicinals.

   Of course, when there is a mixed pattern with signs of stagnation, dampness, heat, etc., and deficiency, there must be some additional considerations. One may merely limit the amount of cloying medicinals or use tricks that allow the body to utilize the medicinals better. For example, one may prescribe Amomi Fructus *(shā rén)* with Rehmanniae Radix preparata *(shú dì huáng)* to aid digestion. Herbal preparation methods can also be considered, such as dry-fried cooked Rehmanniae Radix *(chǎo shú dì huáng)*, or vinegar-fried Testudinis Plastrum *(cù chǎo guī bǎn)*, as used above. Dr. Qin was particularly fond of the preparation method of using Amomi Fructus *(shā rén)* or Asari Radix et Rhizoma *(xì xīn)* fried with dry-fried cooked Rehmanniae Radix *(chǎo shú dì huáng)* to reduce its stickiness.

---

7. Secure and Bind the Essence Gate (固涩精关 *gù sè jīng guān*)

[PRESENTATION] Kidney deficiency with expended essence; nocturnal emissions and leakage and loss (e.g., urine, semen, vaginal discharge, or stool)

Rehmanniae Radix preparata *(shú dì huáng)* 9g

Rosae laevigatae Fructus *(jīn yīng zǐ)* 4.5g

Corni Fructus *(shān zhū yú)* 4.5g

Schisandrae Fructus *(wǔ wèi zǐ)* 1.5g

Mantidis Oötheca *(sāng piāo xiāo)* 4.5g

Calcined Fossilia Dentis Mastodi *(duàn lóng chǐ)* 9g

Nelumbinis Stamen *(lián xū)* 2.4g

COMMENTARY

ADDITIONAL SIGNS AND SYMPTOMS

KEY SIGNS AND SYMPTOMS

- Nocturnal emissions without dreams

If severe:

- Seminal emissions at provocative sights
- White and sticky discharge from penis during bowel movements or after urination
- Morning diarrhea

THERE WILL ALSO BE THE COMMON KIDNEY DEFICIENCY SYMPTOMS SUCH AS

- Fatigue
- Dizziness and vertigo
- Tinnitus
- Lower back pain
- Night and daytime sweating
- Impotence
- Cold hands and feet
- Poor memory
- The pulse is thin and frail
- The tongue is tender, swollen, and pale, or possibly thin, or purple, or dry

DISCUSSION

ETIOLOGY: This commonly occurs from ongoing deficiency and overwork. Furthermore, the nocturnal emissions themselves (as well as the female analogue, continuous vaginal discharge) can further lead to Kidney essence deficiency.

PATTERN: This is Kidney essence deficiency, including both Kidney yin and yang, with a tendency toward yin deficiency. However, there must be some leaking of bodily substance to be in this category.

DIFFERENTIATION: The key sign, nocturnal emissions, not only can occur from deficiency, but also from sovereign and ministerial fire exuberance stirring the essence gate, and should be differentiated appropriately. This latter pattern most likely will have seminal emission with dreams, and a wiry and fast pulse. *Note:* If overabundant ministerial fire is disrupting the essence gate, one must clear heat while still nourishing the yin. However, using the securing and binding method described above is inappropriate. One may consider Anemarrhena and Phellodendron Eight-Ingredient Pill *(zhī bǎi bā wèi wán)*.[28]

TREATMENT PRINCIPLE: Enrich the Kidneys and replenish the essence while simultaneously securing, binding, restraining, and holding back.

---

28. Rehmanniae Radix preparata *(shú dì huáng)*, Dioscoreae Rhizoma *(shān yào)*, Corni Fructus *(shān zhū yú)*, Moutan Cortex *(mǔ dān pí)*, Alismatis Rhizoma *(zé xiè)*, Poria *(fú líng)*, Anemarrhenae Rhizoma *(zhī mǔ)*, and Phellodendri Cortex *(huáng bǎi)*.

MEDICINAL ANALYSIS

ENRICH AND SECURE THE ESSENCE GATE IN ORDER TO REPLENISH THE ROOT:

Rehmanniae Radix preparata *(shú dì huáng)*
Corni Fructus *(shān zhū yú)*
Schisandrae Fructus *(wǔ wèi zǐ)*

Corni Fructus *(shān zhū yú)* and Schisandrae Fructus *(wǔ wèi zǐ)* not only bind fluids (e.g., nocturnal emissions), they also hold in the tonic medicinals so that they can be better utilized. Schisandrae Fructus *(wǔ wèi zǐ)* addresses the various Heart symptoms that can occur in this pattern (e.g., palpitations). Also, see the descriptions of Rehmanniae Radix preparata *(shú dì huáng)* and Corni Fructus *(shān zhū yú)* in the previous method.

RESTRAIN, INHIBIT, SECURE, AND BIND TO TREAT THE BRANCH:

Rosae laevigatae Fructus *(jīn yīng zǐ)*
Mantidis Oötheca *(sāng piāo xiāo)*
calcined Fossilia Dentis Mastodi *(duàn lóng chǐ)*
Nelumbinis Stamen *(lián xū)*

Rosae laevigatae Fructus *(jīn yīng zǐ)* is able to bind any type of leakage or essence, but is especially effective for those occurring from the lower burner. Calcined Fossilia Dentis Mastodi *(duàn lóng chǐ)* is able to connect the Heart and Kidneys. It is more astringing than Fossilia Dentis Mastodi *(lóng chǐ)*. Nelumbinis Stamen *(lián xū)* and Mantidis Oötheca *(sāng piāo xiāo)* merely bind. Mantidis Oötheca *(sāng piāo xiāo)* with other tonifying herbs can aid in augmenting the essence.

Dr. Qin's formula is based on Modified Six-Ingredient Pill with Rehmannia *(jiā jiǎn liù wèi wán)* and Metal Lock Pill to Stabilize the Essence *(jīn suǒ gù jīng wán)*.[29]

Modified Six-Ingredient Pill with Rehmannia *(jiā jiǎn liù wèi wán)*

SOURCE: *Systematized Patterns with Clear-Cut Treatments* (1839)

Rehmanniae Radix preparata *(shú dì huáng)* 60g
Poria *(fú líng)* 60g
Moutan Cortex *(mǔ dān pí)* 60g
Corni Fructus *(shān zhū yú)* 60g
Dioscoreae Rhizoma *(shān yào)* 60g
Nelumbinis Stamen *(lián xū)* 60g
Euryales Semen *(qiàn shí)* 60g
Cuscutae Semen *(tù sī zǐ)* 60g
Fossilia Ossis Mastodi *(lóng gǔ)* 30g
Ostreae Concha *(mǔ lì)* 30g
Alismatis Rhizoma *(zé xiè)* 30g
Schisandrae Fructus *(wǔ wèi zǐ)* 15g

---

29. Can also be thought to be based on Mantis Egg-Case Powder *(sāng piāo xiāo sān)*: Mantidis Oötheca *(sāng piāo xiāo)*, Fossilia Ossis Mastodi *(lóng gǔ)*, Ginseng Radix *(rén shēn)*, Poriae Sclerotium pararadicis *(fú shén)*, Polygalae Radix *(yuǎn zhì)*, Acori tatarinowii Rhizoma *(shí chāng pú)*, vinegar-fried Testudinis Plastrum *(cù chǎo guī bǎn)*, and Angelicae sinensis Radix *(dāng guī)*.

Metal Lock Pill to Stabilize the Essence (*jīn suǒ gù jīng wán*)

SOURCE: *Medical Formulas Collected and Analyzed* (1682)

Dry-fried Astragali complanati Semen (*chǎo shā yuàn zǐ*). 60g
Euryales Semen (*qiàn shí*). 60g
Nelumbinis Stamen (*lián xū*). 60g
Calcined Fossilia Ossis Mastodi (*duàn lóng gǔ*) 30g
Calcined Ostreae Concha (*duàn mǔ lì*) 30g
Nelumbinis Semen (*lián zǐ*). 120g

MODIFICATIONS OF DR. QIN'S FORMULA

Frequent loss of sperm:

    Psoraleae Fructus *(bǔ gǔ zhī)*. 6g

    Calcined Ostreae Concha *(duàn mǔ lì)* 9g

Daybreak diarrhea:

    Chebulae Fructus *(hē zǐ)*. 6g

Premature ejaculation with strong sexual desire:

    Ligustri lucidi Fructus *(nǚ zhēn zǐ)*. 6-9g

    Cuscutae Semen *(tù sī zǐ)*. 6-9g

    Astragali complanati Semen *(shā yuàn zǐ)*. 6-9g

Dizziness:

    Astragali complanati Semen *(shā yuàn zǐ)*. 6-9g

    Tribuli Fructus *(cì jí lí)* 4-6g

    Ligustri lucidi Fructus *(nǚ zhēn zǐ)*. 4-6g

    Ecliptae Herba *(mò hàn lián)*. 4-6g

Tinnitus:

    Salt-fried Anemarrhenae Rhizoma *(yán chǎo zhī mǔ)* 6-9g

    Glycinis Semen *(hēi dòu)* 9-12g

QUESTIONS

1. *Why does Dr. Qin not use Astragali complanati Semen (shā yuàn zǐ) here?*

   Although Astragali complanati Semen *(shā yuàn zǐ)* is in formulas like Metal Lock Pill to Stabilize the Essence *(jīn suǒ gù jīng wán)*, it is not included in this formula because it mainly enters the Liver. Of course, one can add it if the Liver aspect needs to be addressed.

2. *Why does Dr. Qin use Fossilia Dentis Mastodi (lóng chǐ) here instead of Fossilia Ossis Mastodi (lóng gǔ) or Ostreae Concha (mǔ lì)?*

   Fossilia Dentis Mastodi *(lóng chǐ)* not only provides a connecting function between the Kidney and Heart, it has a more tonifying effect. Note its use in the method "sedate floating qi" in Ch. 3 (p. 67), where it sedates floating qi.

3. *Why is there a swollen tongue?*

The swollen tongue shows cold and dampness accumulation that arises from Kidney qi/yang and essence deficiency. The deficiency impairs the circulation of fluids. In this case there will also be symptoms such as a cold sensation in the lower abdomen.

4. *How can there be either a puffy, pale tongue or thin, purple tongue?*

The aspect of the Kidneys that is more deficient (yin or yang) will determine how the tongue looks.

5. *If there is night and daytime sweating, does this imply some heat due to yin deficiency?*

This type of sweating is from essence deficiency. In Ch. 18 of the *Divine Pivot* it states that the protective qi comes from the lower burner/Kidneys. This Kidney essence deficiency results in an inability of the protective qi to hold in the sweat. Therefore, this is not heat forcing out the sweat.

---

8. Warm and Tonify the Lower Base[30] (温补下元 *wēn bû xià yuán*)

[PRESENTATION] Lower burner deficiency cold; Kidney diarrhea[31] and cold limbs

Sliced Cervi Cornu pantotrichum *(lù róng piàn)*	0.9g
Ginseng Radix rubra *(hóng shēn)*	3g
Aconiti Radix lateralis preparata *(zhì fù zǐ)*	3g
Psoraleae Fructus *(bǔ gǔ zhī)*	9g
Rehmanniae Radix preparata *(shú dì huáng)*	9g
Alpiniae oxyphyllae Fructus *(yì zhì rén)*	9g
Juglandis Semen *(hé táo rén)*	2 pieces

COMMENTARY

ADDITIONAL SIGNS AND SYMPTOMS

- Decreased libido
- Impotence
- Low sperm count, decreased sperm activity (motility/speed), or just weak/poor quality sperm (unable to penetrate egg)
- Sensations of cold, or easily feel cold
- Premature ejaculation
- Symptoms are worse in the winter

---

30. "Lower base" refers to the lower burner/Kidneys, encompassing the concept of the *rèn* and *chòng* vessels.

31. This is persistent early morning diarrhea that is accompanied by rumbling intestines.

Other Kidney symptoms such as:

- Low back soreness and pain
- Dizziness
- Fatigue
- Urinary frequency

DISCUSSION

PATTERN: This is essentially a Kidney yang/gate of vitality deficiency and is often called a *dū mài* deficiency.

TREATMENT PRINCIPLE: The Kidney is the grotto of water and fire, therefore one must simultaneously fortify the yang and enrich the yin. Otherwise, exuberant fire will scorch the yin and essence and damage the qi. Zhang Jie-Bin said, "To be good at tonifying the yang one must seek the yang within the yin, and when the yang obtains yin's assistance, there will be birth and transformation without limit." Psoraleae Fructus *(bǔ gǔ zhī)*, Rehmanniae Radix preparata *(shú dì huáng)*, Alpiniae oxyphyllae Fructus *(yì zhì rén)*, and Juglandis Semen *(hé táo rén)* are used for this reason.

MEDICINAL ANALYSIS

- Sliced Cervi Cornu pantotrichum *(lù róng piàn)* is salty and warm to hot. It tonifies the fire, fortifies the yang, and tonifies the essence. It also has a good effect on increasing RBC counts and hemoglobin when these are low, especially from bone marrow dysfunction. It should not be cooked, but instead ground into a fine powder and taken with the decoction. It can also be taken in capsules.

- Aconiti Radix lateralis preparata *(zhì fù zǐ)* is excellent at tonifying fire and is especially effective with Ginseng Radix rubra *(hóng shēn)*, which tonifies both the yang and qi. Both should be pre-cooked for 45-60 minutes. Ginseng Radix rubra *(hóng shēn)* is Ginseng Radix *(rén shēn)* that is processed with other herbs, such as Cinnamomi Cortex *(ròu guì)*, Angelicae sinensis Radix *(dāng guī)*, and Croci Stigma *(zàng hóng huā)*. This increases its warmth and ability to tonify the qi.

- Rehmanniae Radix preparata *(shú dì huáng)* and Psoraleae Fructus *(bǔ gǔ zhī)* both augment the essence. Rehmanniae Radix preparata *(shú dì huáng)* is slightly warm to neutral and is an essential medicinal to tonify and augment the Kidneys and Liver. Not only does it enrich the essence and tonify the marrow, it also supplements the yin and nourishes the blood. It is suitable to use in all patterns of yin deficiency, blood deficiency, and essence depletion. This is a cloying medicinal that should be used with caution when there are digestive issues. (See p. 135, question no. 1, for a discussion of this issue.) Psoraleae Fructus *(bǔ gǔ zhī)* warms and tonifies the fire at the gate of vitality, conserves the lower source, and augments the essence. It is good for daybreak diarrhea and Dr. Qin especially liked it for chronic back pain.

- Juglandis Semen *(hé táo rén)* is sweet and balanced and tonifies the Kidneys yin, yang, and essence as well as the Spleen yang. It strengthens the lower back, secures the urine, and is also good for tinnitus and deafness. Use only the nut, remove the shell and crush.

- Alpiniae oxyphyllae Fructus *(yì zhì rén)* warms, tonifies, and assists the Kidney yang, expels cold, opens the yang of the Heart, returns the yang to its source, secures the urine, and binds the stool.

Dr. Qin's formula is based on Ginseng and Aconite Accessory Root Decoction *(shēn fù tāng)*.

Ginseng and Aconite Accessory Root Decoction *(shēn fù tāng)*

SOURCE: *Classified Compilation of Medical Prescriptions* (1445)

Ginseng Radix *(rén shēn)* 12g
Aconiti Radix lateralis preparata *(zhì fù zǐ)* 9g

---

MODIFICATIONS OF DR. QIN'S FORMULA

Cold limbs:

Cinnamomi Ramulus *(guì zhī)* 4.5g

Eucommiae Cortex *(dù zhòng)* 6g

Low sperm count (50% below normal):

Callorhini Testes et Penis *(hǎi gǒu shèn)* 3g
  (powder, taken with decoction)

Hominis Placenta *(zǐ hé chē)* 5g

Large number of dead sperm:

Vaccariae Semen *(wáng bù liú xíng)* 6g

Corni Fructus *(shān zhū yú)* 9g

Lower back pain:

Dipsaci Radix *(xù duàn)* 4-6g

Dry-fried Eucommiae Cortex *(chǎo dù zhòng)* 4-6g

Cuscutae Semen *(tù sī zǐ)* 4-6g

Cibotii Rhizoma *(gǒu jǐ)* 4-6g

Head symptoms such as dizziness, vertigo, headache, poor memory:

Astragali complanati Semen *(shā yuàn zǐ)* 6-9g

Tribuli Fructus *(cì jí lí)* 3-5g

6

Treatment Guidelines for

Wind 风 *(fēng)*

NATURE

The nature of wind is light and it likes to move around. It can enter even the smallest spaces. It can easily strike humans and its onset of disease is rapid.

The nature of wind in the body produces symptoms that easily move around, switch locations, or are erratic. Examples include some types of arthritis, rashes (most commonly urticaria, eczema, or dermatitis), and even some cases of IBS.

DISEASE LOCATION

Exterior: If mild, there is nasal congestion, raspy voice, occasional clear nasal discharge, cough, and spontaneous sweating. If severe, there is headache, fever, body pain, phlegm gushing upward and wheezing, a hoarse voice, and a dry throat.

Additional signs and symptoms may be sneezing, itchy throat and nose, copious nasal discharge, sore throat, and loss of voice. The headache will usually move around and the feverishness is usually felt as if it exists on the surface of the body. These are all symptoms that indicate wind on the surface. However, wind can mix with heat, cold, dampness, etc., meaning that a combination of treatment methods may be required.

Interior:
Collateral attack: Wind enters the muscles and there will be numbness and paresthesia in the fingers and insensitivity of the muscles.

The patient might describe this as ants or bugs crawling on or under the skin. This may also include deviation of the eyes and mouth. Examples are urticaria, Bell's palsy, or mild stroke.

Channel attack: Nutritive qi and blood are unable to secure the interior and wind enters the channels and collaterals. The body feels heavy and there is difficulty in walking.

Since this is wind affecting the channels, there will be symptoms in the arms and the legs as well as the neck and back. This may manifest as aches or spasms.

From these locations, wind enters deeper.
Yang organ attack: Phlegm-oral mucus ascending and congesting such that it blocks the divine [sensory] orifices,[i] leading to fainting with loss of consciousness.

In addition, one will often hear phlegm in the throat. There may be migraines, low pitched tinnitus, Bell's palsy, or numbness and tingling in the arms and legs. If severe, there will be low levels of consciousness, inability to use the limbs, or possibly unconsciousness. However, the patient will still be continent of urine and bowels and this is easier to cure than a yin organ attack.

Yin organ attack: Spirit radiance[1] is scattered and disorderly, unable to speak, and uncontrolled drooling.

In addition there may be loss of control of the urine and bowels and difficulty opening the mouth. These people may go into a deep coma and be difficult to treat.

SUMMARY OF TREATMENT PRINCIPLES
External wind: Disperse and scatter.

This implies dissipating and resolving the exterior.

Internal wind: Anchor the yang and extinguish the wind.

Depending on the presentation, one may also need to tonify the Liver, clear heat, expel wind, cold, and dampness, or guide phlegm out.

Wind-like attack: Flush away phlegm, direct fire downward, smooth the qi, and unblock the bowels.

This is not really wind and should not be treated as such. Therefore, it is not discussed further in this chapter and one must follow the pattern to successfully treat it. There is usually a mix of pathogens such as heat, fire, or yang rising, as well as deficiency.

For example, if there is:

---

1. See glossary for definition.

- phlegm attack, flush away phlegm;
- fire attack, direct fire downward;
- qi attack, normalize the qi;
- blood stasis, break up the blood stasis;
- food accumulation, open the yang organs;
- blood, fluid, and yin deficiency, nourish the blood and moisten dryness. This is usually applied after the acute condition is under control.
- qi and Kidney essence deficiency, tonify the qi and nurture the base. This is usually applied in conjunction with the above therapies, or following them.

For further information about wind-like attacks, see the addendum on p. 160.

---

1. Diffuse the Lungs and Disperse Wind (宣肺疏风 *xuān fèi shū fēng*)

[PRESENTATION] Wind pathogen common cold and flu; aversion to wind and drafts, fever, dizziness, and headache

Schizonepetae Spica (*jīng jiè suì*)	4.5g
Mori Folium (*sāng yè*)	4.5g
Menthae haplocalycis Herba (*bò hé*)	2.4g
Viticis Fructus (*màn jīng zǐ*)	4.5g
Sojae Semen preparatum (*dàn dòu chǐ*)	9g
Chrysanthemi Flos (*jú huā*)	4.5g
Allii fistulosi Bulbus (*cōng bái*)	2 pieces

COMMENTARY

ADDITIONAL SIGNS AND SYMPTOMS

- Unclear thinking, blurry vision
- Whole body discomfort
- Muscle aches (especially on the back or neck)
- Head distention
- Sneezing
- Itchy or sore throat
- Hoarse or raspy voice
- Slight cough
- May or may not sweat
- Sinus congestion and nasal discharge
- Dry mouth and thirst
- Headache will be dull and distended and not sharp
- Fever and aversion to wind and drafts, if any, will be mild
- Aversion to wind is important for the diagnosis of this pattern

- Pulse: 1. Floating, rapid, slippery, and soft (or larger, if more heat); or
  2. Floating and tight, and perhaps rapid (if more cold)
- Tongue: 1. Normal with a thin white coating; or
  2. Red tip with a slightly yellow and dry coating (if more heat)

DISCUSSION

PATTERN: This is a mild pattern due to damage by external wind. The pathogen resides in the protective aspect and there commonly will be symptoms related to the respiratory system. This formula is thermally balanced, neither too warm nor too cold. However, this formula not only can treat an external wind pattern that does not have a predominance of cold or heat, it can also, when modified, treat wind patterns that tend toward either wind-heat or wind-cold (see question no. 1 below).

TREATMENT PRINCIPLE: Disperse the wind and resolve the exterior. If a wind pathogen is not combined with a cold or warm pathogen, then simply use acrid, balanced medicinals to disperse the wind and resolve the exterior. For a mild illness, one needs only a light treatment and need not make a mountain out of a molehill. Therefore, use medicinals that are balanced, smooth, light, and quick to guide the wind pathogen from the protective aspect to the outside of the body. This formula can produce a light therapeutic sweat; for this condition, a stronger formula that produces a profuse sweat is contraindicated.

DIFFERENTIATION: In the early stages, differentiating between wind damage, cold damage, and wind-heat can be difficult. The following table provides some key points of comparison.

Wind Damage (伤风 *shāng fēng*)	Cold Damage (伤寒 *shāng hán*)
Aversion to wind and drafts (important)	Chills
May feel chilled or warm	Will feel cold Often will have a high temperature
Both can have simultaneous fever and chills, although the severity and nature will vary based on the above differentiation.	
Mild headache (distended feeling)	Sharp headache and body aches
May or may not sweat	Usually no sweating
Uncomfortable throat	Sore throat (tight and sharp)
Overall mild presentation	Overall more severe presentation
Use above formula	Refer to p. 164, "disperse and release exterior cold" method

Wind Damage (伤风 *shāng* fēng)	**Wind Heat** (风热 *fēng rè*)
No thirst	Thirst
No dryness	Dry mouth
Tongue is unremarkable	Tongue is reddish, with possible slight yellow coating
Uncomfortable throat	Very painful sore throat
No bowel or urine changes	Constipation with dark urine (more severe)
Use above formula	1. Modify formula (add Imperatae Rhizoma *(bái máo gēn)* or Phragmitis Rhizoma *(lú gēn)*) 2. If severe (e.g., very achy), add Lonicerae Flos *(jīn yín huā)* etc. or choose a different formula

MEDICINAL ANALYSIS

- Schizonepetae Herba *(jīng jiè)* and Allii fistulosi Bulbus *(cōng bái)* are both acrid and warm and can induce a mild sweat. Schizonepetae Herba *(jīng jiè)* expels wind and cold on the surface of the body, making it effective for eliminating body aches that accompany external wind-cold attacks. It should be noted that Schizonepetae Spica *(jīng jiè suì)* is stronger for expelling cold and inducing sweat, while Schizonepetae Herba *(jīng jiè)* is relatively mild at inducing sweat.

- Allii fistulosi Bulbus *(cōng bái)* is very mild. It releases the exterior, unblocks the yang, and circulates the yang and protective qi. It is especially useful when there is swelling or puffiness accompanying a wind-cold invasion, because it can promote urination.

- Chrysanthemi Flos *(jú huā)*, Mori Folium *(sāng yè)*, Viticis Fructus *(màn jīng zǐ)*, and Menthae haplocalycis Herba *(bò hé)* all cool and dispel wind and heat. Mori Folium *(sāng yè)* is slightly acrid, slightly bitter, slightly sweet, and lightweight. It clears and vents heat from the Lungs and protective aspect, and especially from the head and eyes. Chrysanthemi Flos *(jú huā)* is bitter, sweet, and clears Lung heat. It works especially well with Mori Folium *(sāng yè)* for expelling wind. Both are useful if there are signs of dryness (e.g., thirst and dry mouth). Menthae haplocalycis Herba *(bò hé)* is especially useful for expelling wind and heat from the upper part of the body, for example, manifesting as headache. For this purpose the leaves, Menthae haplocalycis Folium *(bò hé yè)*, are preferred to the stems. Viticis Fructus *(màn jīng zǐ)* is also good for headaches and relieves spasms (in the head).

- Sojae Semen preparatum *(dàn dòu chǐ)* is very mild and neutral. It regulates sweating, and can be used for both wind-heat or wind-cold. For further discussion, see the "disperse and release the exterior cold" method in Ch. 7, p. 164.

- If more expelling and clearing is needed, one can also use Sojae Semen germinatum *(dà dòu juǎn)* 9g. For example, consider this for more severe headache or stiff neck. It is, however, still very mild and can replace Schizonepetae Herba *(jīng jiè)* in debilitated patients, such as the elderly or patients with cancer, HIV, or yin deficiency. Schizonepetae Herba *(jīng jiè)* is inappropriate for these patients because it can cause profuse sweating in weaker people.

This is a very balanced formula and lies somewhere in between the treatment of wind-cold and wind-heat. However, this formula can treat a large spectrum of wind damage, and should be modified as needed. *Note:* This formula should only be cooked for 7-10 minutes.

Dr. Qin's formula is based on Scallion and Prepared Soybean Decoction *(cōng chǐ tāng)* and Schizonepeta and Saposhnikovia Powder to Overcome Pathogenic Influences *(jīng fáng bài dú sǎn)*.

Scallion and Prepared Soybean Decoction *(cōng chǐ tāng)*
SOURCE: *Emergency Formulas to Keep Up One's Sleeve* (3rd century)

Allii fistulosi Bulbus *(cōng bái)*. . . . . 3-5 stalks (9-12g)
Sojae Semen preparatum *(dàn dòu chǐ)*. 12-30g

---

Schizonepeta and Saposhnikovia Powder to Overcome Pathogenic Influences
  (jīng fáng bài dú sǎn)
SOURCE: *Multitude of Marvelous Formulas for Sustaining Life* (1550)

Schizonepetae Herba *(jīng jiè)*. 4.5g
Saposhnikoviae Radix *(fáng fēng)*. 4.5g
Bupleuri Radix *(chái hú)*. 4.5g
Peucedani Radix *(qián hú)*. 4.5g
Chuanxiong Rhizoma *(chuān xiōng)*. 4.5g
Notopterygii Rhizoma seu Radix *(qiāng huó)*. 4.5g
Angelicae pubescentis Radix *(dú huó)*. 4.5g
Poria *(fú líng)*. 4.5g
Platycodi Radix *(jié gěng)*. 4.5g
Aurantii Fructus *(zhǐ ké)*. 4.5g
Glycyrrhizae Radix *(gān cǎo)*. 1.5g
Zingiberis Rhizoma recens *(shēng jiāng)*. . . . . 3 pieces

---

MODIFICATIONS OF DR. QIN'S FORMULA

Sinus blockage:

  Magnoliae Flos *(xīn yí)* 4.5g

  Xanthii Fructus *(cāng ěr zǐ)* 6g

Rhinitis/runny nose, sinus pain, and sticky white or slightly yellow discharge:

  Angelicae dahuricae Radix *(bái zhǐ)*. 3g

Cough:

  Fritillariae thunbergii Bulbus *(zhè bèi mǔ)*. 6g

  Armeniacae Semen amarum *(kǔ xìng rén)*. 9g

Head distention (severe):

Increase the dosages of Chrysanthemi Flos *(jú huā)* and Viticis Fructus *(màn jīng zǐ)*

Vertex headache:

Ligustici Rhizoma *(gǎo běn)* 4.5g

Sore muscles or joints affecting the neck, shoulder, or upper back:

Notopterygii Rhizoma seu Radix *(qiāng huó)* 4.5g

Cinnamomi Ramulus *(guì zhī)* 4.5g

Easily sweats (e.g., after drinking hot beverages):

Saposhnikoviae Radix *(fáng fēng)* 4.5g

Sore throat, swollen lymph nodules (severe):

Isatidis/Baphicacanthis Radix *(bǎn lán gēn)* 3-5g

Isatidis Folium *(dà qīng yè)* 3-5g

Note: Acrid, warm medicinals such as Ligustici Rhizoma *(gǎo běn)*, Notopterygii Rhizoma seu Radix *(qiāng huó)*, and Angelicae pubescentis Radix *(dú huó)* should not be used in large dosages and only added if specifically indicated, such as for headache, neck pain, etc.

It is inappropriate to use medicinals such as Coptidis Rhizoma *(huáng lián)* or Gypsum fibrosum *(shí gāo)* here. One may use a small dose of Scutellariae Radix *(huáng qín)* if there is some heat in the Lungs, for example, if there is sore throat and cough with yellow phlegm.

QUESTIONS

1. *How can the same formula treat both a wind-cold and wind-heat presentation, and what does that mean?*

This treatment principle is suitable for relatively mild presentations of wind damage. This wind comes from the exterior and accosts the exterior of the body. Although many books make a clear distinction between wind-heat and wind-cold, many real life clinical presentations, especially in modern times, are actually a combination of wind-cold and wind-heat, or not far enough to one side to clearly differentiate. For example, one may have chills, headache, sore throat, and a red tongue. This is a combination of heat and cold signs in a pattern that is primarily due to wind. Being balanced, rather than warm or cold, this formula can treat both together; or said another way, it can treat a condition that resides in the middle.

However, if there is a predominance of heat (more thirst, dry mouth, and thick and colored nasal discharge) or cold (no thirst, runny nose), then one should modify the formula. For example, if there is more heat, one should remove Allii fistulosi Bulbus *(cōng bái)* and add Sojae Semen germinatum *(dà dòu juǎn)*, and include Imperatae Rhizoma *(bái máo gēn)* and Phragmitis Rhizoma *(lú gēn)* if there is thirst and dry mouth. Of course, as the heat becomes more severe, one will add stronger medicinals, such as Lonicerae Flos *(jīn yín huā)*, transforming the formula into a more typical wind-heat formula. If there is a clear wind-cold presentation, one should refer to the method "disperse and release the exterior cold" in Ch. 7.

Essentially, one must gauge how much heat or cold is combined with the wind and adjust the dosage and herb selection accordingly. If there are both minor heat and cold symptoms that are relatively equal, one can choose Dr. Qin's balanced formula as is.

It should be noted that for most common colds and flus, Ephedra Decoction *(má huáng tāng)*, Cinnamon Twig Decoction *(guì zhī tāng)*, and Schizonepeta and Saposhnikovia Powder to Overcome Pathogenic Influences *(jīng fáng bài dú sǎn)* are too warm and drying. Even when a patient has symptoms of heat, Mulberry Leaf and Chrysanthemum Drink *(sāng jú yǐn)* and Honeysuckle and Forsythia Powder *(yín qiáo sǎn)* are also usually inappropriate because they do not create enough of a sweat.

2. *Could this formula be used for a wind-heat attack?*

As the above table suggests, this formula may be used for some wind-heat attacks. However, as the previous answer illustrates, proper treatment depends on the degree of severity. For this method to be useful, the presentation still must be fairly mild. Essentially, wind-heat is a wind pathogen that is simultaneously confined with a warm-heat pathogen. When the presentation becomes more serious (e.g., higher fever, dark urine, constipation, thirst, dry mouth, and aversion to wind), the formula is no longer appropriate and one should switch to a more standard wind-heat approach, such as Honeysuckle and Forsythia Powder *(yín qiáo sǎn)*, or heavily modify the formula above. There is no magic point at which this occurs. One's thinking should reflect an understanding of a continuum. This allows for a flexible treatment approach.

One should keep in mind that as long as there is some aversion to wind (even with heat signs), one must retain medicinals such as Schizonepetae Herba *(jīng jiè)* or Saposhnikoviae Radix *(fáng fēng)*.

3. *What does it mean that Sojae Semen preparatum (dàn dòu chǐ) can regulate sweating?*

The tonifying quality of Sojae Semen preparatum *(dàn dòu chǐ)*, especially on the Spleen, allows it to stop sweating in deficient patients, while its slightly dispersing nature can also expel external wind by causing a mild sweat.

2. Harmonize the Nutritive and Protective (调和营卫 *tiáo hé yíng wèi*)

[PRESENTATION] Wind damages the muscle layer; collateral attack and/or channel attack

Notopterygii Rhizoma seu Radix *(qiāng huó)*	2.4g
Saposhnikoviae Radix *(fáng fēng)*	3g
Cinnamomi Ramulus *(guì zhī)*	2.4g
Dry-fried Angelicae sinensis Radix *(chǎo dāng guī)*	4.5g
Paeoniae Radix alba *(bái sháo)*	4.5g
Mori Ramulus *(sāng zhī)*	9g
Zingiberis Rhizoma recens *(shēng jiāng)*	2 slices

COMMENTARY

ADDITIONAL SIGNS AND SYMPTOMS

- Easily fatigued
- Sweats easily
- Sometimes feels hot on the surface
- Easily contracts externally-contracted disorders
- Aversion to wind and drafts
- Mood swings
- Pale face
- Insomnia
- The pulse is soft, soggy, moderate, and/or floating
- The tongue is pale, puffy, swollen with teeth marks, wet, and tender

DISCUSSION

ETIOLOGY AND PATHODYNAMIC: Although many issues can bring about a protective qi deficiency, overwork is a common cause. This occurs through a weakening of the Spleen qi (specifically middle burner deficiency cold), which leads to a nutritive and protective disharmony. (*See* the discussion below for further explanation of nutritive and protective disharmony.)

DURATION: This can be an acute or chronic presentation. In addition to the specific symptoms below, both acute and chronic presentations will have aspects from the above signs and symptoms.

- ACUTE

Wind attack: sweating, fever, and aversion to wind, as well as possible acute symptoms from the painful obstruction syndrome section below, such as aching joints.

Wind striking the collaterals: skin and muscle insensitivity and deviated mouth and eyes. Many times this is an acute flare-up of a chronic disease, which is precipitated by a change in weather.

Note: For patterns that are acute, one should use the traditional method of eating warm porridge and covering up to induce a mild sweat to aid in evicting the pathogen.

- CHRONIC

Painful obstruction: tight and achy muscles (e.g., backache) or achy joints (e.g., knees may be stiff after sitting for a while). This is from stagnation of qi and blood resulting from nutritive and protective disharmony. The base prescription above can be used for conditions such as chronic osteoarthritis, rheumatoid arthritis, and carpal tunnel syndrome.

Disharmony of the nutritive and protective: The patient may have only mild aches and pains, as in painful obstruction above, but will primarily present with middle burner deficiency and a chief complaint of being easily fatigued or readily contracting externally-contracted disorders. (*See* discussion below on differentiating this pattern from a Jade Windscreen Powder *(yù píng fēng sǎn)* pattern.)

One should modify the base prescription depending on the above differentiations. For example, when painful obstruction or wind striking the collaterals predominates, one should include (or increase) medicinals that directly remove the pathogen/stagnation and work on the protective level such as Notopterygii Rhizoma seu Radix *(qiāng huó)*, Saposhnikoviae Radix *(fáng fēng)*, and Mori Ramulus *(sāng zhī)*. For a chronic presentation with less stagnation and fewer aches and pains, one may reduce or omit those medicinals and focus more on those that strengthen the middle and harmonize the nutritive and protective aspects by adding more Spleen-tonifying medicinals such as Jujubae Fructus *(dà zǎo)*. It is important to properly gauge the relative importance of the underlying deficiency versus the strength of the pathogenic influence (excess/stagnation).

MEDICINAL ANALYSIS

SUMMARY

- Cinnamomi Ramulus *(guì zhī)*, Zingiberis Rhizoma recens *(shēng jiāng)*, Paeoniae Radix alba *(bái sháo)*, and Angelicae sinensis Radix *(dāng guī)* harmonize the nutritive and protective aspects.

- Cinnamomi Ramulus *(guì zhī)* and Zingiberis Rhizoma recens *(shēng jiāng)* strengthen the protective aspect and tonify the middle qi.

- Paeoniae Radix alba *(bái sháo)* and Angelicae sinensis Radix *(dāng guī)* strengthen the nutritive qi.

- Notopterygii Rhizoma seu Radix *(qiāng huó)* and Saposhnikoviae Radix *(fáng fēng)* strengthen the protective qi.

- Notopterygii Rhizoma seu Radix *(qiāng huó)*, Saposhnikoviae Radix *(fáng fēng)*, and Mori Ramulus *(sāng zhī)* unblock and dispel the pathogen.

INDIVIDUAL CHARACTERISTICS

- Cinnamomi Ramulus *(guì zhī)* and Paeoniae Radix alba *(bái sháo)* are the fundamental pair for harmonizing the nutritive and protective aspects.

- Cinnamomi Ramulus *(guì zhī)* is acrid and warm. It strengthens the protective aspect, penetrates the yang, expels wind and cold from the muscle layer, and warms the channels. It does not create a sweat on its own.

- Paeoniae Radix alba *(bái sháo)* is slightly sour, and neutral to cool. It augments the yin and harmonizes the blood. Its sour, astringent nature helps restrain the more acrid medicinals from excessive scattering.

- Angelicae sinensis Radix *(dāng guī)* is acrid, aromatic, and warm. It tonifies and moves the blood. Together with Paeoniae Radix alba *(bái sháo)*, they strengthen the nutritive qi.

- Notopterygii Rhizoma seu Radix *(qiāng huó)*, Saposhnikoviae Radix *(fáng fēng)*, and Mori Ramulus *(sāng zhī)* unblock the collaterals and dispel wind.

- Notopterygii Rhizoma seu Radix *(qiāng huó)* is acrid, bitter, and warm. It expels wind, cold, and dampness, and can promote a sweat.

- Saposhnikoviae Radix *(fáng fēng)* is bitter and slightly warm. It is able to scatter wind, cold, and dampness. It is very mild and can strengthen the protective qi.

- Mori Ramulus *(sāng zhī)* is sweet and cool and enters the joints and muscles.

- Zingiberis Rhizoma recens *(shēng jiāng)* and Cinnamomi Ramulus *(guì zhī)* assist in both tonifying the middle qi as well as strengthening the protective level.

Dr. Qin's formula is based on Cinnamon Twig Decoction *(guì zhī tāng)*.

Cinnamon Twig Decoction *(guì zhī tāng)*
SOURCE: *Discussion of Cold Damage* (c. 220)

Cinnamomi Ramulus *(guì zhī)* 9g
Paeoniae Radix alba *(bái sháo)* 9g
Zingiberis Rhizoma recens *(shēng jiāng)* 9g
Jujubae Fructus *(dà zǎo)* 12p
Glycyrrhizae Radix preparata *(zhì gān cǎo)* 6g

---

MODIFICATIONS OF DR. QIN'S FORMULA

Achy muscles (especially in the neck region):

Puerariae Radix *(gé gēn)* 6g

Sneezing with mucus (chronic or acute):

Xanthii Fructus *(cāng ěr zǐ)* 6g

Magnoliae Flos *(xīn yí)* 4.5g

Easily fatigued, pale face, poor appetite, and prolapse of organs
(mild pathogen, mostly deficiency):

Astragali Radix *(huáng qí)* 6g

Dry-fried Atractylodis macrocephalae Rhizoma *(chǎo bái zhú)* 6g

Headache (ongoing and heavy sensation, especially in the back of the head):

Ligustici Rhizoma *(gǎo běn)* 4.5g

Tribuli Fructus *(cì jí lí)* 6g

Headache (frontal):

Angelicae dahuricae Radix *(bái zhǐ)* 4.5g

Significantly weakened patient who sweats easily
(e.g., after drinking hot tea) **and profusely:**

Tritici Fructus levis *(fú xiǎo mài)* 9g

Oryzae glutinosae Radix *(nuò dào gēn xū)* 6g

Poor digestion with insomnia

(Spleen dampness with poor circulation of the Stomach qi):

Sorghum or millet 12g

Pinelliae Rhizoma preparatum *(zhì bàn xià)* 6g

Yin deficiency:

Ophiopogonis Radix *(mài mén dōng)* 6g

Schisandrae Fructus *(wǔ wèi zǐ)* 3g

Weak cardiac function, such as shortness of breath and palpitations after walking:

Ginseng Radix *(rén shēn)* 4.5g

Cold hands and feet (frequent):

Spatholobi Caulis *(jī xuè téng)* 6g

Trachelospermi Caulis *(luò shí téng)* . . . . 6g[ii]

QUESTIONS

1. What is a nutritive and protective disharmony? [2]

Key points of nutritive and protective disharmony

- Middle burner deficiency of qi and yang
- Pathogen lodged in the superficial layers of the body
- Acute or chronic

In normal physiology, the middle burner qi generates the nutritive qi and this supports and nourishes the protective qi. Pathology occurs when the middle burner does not fulfill its role in nourishing the protective qi, which then allows the penetration of a pathogen. In addition, the protective qi becomes occupied in battling the pathogen and thus is unable to fulfill its normal function of distributing warmth to the flesh, filling the skin, fattening the pores, and taking charge of opening and closing the interstices. This may result in symptoms such as sweating, aversion to cold, frequent externally-contracted disorders, and a lax and weak pulse. Fundamentally, a nutritive and protective disharmony has its root in a deficiency of the middle burner.

Although the deficiency creates a disharmony, fundamental to a nutritive and protective disharmony (for Dr. Qin's formula) is the involvement of a pathogen. This pathogen lodges itself in the superficial layers of the body. The deeper the pathogen resides, the more severe the problem. A pathogen in the muscle layer can result in an acute cold or flu presentation (such as a wind-cold deficiency pattern); however, if the pathogen enters into the channels and collaterals, one can have a more serious stroke-like condition. It should be noted that, if the pathogen enters deeper into the organ system, it is no longer a nutritive and protective disharmony.

Treatment of nutritive and protective disharmony

Harmonization of the nutritive and protective levels is done by strengthening the nutri-

---

2. There are many viewpoints regarding the meaning and clinical application of a nutritive and protective disharmony. The presentation here is based on Dr. Wu's understanding.

tive and protective qi, allowing the body to eliminate the pathogen. Dr. Qin's prescription is a modification of Cinnamon Twig Decoction *(guì zhī tāng)* with other medicinals to better accommodate the full spectrum of problems that can arise out of nutritive and protective disharmony. Dr. Qin's additions allow the formula to more forcefully eliminate pathogens and strengthen the nutritive qi. Understanding the level on which each herb acts allows one to tailor the prescription for the individual. For example, if there is more deficiency and a weaker pathogen, one would reduce or omit medicinals like Notopterygii Rhizoma seu Radix *(qiāng huó)*, Saposhnikoviae Radix *(fáng fēng)*, and Mori Ramulus *(sāng zhī)*.

2. *How can the same formula treat an acute external condition and chronic deficiency condition?*

To understand this question we must first look closely at Cinnamon Twig Decoction *(guì zhī tāng)*. It is essentially a treatment for middle burner deficiency (yang or qi deficiency with cold). From the medicinal analysis above, one will note that the principal medicinals, Cinnamomi Ramulus *(guì zhī)* and Paeoniae Radix alba *(bái sháo)*, both have an effect on the middle burner. Furthermore, it is not really a diaphoretic formula that has as its main purpose the releasing of the exterior.

To understand the full potential of Cinnamon Twig Decoction *(guì zhī tāng)*, it is useful to grasp how it eliminates a pathogen and how this differs from the method of Ephedra Decoction *(má huáng tāng)*. Cinnamon Twig Decoction *(guì zhī tāng)* does not release the exterior, open the pores, and create a sweat like Ephedra Decoction *(má huáng tāng)*. Cinnamon Twig Decoction *(guì zhī tāng)* eliminates the pathogen by strengthening the protective qi through the middle burner, which then allows the body's protective qi to push out the pathogen. The protective qi may then return to fulfilling its normal functions, such as controlling the pores.

Consequently, Cinnamon Twig Decoction *(guì zhī tāng)* is often used as a basic tonifying formula to resist pathogens and can be used when there is pure deficiency without any pathogen. Dr. Qin's formula does add medicinals to specifically address a pathogen, either newly acquired or lurking. However, both of these formulas can be used for a pattern without any external presentation and can address a multitude of chronic internal complaints (e.g., sweating issues, fatigue, easily catching colds, or feeling cold) as well as acute colds and flus.

A key point for Dr. Qin's formula is that it is not for a mere deficiency pattern, but a deficiency pattern with a pathogen that is retained in the superficial aspects of the body. This situation can persist for days or years.

3. *If this is essentially Spleen deficiency leading to protective qi deficiency, then what is the difference between this approach, Cinnamon Twig Decoction (guì zhī tāng), and a Jade Windscreen Powder (yù píng fēng sǎn) approach?*

All of these conditions have middle burner deficiency with such symptoms as sweating, frequent colds, or fatigue, and all of them can be used for a chronic presentation and for the prevention of colds. However, there are some subtle differences. First, let us look at an unmodified Cinnamon Twig Decoction *(guì zhī tāng)* formula.

Cinnamon Twig Decoction *(guì zhī tāng)* is indicated when there is a chronic history of frequent externally-contracted disorders with middle burner deficiency. It is best given as a preventative measure and can be combined with Astragali Radix *(huáng qí)*, which secures the exterior, for this purpose.

Jade Windscreen Powder *(yù píng fēng sǎn)* treats deficient patients who contract a pathogen which lingers without resolution. The pathogen is eliminated by augmenting the qi. Using Saposhnikoviae Radix *(fáng fēng)* prevents the pathogen from being locked in. Actually, there is tonification in the midst of dispersion, and dispersion within tonification. This is different than supporting the normal and securing the exterior, which is what Cinnamon Twig Decoction *(guì zhī tāng)* plus Astragali Radix *(huáng qí)* does. For this reason, if the body does not have an exterior pathogen and one frequently gives Saposhnikoviae Radix *(fáng fēng)* or other dispersing medicinals to disperse and scatter, this will perversely provide a pathogen with the opportunity to invade.

Dr. Qin's formula above combines all of these ideas. To use this formula for any type of chronic presentation there must be a pathogen trapped in the superficial layers of the body. This often manifests as a painful obstruction type condition with such symptoms as muscle aches or joint pain. This is why Dr. Qin has included medicinals such as Notopterygii Rhizoma seu Radix *(qiāng huó)*, Saposhnikoviae Radix *(fáng fēng)*, and Mori Ramulus *(sāng zhī)*. Although Jade Windscreen Powder *(yù píng fēng sǎn)* embodies a similiar strategy, it really only addresses a deficient pattern with mild pathogenic involvement. By contrast, Dr. Qin's formula can address much more severe pathogenic involvement.

All of these formulas and ideas can be combined. For example, Cinnamon Twig Decoction *(guì zhī tāng)* and Jade Windscreen Powder *(yù píng fēng sǎn)* can be used together to prevent allergic rhinitis or urticaria conditions that easily occur with exposure to wind.

In summary, the amount of dispersing medicinals must be tempered by tonification while paying attention to not overly disperse the exterior, which will further weaken the patient.

4. *What does it mean that Cinnamomi Ramulus (guì zhī), Zingiberis Rhizoma recens (shēng jiāng), Notopterygii Rhizoma seu Radix (qiāng huó), and Saposhnikoviae Radix (fáng fēng) strengthen the protective qi?*

Protective qi is yang in nature and thus often is called protective yang. When there is a nutritive and protective disharmony, the protective qi is weak and essentially lacks yang, diminishing its movement and warming function. All of these medicinals provide some bit of movement and warmth to the protective yang, which in turn help eliminate the pathogen. Once the pathogen is eliminated, the protective qi is less burdened and can more easily function. Since the problem is also a lack of support from the middle burner, one cannot utilize such medicinals alone for a successful treatment.

3. Pursues Wind and Thrusts Out the Pathogen (追风达邪 *zhuī fēng dá xié*)

[PRESENTATION] Wind pathogen penetrates deeply; impaired consciousness with collapse and inability to be aroused

Prepared Ephedrae Herba *(zhì má huáng)*	1.5g
Notopterygii Rhizoma seu Radix *(qiāng huó)*	2.4g
Angelicae pubescentis Radix *(dú huó)*	2.4g
Cinnamomi Ramulus *(guì zhī)*	2.4g
Bombyx batryticatus *(bái jiāng cán)*	9g
Saposhnikoviae Radix *(fáng fēng)*	4.5g
Gastrodiae Rhizoma *(tiān má)*	4.5g
Acori tatarinowii Rhizoma *(shí chāng pǔ)*	2.4g

COMMENTARY

ADDITIONAL SIGNS AND SYMPTOMS

- Spasms
- Numbness and tingling
- One-sided paralysis
- Profuse phlegm
- Chills (predominant) and fever (low-grade)
- Absence of sweating
- Dark face
- Lack of mental clarity
- Dizziness/vertigo
- Nausea/vomiting
- Muddled consciousness
- If severe, loss of consciousness/coma, clenched jaw, and urinary and bowel incontinence
- The pulse is slippery (or soggy), rapid, tight, stagnant, and floating or hidden
- The tongue has a dark pale or dark red body with a white greasy or sticky coating. The coating may or may not be thick.

DISCUSSION

PATTERN: This is a genuine wind attack (stroke) or external wind attack (stroke) pattern and is a serious condition. It is relatively uncommon today where wind-like attack and internal wind attacks are more common. It occurred more frequently in the past because people were more exposed to the environment and weather. The use of this formula was originally utilized for very serious conditions such as coma or stroke and can still be used to revive such patients. However, at present, it is more commonly used for less severe problems such as Bell's palsy.

PATHODYNAMIC AND ETIOLOGY: This pattern is caused by a severe invasion of a wind-cold-damp turbid pathogen. The important feature of this pattern is an external invasion that penetrates deeply into the yin and yang organs. There may or may not be an obvious underlying deficiency that allows for external wind to attack, although people with qi and yang deficiencies are more commonly affected than those with blood and yin deficiencies. Of course, the stronger the pathogen, the more likely it will affect those without significant underlying deficiencies. One can often trace the occurrence to some environmental exposure coupled with fatigue. This condition occurs especially in wet and damp areas such as swamps. There may be a biomedical correlation to some diseases from viral or insect exposure.

DURATION: This is an acute illness with sudden onset. One would usually not use this method if the problem has persisted for more than a week. If untreated, the condition may persist for many years, but a different formula is needed for a chronic presentation.

DEPTH: The severity will be dependent on the depth to which the pathogen enters. For example, in a very serious and deep penetration one may see loss of consciousness, while a more mild one will look something like Bell's palsy.

Below are general guidelines to help determine the level that the pathogen has entered.

If the pathogen enters the yang organs (more mild):

- Low levels of consciousness
- Limbs and joints will be useless (unable to work)
- Use Dr. Qin's formula as is.

If the pathogen enters the yin organs (more serious):

- Difficulty in speaking
- Uncontrolled drooling
- One may add Scorpio (*quán xiē*) or Scolopendra (*wú gōng*) to Dr. Qin's formula.

TREATMENT PRINCIPLE: vent and thrust out the pathogen from the deep layers of the organs. Usually 1-2 bags is adequate, which typically induces a sweat and arouses the patient. One may then follow up with a formula such as Flushing Away Roiling Phlegm Pill (*gǔn tán wán*) or Three-Seed Decoction (*sān rén tāng*). After the acute situation has resolved, one may need to tonify with something like Tonify the Yang to Restore Five-tenths Decoction (*bǔ yáng huán wǔ tāng*).[3]

DIFFERENTIATION: This condition should be differentiated from internally-generated ones with similar presentations. For example:

1. Yin or essence deficiency causing yang rising; or
2. Internal heat leading to wind, phlegm, and fire rising, clogging up the brain.

These are commonly seen in strokes from chronic heart disease or hypertension, which

---

3. Astragali Radix *(huáng qí)*, Angelicae sinensis Radix *(dāng guī)*, Chuanxiong Rhizoma *(chuān xiōng)*, Paeoniae Radix rubra *(chì sháo)*, Persicae Semen *(táo rén)*, Carthami Flos *(hóng huā)*, and Pheretima *(dì lóng)*.

may be triggered from etiological factors such as stress, sudden bad news, or overwork. These conditions may manifest with a similar presentation to this pattern with sudden loss of consciousness, although one will also see signs and symptoms such as red face and eyes, profuse amounts of phlegm, a wiry, forceful, and rapid pulse, and a fresh red or purplish red tongue (and lips) with a thick, yellow coating. This all corresponds to a wind-like attack (internal wind-stroke) and is not a genuine wind-attack (external wind-stroke) for which Dr.Qin's method above would be appropriate.

MEDICINAL ANALYSIS

- Prepared Ephedrae Herba *(zhì má huáng)* (processed by water frying) vents the pathogen from the muscles and interstices. If the condition is serious, for example, the patient is very cold with an absence of sweating, severe headache, or is unconscious, unprocessed Ephedrae Herba *(má huáng)* may be used.

- Cinnamomi Ramulus *(guì zhī)* thrusts out the pathogen from the blood collaterals.

- Notopterygii Rhizoma seu Radix *(qiāng huó)* disperses wind from the *tài yáng*.

- Angelicae pubescentis Radix *(dú huó)* eliminates wind from the *shào yīn*.

- Saposhnikoviae Radix *(fáng fēng)* eliminates wind from the channels.

- Bombyx batryticatus *(bái jiāng cán)* eliminates wind-phlegm from the collaterals.

- Gastrodiae Rhizoma *(tiān má)* eliminates phlegm and extinguishes wind.

- Acori tatarinowii Rhizoma *(shí chāng pǔ)* awakens the Spleen and open the orifices.

Dr. Qin's formula is based on Minor Extend Life Decoction *(xiǎo xù mìng tāng)*.

Minor Extend Life Decoction *(xiǎo xù mìng tāng)*

SOURCE: *Formulas with Short Articles* (Eastern Jin, 4th century)

Ephedrae Herba *(má huáng)* 3g
Stephaniae tetrandrae Radix *(hàn fáng jǐ)*[4] 3g
Ginseng Radix *(rén shēn)* 3g
Scutellariae Radix *(huáng qín)* 3g
Cinnamomi Cortex *(ròu guì)* 3g
Glycyrrhizae Radix *(gān cǎo)* 3g
Paeoniae Radix alba *(bái sháo)* 3g
Chuanxiong Rhizoma *(chuān xiōng)* 3g
Armeniacae Semen *(xìng rén)* 3g
Aconiti Radix lateralis preparata *(zhì fù zǐ)* 1p
Saposhnikoviae Radix *(fáng fēng)* 4.5g
Zingiberis Rhizoma recens *(shēng jiāng)* 15g

---

MODIFICATIONS OF DR. QIN'S FORMULA

Profuse phlegm (e.g., in the throat):

---

4. The original ingredient listed in this formula is Aristolochiae fangchi Radix *(guǎng fáng jǐ)*, which is now an obsolete toxic substance and therefore no longer used.

Polygalae Radix *(yuǎn zhì)* 4.5g

Fritillariae thunbergii Bulbus *(zhè bèi mǔ)* 6g

If there is sweating:

Consider reducing or omitting Ephedrae Herba *(má huáng)* and
Cinnamomi Ramulus *(guì zhī)*

QUESTIONS

1. Why does Dr. Qin not use Ginseng Radix (rén shēn) and other tonifying medicinals when the original Minor Extend Life Decoction (xiǎo xù mìng tāng) utilizes this approach?

Quite simply, one must first expel the wind pathogen. Tonifying medicinals can reduce the speed in which this formula needs to work. As mentioned above, if necessary, one can follow up with a formula that contains more tonics.

2. Why does Dr. Qin mention 'wind-like attack' in the introduction to the chapter, yet not supply a treatment principle or formula for it?

One reason is that this is a classic disease category and is included for completeness, but the principles needed to treat this pattern are made up of many other principles based on the presenting pattern. For example, one may choose principles such as direct fire downward, flush away phlegm, nourish the yin, smooth the flow of qi, unblock the bowels, or others. See the following addendum.

ADDENDUM: WIND-LIKE ATTACK

PATTERN: Following are some strategies for the treatment of wind-like attack. This presentation may be similar to genuine wind-attack, such as sudden loss of consciousness, hemiplegia, deviated eyes and mouth, or difficult speech. However, its cause is from internal wind and one should look for internal imbalances and etiological factors that support this pattern. Furthermore, there will not be external signs and symptoms (as above) such as fever and chills, etc. For example, with a Liver fire and phlegm pattern that generates ascendant wind, fire, and phlegm, one may also see red face and eyes, profuse phlegm, a very wiry, forceful, and rapid pulse, and a very red or fresh or purple red tongue (and lips), with a thin, yellow coating. It should be noted that any pattern that can give rise to internal wind can be responsible for a wind-like attack, such as Liver-Kidney yin deficiency, etc.

TREATMENT PRINCIPLE: Quickly direct the fire/yang and wind downward, flush away the phlegm, smooth the flow of qi, and unblock the bowels.

Possible formulas include Antelope Horn and Uncaria Decoction *(líng jiǎo gōu téng tāng)*,[5]

---

5. Saigae tataricae Cornu *(líng yáng jiǎo)*, Uncariae Ramulus cum Uncis *(gōu téng)*, Mori Folium *(sāng yè)*, Chrysanthemi Flos *(jú huā)*, Paeoniae Radix alba *(bái sháo)*, Rehmanniae Radix *(shēng dì huáng)*, Fritillariae cirrhosae Bulbus *(chuān bèi mǔ)*, Bambusae Caulis in taeniam *(zhú rú)*, Poriae Sclerotium pararadicis *(fú shén)*, and Glycyrrhizae Radix *(gān cǎo)*.

Gastrodia and Uncaria Drink *(tiān má gōu téng yǐn)*,[6] and Five Stone Drink *(wǔ shí yǐn)*.[7]

MODIFICATIONS OF DR. QIN'S FORMULA

Tonify the yin to guide down the yang:

Rehmanniae Radix *(shēng dì huáng)* and/or
Rehmanniae Radix preparata *(shú dì huáng)* 6-9g

Scrophulariae Radix *(xuán shēn)* 6-9g

Anemarrhenae Rhizoma *(zhī mǔ)* 6-9g

Asparagi Radix *(tiān mén dōng)* and/or
Ophiopogonis Radix *(mài mén dōng)* 6-9g

If there is visible phlegm:

Chloriti Lapis *(qīng méng shí)* 9-12g

Bambusae Concretio silicea *(tiān zhú huáng)* 4-6g

Bambusae Succus *(zhú lì)* 20cc
(10cc twice per day, directly swallowed)

Bambusae Caulis in taeniam *(zhú rú)* 4-6g

Constipation:

Rhei Radix et Rhizoma *(dà huáng)* 4-6g

Natrii Sulfas *(máng xiāo)* 3-5g
(dissolved into strained decoction)

EMERGENCY STRATEGIES

If there is a coma, one must use a strategy to first revive the patient:

Calm the Palace Pill with Cattle Gallstone *(ān gōng niú huáng wán)* (1/16 a dose, qid.
One can mash and mix with liquid and feed through a nasogastric tube if needed).
If unavailable, one can use the patent medicine Clear and Open the Spirit *(qīng kāi
líng)*. These can save people's lives.

Loss of consciousness, but with restlessness and spasms:

Purple Snow Special Pill *(zǐ xuě dān)*

Sometimes clear minded, sometimes muddled (e.g., after a meal, cannot remember
what they ate, can sometimes recognize people and sometimes cannot):

Greatest Treasure Special Pill *(zhì bǎo dān)*

This strategy can also be applied to some severe situations of Alzheimer's, epilepsy,
or Tourette's syndrome that manifest on the colder side. Since many modern

---

6. Gastrodiae Rhizoma *(tiān má)*, Uncariae Ramulus cum Uncis *(gōu téng)*, Haliotidis Concha *(shí jué míng)*, Gardeniae
Fructus *(zhī zǐ)*, Scutellariae Radix *(huáng qín)*, Leonuri Herba *(yì mǔ cǎo)*, Cyathulae Radix (chuān niú xī), Eucommiae Cortex (dù zhòng), Taxilli Herba (sāng jì shēng), Polygoni multiflori Caulis *(yè jiāo téng)*, and Poriae Sclerotium
pararadicis *(fú shén)*.

7. Haliotidis Concha *(shí jué míng)* 9-12g, unprepared Ostreae Concha *(shēng mǔ lì)* 9-12g, Glauberitum *(hán shuî shí)*
9-12g, blue-green Fossilia Dentis Mastodi *(qīng lóng chǐ)* 6-9g, and Margaritiferae Concha usta *(zhēn zhū mǔ)* 9-12g.

day presentations manifest more on the hot side, one may consider adding these additional herbs:

- Saigae tataricae Cornu *(líng yáng jiǎo)* (cold)
- Bovis Calculus *(niú huáng)* (cold)
- Margarita *(zhēn zhū)* (cold)
- Bufonis Venenum *(chán sū)* (warm)
- Acori tatarinowii Rhizoma *(shí chāng pǔ)* (warm)

7

Treatment Guidelines for

Cold 寒 *(hán)*

DISEASE LOCATION

Exterior: Chills, fever, and absence of sweating

Fever here means an objective rise in body temperature and may be quite high compared to other externally-contracted diseases, particularly wind-attack. This is because the external cold pathogen attacks the body's normal qi, and the resulting fight between the normal and pathogenic raises the temperature of the body.

The chills are also relatively severe, where blankets do not help warm the body. This means that the cold pathogen resides in the body's channel system. This is deeper than just the surface of the body and includes the muscles, tendons, and bones. By contrast, chills from yang deficiency will lessen when one is covered with blankets.

Other common symptoms include sharp headache, tight neck, and painful joints, muscles, and bones. The pulse is usually floating and tight and may be rapid. The tongue usually does not exhibit much change, for example, a thin, white coating is common. The *tài yáng* warp discussed in the *Discussion of Cold Damage* is an example of this.

Exterior cold is usually of short duration, the pain is worse during the day, and promotion of sweating relieves the symptoms.

Interior: Rigid and tight body, clenched jaw preventing speech, severe shivering of the extremities, chills as after a soaking,[1] sudden attacks of dizziness, absence of sweating, cavernous diarrhea[2] with incontinence, and a sinking and tight pulse

---

1. These are chills that feel like one has been sprinkled with cold water. Although this corresponds to internal cold, the body's exterior nonetheless feels like it is permeated with cold water.

2. This is diarrhea that occurs after eating and contains undigested food.

163

Interior cold can occur at many levels of the body. The location of the symptoms are reflective of where the cold is lodged. For example, cold in the joints and muscles will manifest as tightness or spasm of the muscles and stiff or achy joints. Cold in the Stomach may manifest as stomach pain, diarrhea, and cramping. Cold in the lower abdomen will manifest with tightness and spasm in the lower abdomen (e.g., hernia). Interior cold will usually be of long duration, present with pain that is worse at night, and promotion of sweating does not relieve the symptoms. There may also be symptoms such as skin that is cold to the touch.

> **METHOD OF TREATMENT**
> When cold attacks the exterior, simply induce sweating; when it attacks the interior, one must differentiate among the three yin warps.

COMMENTARY

Location	Six Warps	Treatment Method	Sample Formula
Cold in the Spleen	*tài yīn*	Warm and move	Regulate the Middle Pill (*lǐ zhōng wán*)
Cold in the Kidney	*shào yīn*	Warm and tonify	True Warrior Decoction (*zhēn wǔ tāng*)
Cold in the Liver	*jué yīn*	Warm and direct downward	Evodia Decoction (*wú zhū yú tāng*)

1. Disperse and Release the Exterior Cold (疏解表寒 *shū jiê biâo hán*)

[PRESENTATION] External contraction of a cold pathogen; simultaneous fever and chills without sweating

Prepared Ephedrae Herba *(zhì má huáng)* 1.5g
Notopterygii Rhizoma seu Radix *(qiāng huó)* 2.4g
Perillae Folium *(zǐ sū yè)* 4.5g
Cinnamomi Ramulus *(guì zhī)* 2.4g
Sojae Semen preparatum *(dàn dòu chǐ)* 4.5g
Platycodi Radix *(jié gěng)* 2.4g
Zingiberis Rhizoma recens *(shēng jiāng)* . . . . 2 slices

COMMENTARY

ADDITIONAL SIGNS AND SYMPTOMS

- Chills or aversion to cold that is usually strong and will predominate over the fever, although the actual temperature of the body can be very high. The patient will want to be covered up.

- Headache that is usually sharp and very painful, accompanied by tight and achy muscles of the head
- Dry skin
- Dry or barking cough
- Difficulty obtaining a sweat
- The pulse is floating and tight; possibly slippery and/or rapid
- The tongue is unremarkable

DISCUSSION

ETIOLOGY: Exposure to cold and/or wet conditions such as rain, or just getting wet in the winter time. Although this pattern can occur in any of the four seasons, it is most likely to occur in the winter.

TREATMENT PRINCIPLE: Use acrid warm medicinals to induce a sweat. After taking the formula, one should keep warm to assist the sweating process; this is important to bring about a cure. However, one should be cautious not to create too much of a sweat, as this can lead to depletion of the qi, fluids, and yang.

Proper differentiation is important to distinguish this from a wind-attack, which requires an acrid and balanced method, and wind-warmth, which requires an acrid, cool approach.

This presentation is often accompanied by dampness, as evidenced by such symptoms as tight and achy muscles and neck. This is not an external invasion of dampness (e.g., from humid weather), but dampness that is caused from cold restricting the flow of the normal body fluids in the affected areas.

MEDICINAL ANALYSIS

- Prepared Ephedrae Herba *(zhì má huáng)*, Notopterygii Rhizoma seu Radix *(qiāng huó)*, Perillae Folium *(zǐ sū yè)*, Zingiberis Rhizoma recens *(shēng jiāng)*, and Cinnamomi Ramulus *(guì zhī)* are all acrid and warm.

- Prepared Ephedrae Herba *(zhì má huáng)* (processed by water frying) acts on the surface/ protective level and releases the exterior. Cinnamomi Ramulus *(guì zhī)* acts on a deeper level and releases the muscle layer. When these two medicinals are combined, they create a sweat, expelling cold from the muscles and the body's surface.

- Perillae Folium *(zǐ sū yè)* scatters wind-cold, disperses and resolves the exterior, transforms the upper burner, and diffuses the Lungs. It is suitable for relatively severe exterior contractions of wind-cold with phlegm or dampness that readily combines with a cold pathogen.

- Notopterygii Rhizoma seu Radix *(qiāng huó)* enters the Bladder channel, expels wind-cold-dampness, and is specific for upper body (e.g., neck, back, shoulder) tightness, achiness, and pain. It also promotes sweating.

- Platycodi Radix *(jié gěng)* is neutral, ascends, and opens the Lungs. Thus, if there is nausea or vomiting, it should not be used. In such a case, one may choose to use dry-fried Arctii

Fructus *(chǎo niú bàng zǐ)*, which opens the Lungs and calms the Lung qi, without the potential of aggravating the rebellious Stomach qi.

- Sojae Semen preparatum *(dàn dòu chǐ)* expels wind-cold (see question no. 1 below).
- Zingiberis Rhizoma recens *(shēng jiāng)* scatters wind and cold pathogens on the surface and releases the exterior.

There are various degrees of severity based on the intensity of the pathogen and the debilitation of the body. Thus, depending on the particularities of the presentation, different medicinals should be emphasized; that is, one may increase or reduce their dosage or even eliminate other medicinals in the formula. For example:

— For a mild presentation, one can emphasize medicinals such as Sojae Semen preparatum *(dàn dòu chǐ)* and Allii fistulosi Bulbus *(cōng bái)*, as in Scallion and Prepared Soybean Decoction *(cōng chǐ tāng)*.

— For moderate presentations, emphasize Perillae Folium *(zǐ sū yè)* and Notopterygii Rhizoma seu Radix *(qiāng huó)*.

— For severe presentations, emphasize Ephedrae Herba *(má huáng)* and Cinnamomi Ramulus *(guì zhī)*.

Dr. Qin's formula is based on Ephedra Decoction *(má huáng tāng)* and Notopterygium Decoction to Overcome Dampness *(qiāng huó shèng shī tāng)*.

Ephedra Decoction *(má huáng tāng)*
SOURCE: *Discussion of Cold Damage* (c. 220)

Ephedrae Herba *(má huáng)*. 9g
Cinnamomi Ramulus *(guì zhī)*. 6g
Armeniacae Semen *(xìng rén)* 9-12g
Glycyrrhizae Radix preparata *(zhì gān cǎo)*. 3g

---

Notopterygium Decoction to Overcome Dampness *(qiāng huó shèng shī tāng)*
SOURCE: *Clarifying Doubts about Damage from Internal and External Causes* (1247)

Notopterygii Rhizoma seu Radix *(qiāng huó)* 3g
Angelicae pubescentis Radix *(dú huó)*. 3g
Ligustici Rhizoma *(gǎo běn)* 1.5g
Chuanxiong Rhizoma *(chuān xiōng)* 1.5g
Viticis Fructus *(màn jīng zǐ)* 0.9g
Glycyrrhizae Radix preparata *(zhì gān cǎo)*. 1.5g

---

MODIFICATIONS OF DR. QIN'S FORMULA

Cough:

Fritillariae thunbergii Bulbus *(zhè bèi mǔ)*. 6g
Armeniacae Semen amarum *(kǔ xìng rén)*. 6-9g
Dry-fried Arctii Fructus *(chǎo niú bàng zǐ)*. 6-9g

Cough with profuse phlegm:

Citri reticulatae Exocarpium rubrum *(jú hóng)* 3-5g

Pinelliae Rhizoma preparatum *(zhì bàn xià)* 6-9g

Severe cough and unable to lie flat:

Peucedani Radix *(qián hú)* 4.5g

Dry-fried Arctii Fructus *(chǎo niú bàng zǐ)* 9g

Sticky, glue-like phlegm that is hard to expectorate (this is from cold-dampness):

Pinelliae Rhizoma preparatum *(zhì bàn xià)* 6g

Citri reticulatae Pericarpium *(chén pí)* 3-5g

Magnoliae officinalis Cortex *(hòu pò)* 3-5g

▶ Do *not* use cold medicinals such as Bambusae Concretio silicea *(tiān zhú huáng)* or Mori Cortex *(sāng bái pí)*.

Chronic asthma:

Asari Radix et Rhizoma *(xì xīn)* 1g

Zingiberis Rhizoma *(gān jiāng)* 2g

Schisandrae Fructus *(wǔ wèi zǐ)* 3g

▶ This then becomes a modified Minor Bluegreen Dragon Decoction *(xiǎo qīng lóng tāng)*. With simultaneous internal heat, such as yellow tongue coating, dry mouth, and sore throat (a very common pattern), add:

Gypsum fibrosum *(shí gāo)* 9-12g

Cold phlegm (e.g., mucus in the throat or the sensation of water in the epigastrium):

Atractylodis macrocephalae Rhizoma *(bái zhú)* 6g

Citri reticulatae Pericarpium *(chén pí)* 4.5g

Headache:

Angelicae dahuricae Radix *(bái zhǐ)* 4.5g

Chuanxiong Rhizoma *(chuān xiōng)* 3g

QUESTIONS

1. *Why does Dr. Qin include Sojae Semen preparatum (dàn dòu chǐ) in this formula?*

   Qin Bo-Wei was very fond of using Sojae Semen preparatum *(dàn dòu chǐ)* for external attacks. Among his reasons:

   • It assists other herbs to expel the pathogen outward, no matter if it is wind-heat or wind-cold.

   • It has some Spleen-tonifying qualities and is appropriate when the patient feels exhausted. Codonopsis Radix *(dǎng shēn)* or Astragali Radix *(huáng qí)* should not be used in the above presentation.

   • It harmonizes the Stomach, which also can assist in relieving nausea.

   • It is very mild and good for older or weak people.[i]

2. *Why does Dr. Qin use prepared Ephedrae Herba (zhì má huáng) and not unprocessed Ephedrae Herba (má huáng)?*

Prepared Ephedrae Herba *(zhì má huáng)* is Ephedrae Herba *(má huáng)* that has been stir-fried with water to moderate its diaphoretic effects, although it will still promote a little sweating. Dr. Qin by nature had a predilection to use mild medicinals to avoid side effects. Its use here also allows the formula more versatility: it can be prescribed for weaker individuals. If the patient is very robust, and the presentation is very severe, one can use unprocessed Ephedrae Herba *(má huáng)*.

---

2. Warm and Promote the Transportation Function of the Middle Palace[ii]
(温运中宫 *wēn yùn zhōng gōng*)

[PRESENTATION] Cold in the *tài yīn*; abdominal pain and diarrhea

Codonopsis Radix *(dǎng shēn)*	4.5g
Amomi Fructus *(shā rén)*	2.4g
charred Zingiberis Rhizoma preparata *(páo jiāng tàn)*	2.4g
Pinelliae Rhizoma preparatum *(zhì bàn xià)*	4.5g
Atractylodis macrocephalae Rhizoma *(bái zhú)*	4.5g
baked Aucklandiae Radix *(wēi mù xiāng)*	2.4g
Citri reticulatae Pericarpium *(chén pí)*	4.5g

COMMENTARY

ADDITIONAL SIGNS AND SYMPTOMS

- Poor digestion
- Reduced appetite
- Generalized sense of fatigue
- Possibly constipation (from cold stagnation)
- Pale face
- Lack of warmth in the extremities (or just the hands and feet)
- Palmar surface of the forearm feels cold, even after pressing for a few minutes
- Desire for warmth (e.g., heating pad on abdomen)
- Strong aversion to drafts coming through narrow cracks
- Absence of thirst
- Easily develops abdominal cramping after consumption of cold beverages
- The pulse is deep, thin, slow, and faint; the right middle position may be especially deep
- The tongue is pale-dark, wet, with a greasy grey or black coating; the coating should not be yellow

DISCUSSION

PATTERN: Cold in the middle burner with middle burner/Spleen deficiency

ETIOLOGY AND PATHODYNAMIC: This pattern can arise from both internal and external causes. The Spleen can become cold and deficient after a common cold or flu, from excessive consumption of cold foods, exposure to the elements (e.g., being out in a cold rain/catching a chill), or cold that arises from within (e.g., internal cold/yang deficiency).

When a cold pathogen strikes the interior, it frequently influences the Spleen and Stomach. This constrains and hinders the yang qi, which further leads to deficiency. This, in turn, will usually lead to the formation of dampness.

TREATMENT PRINCIPLE: Warm the middle, drive out the cold, and transform dampness. Promoting the movement of qi is also an important secondary principle.

DURATION: This condition may be acute or chronic.

MEDICINAL ANALYSIS

All the medicinals are warm.

- Codonopsis Radix *(dǎng shēn)* and Atractylodis macrocephalae Rhizoma *(bái zhú)* warm the middle and tonify Spleen qi and yang. Atractylodis macrocephalae Rhizoma *(bái zhú)* has the additional ability to stop diarrhea.
- Charred Zingiberis Rhizoma preparata *(páo jiāng tàn)* warms the Spleen and eliminates dampness. It also has the ability to stop diarrhea.
- Pinelliae Rhizoma preparatum *(zhì bàn xià)* is acrid and bitter. It disperses and opens, and dries dampness.
- Citri reticulatae Pericarpium *(chén pí)* is acrid, bitter, and drying, which enables it to transform dampness and aromatically regulate qi, especially in the Spleen and Stomach.
- Aucklandiae Radix *(mù xiāng)* and Amomi Fructus *(shā rén)* are acrid and are able to promote the movement of the qi dynamic, awaken the Spleen, regulate the Stomach, and dry dampness.

Dr. Qin's formula is based on Six-Gentleman Decoction with Aucklandia and Amomum *(xiāng shā liù jūn zǐ tāng)*.

Six-Gentleman Decoction with Aucklandia and Amomum *(xiāng shā liù jūn zǐ tāng)*

SOURCE: *Comprehensive Medicine According to Master Zhang* (1695)

Ginseng Radix *(rén shēn)* 3g
Atractylodis macrocephalae Rhizoma *(bái zhú)* 6g
Poria *(fú líng)* 6g
Glycyrrhizae Radix preparata *(zhì gān cǎo)* 2.1g
Citri reticulatae Pericarpium *(chén pí)* 2.4g
Pinelliae Rhizoma preparatum *(zhì bàn xià)* 3g
Amomi Fructus *(shā rén)* 2.4g
Aucklandiae Radix *(mù xiāng)* 2.1g

MODIFICATIONS OF DR. QIN'S FORMULA

ACCORDING TO ETIOLOGY:

For an external invasion of a cold pathogen in a patient with long-term middle burner cold (commonly manifesting as diarrhea, aversion to wind and drafts, and abdominal pain), add:

Dry-fried Saposhnikoviae Radix *(chǎo fáng fēng)* 4.5g

Perillae Folium *(zǐ sū yè)* 4.5g

For internally-generated cold (e.g., daybreak diarrhea), add:

Cinnamomi Cortex *(ròu guì)* 2.4g

Roasted Myristicae Semen *(wēi ròu dòu kòu)* 3g

OTHER:

Readily contracts externally-contracted disorders or cramps, burping, or stomachache after ingesting food or drink that is cold in nature, with aversion to wind and drafts:

Perillae Folium *(zǐ sū yè)* 4.5g

Dry-fried Saposhnikoviae Radix *(chǎo fáng fēng)* 4.5g

Zingiberis Rhizoma recens *(shēng jiāng)* 3-5s

More severe cramping:

Charred Paeoniae Radix alba *(bái sháo tàn)* 6-9g

plus Glycyrrhizae Radix preparata *(zhì gān cǎo)* 4-6g

More severe abdominal cold, with stagnation (e.g., cramping) **but no gas:** [iii]

Zingiberis Rhizoma *(gān jiāng)* 3g

Poor digestion:

Dry-fried Massa medicata fermentata *(chǎo shén qū)* 9g

Dry-fried Hordei Fructus germinatus *(chǎo mài yá)* 9g

Spitting up frothy saliva:

Evodiae Fructus *(wú zhū yú)* 1g

Watery diarrhea:

Baked Chebulae Fructus *(wēi hē zǐ)* 6g

Abdominal pain with diarrhea, with possible sore back and neck:

Roasted Puerariae Radix *(wēi gé gēn)* 9g

Constipation (from cold stagnation):

Aconiti Radix lateralis preparata *(zhì fù zǐ)*[3] 3-5g

plus steamed Rhei Radix et Rhizoma *(shú dà huáng)* 4-6g

---

3. If Aconiti Radix lateralis preparata *(zhì fù zî)* is unavailable, one can substitute Zingiberis Rhizoma *(gān jiāng)*.

2. Warm and Promote the Transportation Function of the Middle Palace

▶ If there is also periumbilical cold, add Cinnamomi Cortex *(ròu guì)* and steamed Rhei Radix et Rhizoma *(shú dà huáng).*[iv]

Bloating and gas:

Arecae Pericarpium *(dà fù pí)* 6g

Dry-fried Aurantii Fructus immaturus *(chǎo zhǐ shí)* 6g

Scorched Arecae Semen *(jiāo bīng láng)* 9g

Constipation, low back pain, and cold hands and feet:

Cistanches Herba *(ròu cōng róng)* 6g

QUESTIONS

1. *Why does Dr. Qin use charred Zingiberis Rhizoma preparata (páo jiāng tàn) instead of Zingiberis Rhizoma (gān jiāng) or Zingiberis Rhizoma recens (shēng jiāng)?*

In general, Zingiberis Rhizoma recens *(shēng jiāng)* is best for upper burner problems, Zingiberis Rhizoma *(gān jiāng)* for those of the middle burner, and charred Zingiberis Rhizoma preparata *(páo jiāng tàn)* for those of the lower. In this presentation, abdominal pain is the chief complaint. Zingiberis Rhizoma *(gān jiāng)*, compared to charred Zingiberis Rhizoma preparata *(páo jiāng tàn)*, is more acrid and warm and can actually cause more stomach pain due to its harshness, aggravating the mucus membranes of the stomach. It is not as good for Spleen and Stomach deficiency with abdominal pain and diarrhea. For the same reason, other acrid foods and medicinals, such as peppers and garlic, although warm in nature, should be avoided in this pattern. Zingiberis Rhizoma recens *(shēng jiāng)*, compared to charred Zingiberis Rhizoma preparata *(páo jiāng tàn)*, is more mobile and does not have the ability to conserve. If there is diarrhea, one needs to bind things up.

2. *Why does Dr. Qin use charred Zingiberis Rhizoma preparata (páo jiāng tàn) instead of Zingiberis Rhizoma preparata (páo jiāng)?*

Charred Zingiberis Rhizoma preparata *(páo jiāng tàn)* is better at strengthening the middle and stopping diarrhea. In addition, a mild approach may be needed, because of possible underlying deficiency or the tendency for these patients to have sensitive stomachs. Zingiberis Rhizoma preparata *(páo jiāng)* can irritate the Stomach, resulting in abdominal pain, and is considered more acrid and dispersing than charred Zingiberis Rhizoma preparata *(páo jiāng tàn)*. However, if there is a significant amount of dampness, one can make use of this additional acrid quality and use Zingiberis Rhizoma preparata *(páo jiāng)*.

3. *Why does Dr. Qin not use dry-fried Atractylodis macrocephalae Rhizoma (chǎo bái zhú) or dry-fried Codonopsis Radix (chǎo dǎng shēn)?*

As noted in previous chapters, dry-fried Atractylodis macrocephalae Rhizoma *(chǎo bái zhú)* and dry-fried Codonopsis Radix *(chǎo dǎng shēn)* are best for dampness. However, this illustrates the eloquent thinking of Dr. Qin. He realized that there are already enough aromatic drying herbs present in the formula and therefore used the unprocessed form of these herbs so as not to damage the Spleen yin by overdrying. In their unprocessed forms, they are actually considered to be slightly moist.

3. Warm the Lower Burner (温暖下焦 *wēn nuán xià jiāo*)

[PRESENTATION] Cold in the *shào yīn*; cold inversion of the extremities

Aconiti Radix lateralis preparata *(zhì fù zǐ)*	6g
Poria *(fú líng)*	9g
Cinnamomi Cortex *(ròu guì)*[4]	1.5g
Trigonelle Semen *(hú lú bā)*	2.4g
bland Zingiberis Rhizoma *(dàn gān jiāng)*	2.4g
Glycyrrhizae Radix preparata *(zhì gān cǎo)*	4.5g
Allii fistulosi Bulbus *(cōng bái)*	2 pieces

COMMENTARY

ADDITIONAL SIGNS AND SYMPTOMS

- Chills, a body that is cold to the touch, and a lower back that feels cold
- Lower back and knee pain
- Moist genital area
- Pale face
- Abdominal pain and cramping that improves with pressure
- Loud intestinal sounds (borborygmus)
- Daybreak diarrhea or infrequent, but loose, stools
- Frequent urination, especially at night
- Lower sex drive
- Women: watery discharge
- The pulse is deep, thin, and weak; the proximal position is difficult to find
- The tongue is pale, puffy, swollen, with a grey and wet coating on the root

Note: The pulse and tongue are crucial for diagnosing this pattern.

DISCUSSION

PALPATION: Further confirmation can be obtained by palpating the palmar surface of the forearm and the periumbilical area and see if they are cold.

PATTERN: This treatment principle addresses a problem that is deeper than those addressed by the previous methods and has a component of deficiency of Kidney yang and the fire at

---

4. The original text prescribed cinnamon heart *(ròu guì xīn)* 1.5g.

the gate of vitality. A cold pathogen has penetrated deeply and one must use acrid and warm medicinals to thrust it out. However, the deficiency is still relatively mild, and the pattern centers around cold. Thus, this is more Kidney *(shào yīn)* cold then Kidney deficiency cold. For more prominent deficiency—fatigue, low libido, back pain, and desire to sleep—one must incorporate a more comprehensive plan, including medicinals such as Rehmanniae Radix preparata *(shú dì huáng)*, Corni Fructus *(shān zhū yú)*, and Dioscoreae Rhizoma *(shān yào)*. These address not only the fire at the gate of vitality, but also yin-essence. For further discussion, see the method "warm and tonify the lower base" in Ch. 5, p. 139.

LOCATION: This pathology is primarily in the foot *shào yīn* (Kidneys). However, there is often some hand *shào yīn* (Heart) involvement as well, such as with palpitations.

DURATION AND ETIOLOGY: This can be either acute or chronic. For example, acute situations can occur after exposure to a cold, damp environment, such as falling in a river. This, of course, only occurs when the cold pathogen is able to enter the body deeply; thus, there is usually a preexisting Spleen and Kidney yang deficiency. This type scenario does not mean that the layers above the *shào yīn* (*tài yáng* or *shào yáng*) are necessary weak, but that the *shào yīn* itself is vulnerable and allows the pathogen to enter. Chronic situations can occur from yang deficiency or a lingering cold pathogen that damages the yang. For example, patients with chronic nephritis frequently have this pattern.

MEDICINAL ANALYSIS

- Aconiti Radix lateralis preparata *(zhì fù zǐ)*, Cinnamomi Cortex *(ròu guì)*, bland Zingiberis Rhizoma *(dàn gān jiāng)*, and Trigonelle Semen *(hú lú bā)* expel cold and rescue the yang.

- Aconiti Radix lateralis preparata *(zhì fù zǐ)*, bland Zingiberis Rhizoma *(dàn gān jiāng)*, and Glycyrrhizae Radix preparata *(zhì gān cǎo)* together drive out cold while simultaneously unblocking the yang. They are especially useful when the cold pathogen is rampant and yang qi verges on expiration.

- Aconiti Radix lateralis preparata *(zhì fù zǐ)* warms and drives out cold from the qi aspect and should be pre-cooked.

- Cinnamomi Cortex *(ròu guì)* enters the Kidney, Spleen, and Heart and warms and penetrates through cold in the blood aspect. It can be ground into powder and either dissolved into the decoction or chased with the strained decoction.

- Bland Zingiberis Rhizoma *(dàn gān jiāng)* is hot, acrid, and expelling, and has an affinity for the Spleen. It warms the yang and eliminates cold. It is indicated for symptoms such as diarrhea, nausea, vomiting, cough, and wheezing. Bland Zingiberis Rhizoma *(dàn gān jiāng)* is milder than Zingiberis Rhizoma *(gān jiāng)*.

- Poria *(fú líng)* is sweet and neutral. It tonifies the Spleen circulation, moves dampness, and promotes urination. It is important because there is usually some accumulation of dampness from the cold, often manifested as difficulty finishing urination.

- Trigonelle Semen *(hú lú bā)* is bitter and salty. It warms and tonifies the fire of the lower burner, is very dry, and binds diarrhea. It is also very useful for lower back pain and frequent urination. If unavailable, one can substitute Morindae officinalis Radix *(bā jǐ tiān)* 2.4g.

- Allii fistulosi Bulbus *(cōng bái)* is acrid. It scatters cold and opens the yang, promoting the circulation and linking of the body's yang qi. It is able to enter the deep regions of the body, specifically the deep collaterals.

Dr. Qin's formula is based on True Warrior Decoction *(zhēn wǔ tāng)*, Frigid Extremities Decoction *(sì nì tāng)*, and White Penetrating Decoction *(bái tōng tāng)*.

SOURCE: All three formulas are from *Discussion of Cold Damage* (c. 220)

True Warrior Decoction *(zhēn wǔ tāng)*

Aconiti Radix lateralis preparata *(zhì fù zǐ)* 9g
Atractylodis macrocephalae Rhizoma *(bái zhú)* 6g
Poria *(fú líng)*. 9g
Zingiberis Rhizoma recens *(shēng jiāng)*. 9g
Paeoniae Radix alba *(bái sháo)* 9g

Frigid Extremities Decoction *(sì nì tāng)*

Aconiti Radix lateralis preparata *(zhì fù zǐ)* 6-9g
Zingiberis Rhizoma *(gān jiāng)*. 4.5g
Glycyrrhizae Radix preparata *(zhì gān cǎo)*. 6g

---

White Penetrating Decoction *(bái tōng tāng)*

Allii fistulosi Bulbus *(cōng bái)*. 4p
Zingiberis Rhizoma *(gān jiāng)*. 3g
Aconiti Radix lateralis preparata *(zhì fù zǐ)* 4.5-9g

---

MODIFICATIONS OF DR. QIN'S FORMULA

Simultaneous Kidney yin deficiency:

Rehmanniae Radix preparata *(shú dì huáng)*[5]. 6g

Corni Fructus *(shān zhū yú)* 6g

Lower sexual desire, impotence, and fatigue:

Epimedii Herba *(yín yáng huò)*. 4.5g

Morindae officinalis Radix *(bā jǐ tiān)*. 4.5g

Lower back pain:

Psoraleae Fructus *(bǔ gǔ zhī)*. 4.5g

---

5. Rehmanniae Radix preparata *(shú dì huáng)* can sometimes be too sticky and cold, therefore Dr. Qin likes the prepared form, Asarum prepared rehmannia (细辛熟 *xì xīn shú*), better. This is 100g Rehmanniae Radix preparata *(shú dì huáng)* plus 20g Asari Radix et Rhizoma *(xì xīn)* fried together. This activates the Rehmanniae Radix preparata *(shú dì huáng)*.

Cold-dampness (e.g., feeling of a surfeit of fluids in the body, such as puffy, swollen hands or legs, wet tongue, and profuse saliva):

Curculiginis Rhizoma *(xiān máo)* 4.5g

Atractylodis Rhizoma *(cāng zhú)* 4.5g

Cough induced by cold and a strong sensation of cold:

Asari Radix et Rhizoma *(xì xīn)* 1.5g

QUESTIONS

1. *Why does Dr. Qin use bland Zingiberis Rhizoma (dàn gān jiāng) here instead of Zingiberis Rhizoma preparata (páo jiāng) or Zingiberis Rhizoma recens (shēng jiāng)?*

    Whenever there is Kidney yang deficiency there is almost always some influence on the Spleen. Thus, bland Zingiberis Rhizoma *(dàn gān jiāng)* is used to address the Spleen, since all the other herbs in the formula are essentially *shào yīn* (Kidney) herbs. One can see this idea used in classic formulas such as Frigid Extremities Decoction *(sì nì tāng)*.

2. *How can Allii fistulosi Bulbus (cōng bái), which enters the deep regions of the body in this formula and in other formulas, be used to release the exterior?*

    Allii fistulosi Bulbus *(cōng bái)* is a very versatile herb that can enter many layers of the body depending on with which other medicinals it is paired. For example, if paired with Schizonepetae Herba *(jīng jiè)*, as in the method "diffuse the Lungs and disperse wind" in Ch. 6 (p. 145), it works more on the surface. Here, the deep *shào yīn* herbs guide it to that layer.

---

4. Warm and Direct the *jué yīn* Downward (溫降厥陰 *wēn jiàng jué yīn*)

[PRESENTATION] Cold in the *jué yīn*; abdominal pain and acid regurgitation

Evodiae Fructus *(wú zhū yú)* 2.4g

Foeniculi Fructus *(xiǎo huí xiāng)* 1.5g

Cinnamomi Cortex *(ròu guì)*[6] 1.5g

Corydalis Rhizoma *(yán hú suǒ)* 4.5g

Dry-fried Zanthoxyli Pericarpium *(chǎo huā jiāo)* 1.5g

Linderae Radix *(wū yào)* 4.5g

Zingiberis Rhizoma recens *(shēng jiāng)* . . . . 2 slices

---

COMMENTARY

ADDITIONAL SIGNS AND SYMPTOMS

- Indefinable epigastric discomfort, or a cold, tight, and spasmodic abdomen (especially the lower part), which feels better with warmth and pressure

---

6. The original text prescribed Cinnamon heart *(ròu guì xīn)* 1.5g.

- Poor digestion
- Reduced appetite
- After eating there is a desire to vomit, or vomiting of thin, cold mucus accompanied by an upwelling sensation from the epigastrium
- Regurgitation of frothy, profuse, thin, cold fluids, which may be only slightly acidic but not burning; this especially occurs after drinking cold liquids, and is often preceded by borborygmus
- Diarrhea or irregular bowels (alternating constipation with loose stools)
- Icy cold extremities
- Hernia
- Contractions and pain in the groin
- Pain may be more severe when barefoot on cold surfaces
- General sense of coldness in the perineum
- Testicular infection (e.g., epididymitis)
- Headache, especially around the vertex, that feels deep in the head, slightly cold, and tight
- Emotionally sad or depressed
- Difficulty concentrating
- Lots of dreams (especially sad dreams)
- Edema
- This formula may also be used for gynecological conditions such as infertility or painful menses where the tight sensation in the lower back and lower abdomen is relieved by heat.
- The pulse is deep, wiry, slow, and thin
- The tongue has a thin, dark pale body, with a white or grey and wet (or sticky) coating

DISCUSSION

LOCATION, PATTERNS, AND PATHODYNAMICS: This pattern usually starts with *jué yīn* weakness, meaning Liver qi, yang, and blood deficiency, which then allows an invasion of cold into the lower burner. This may occur from such things as drinking cold beverages or exposure to a cold environment. This leads to cold stagnation and then Liver qi and blood stasis. Thus, there is a component of stagnation due to deficiency. Usually, but not always, this results in some floating or counterflow signs and symptoms.

Although this pattern essentially starts from cold in the *jué yīn* channel, there are a few secondary patterns that help explain the complex array of symptoms. However, eliminating the root—cold in the *jué yīn*—treats all of them:

- Liver and Stomach deficiency cold
- Impaired harmonious descent of the Stomach leading to ascending turbid yin counterflow
- Cold pathogen encroaches upon the middle so that the clear yang is unable to ascend
- Yang qi is deficient and cannot distribute and spread out to the extremities.

- Yin cold attacks the collaterals of the *jué yīn*

TREATMENT PRINCIPLES: Tonify the Liver yang and expel the cold. This method treats the root of the problem.

MEDICINAL ANALYSIS

- Evodiae Fructus *(wú zhū yú)* is acrid and hot. It enters the Liver and Stomach, and re-directs qi counterflow downward.

- Zingiberis Rhizoma recens *(shēng jiāng)* is acrid and dispersing. It warms the Stomach and redirects counterflow in the Stomach downward, especially in a pattern of Stomach cold turbid yin with qi ascending counterflow.

- Zanthoxyli Pericarpium *(chǎo huā jiāo)*, Foeniculi Fructus *(xiǎo huí xiāng)*, Linderae Radix *(wū yào)*, and Cinnamomi Cortex *(ròu guì)* all warm the Liver and Stomach, redirect counterflow downward, and calm the *chōng* vessel.

- Zanthoxyli Pericarpium *(chǎo huā jiāo)* is acrid, warm, and dry. It enters the *jué yīn* and is able to separate and expel cold and dampness. It also tonifies the Liver yang.

- Foeniculi Fructus *(xiǎo huí xiāng)* is acrid and warm. It relieves pain in the *jué yīn*/lower abdomen (e.g., from hernia or testicular inflammation) and is useful for gynecological disorders due to cold and dampness.

- Linderae Radix *(wū yào)* is aromatic. It warms the Liver qi, circulates the *jué yīn*/Liver qi in the groin area, and warms the *shào yīn*.

- Cinnamomi Cortex *(ròu guì)* warms and unblocks cold from the blood aspect, specifically in the Liver and Kidneys. Because it enters the blood aspect of the Liver, it is able to assist in the production of qi. It also tonifies the Liver yang. It can be ground into powder and added to a strained decoction or taken with the decoction.

- Corydalis Rhizoma *(yán hú suǒ)* is acrid and slightly warm. It enters the Liver channel, moves the qi and blood, stops pain, and relaxes spasmodic tension throughout the entire trunk. It is especially useful for patterns of Liver invading the Stomach.

Dr. Qin's formula is based on Evodia Decoction *(wú zhū yú tāng)*.

Evodia Decoction *(wú zhū yú tāng)*

SOURCE: *Discussion of Cold Damage* (c. 220)

Evodiae Fructus *(wú zhū yú)* 9-12g
Zingiberis Rhizoma recens *(shēng jiāng)* 18g
Ginseng Radix *(rén shēn)* 9g
Jujubae Fructus *(dà zǎo)* 12p

MODIFICATIONS OF DR. QIN'S FORMULA

Hernia:

Litchi Semen *(lì zhī hé)* 6-9g

Citri reticulatae Semen *(jú hé)* 4.5g

Allii macrostemi Bulbus *(xiè bái)* 6g

   (especially good if there is cramping, as it relaxes spasms)

Dry-fried Toosendan Fructus *(chǎo chuān liàn zǐ)* 4-6g

Lower back pain:

Eucommiae Cortex *(dù zhòng)* 6g

Dipsaci Radix *(xù duàn)* 4.5g

For additional tonification of Liver blood and yang (e.g., fatigue
   with a wiry, weak, and deep pulse, and a pale dark face):

Astragali complanati Semen *(shā yuàn zǐ)* 4-6g

Angelicae sinensis Radix *(dāng guī)* 3-5g

Additional therapeutic considerations:

- Moxa Liv-1 *(dà dūn):* Use either a moxa stick or cones, although cones have a quicker effect. For a hernia, burn moxa on the contralateral side or bilaterally. A slight variation is to burn 9 cones on a slice of ginger placed over this point.
- Make a paste of Evodiae Fructus *(wú zhū yú)*, Cinnamomi Cortex *(ròu guì)*, and Zingiberis Rhizoma *(gān jiāng)* (equal amounts) and place on CV-8 *(shén què)*.
- In general, one should pay attention to keeping the lower abdomen and perineum warm.

QUESTIONS

1. *If Dr. Qin's formula is based on Evodia Decoction (wú zhū yú tāng), why does he omit Ginseng Radix (rén shēn)?*

   Ginseng Radix *(rén shēn)* does not enter the *jué yīn*. This formula is very precise in focusing on the pathodynamic and root cause of the problem. Even though Ginseng Radix *(rén shēn)* tonifies Liver yang and can treat some cases of stomach pain, it is not the best choice here. Ginseng Radix *(rén shēn)* can be added if the patient has a severe deficiency (e.g., of the ancestral qi or middle burner), if there is a loss of fluids from vomiting, or if there is a need to moderate the formula (see following question).

2. *How strong is this formula?*

   This formula is quite strong and thus the presentation would have to match. However, if the patient's presentation is milder, one can either reduce the dosage of the hotter medicinals or remove them altogether. In addition, to moderate the effects, one can add Ginseng Radix *(rén shēn)* or dry-fried Atractylodis macrocephalae Rhizoma *(chǎo bái zhú)*.

3. *There are many signs and symptoms listed, how does one make sense of it all?*

   The large number of symptoms demonstrates the many ways in which this pattern may branch off from cold in the *jué yīn*. One may actually only see something like acute hernia or painful menses and treat it with this method. Staying focused on the relationship between the symptoms and the core pathodynamic will help make sense of the diverse possibilities.

4. *Can one use Zingiberis Rhizoma (gān jiāng) or Zingiberis Rhizoma preparata (páo jiāng) instead of Zingiberis Rhizoma recens (shēng jiāng)?*

One should not use Zingiberis Rhizoma *(gān jiāng)* because its ability to redirect counterflow downward is relatively weak. Nor should one use Zingiberis Rhizoma preparata *(páo jiāng)* because the processing has taken away the most important function of Zingiberis Rhizoma recens *(shēng jiāng)*, to deal with the nausea and to expel the cold and dampness. However, if one were using this formula for a condition like infertility (as noted above), with no digestive issues, then of course one may use Zingiberis Rhizoma preparata *(páo jiāng)* or charred Zingiberis Rhizoma preparata *(páo jiāng tàn)*.

5. *How does Liver yang deficiency relate to this pattern?*

Liver yang, as discussed here, is a physiological functional component of the Liver and is the foundation of Liver qi. Liver qi is essential for the proper functioning of other organs. For example, if the Liver is healthy, the Liver's qi and yang assist in the earth's normal function. However, if the yang is deficient, then 'wood is unable to restrain earth,' which is also called 'wood is unable to disseminate earth.' Here, the Liver qi has lost its free coursing and consequently slows the function of the Spleen and Stomach. This manifests as depression, fullness and stifling sensation in the chest and flanks, reduced appetite with difficult digestion, abdominal distention, constipation, or sloppy stools. It should be noted that this pattern arises from Liver qi constraint, which can come about from a multitude of underlying patterns such as blood deficiency or, as here, yang deficiency.

However, the above treatment method is for excess cold with underlying deficiency. The more acute the presentation, the more likely excess predominates, whereas the more chronic the situation, the more likely deficiency predominates. It is worth understanding Dr. Qin's differentiation of Liver cold in isolation to help in understanding these patterns in combination:

- Liver cold can arise from a direct attack of a cold pathogen causing the acute presentation of inversion with very cold extremities, abdominal pain, purplish green-blue nails, a thin and wiry pulse, or a deep, thin pulse on the verge of being impalpable. This requires that one select the method of using acrid and warm medicinals to unblock the yang.

- However, it may also occur from the more gradual process of the Liver organ itself becoming deficient, and thus its function weakening. This manifests as lassitude and an inability to endure hard work, melancholy, timidity, lack of warmth in the extremities, and a pulse that is deep, thin, and slow. This requires a tonifying, warming, and nourishing treatment strategy.

Also worth noting are the symptoms associated with a pattern of Liver yang and Liver qi deficiency that has not necessarily affected the middle burner. These include lassitude, melancholy, timidity, headache, numbness and tingling, and lack of warmth in the extremities.

Dr. Qin's formula contains herbs that address all of these issues, and one can alter them accordingly. According to Dr. Qin:

- Herbs to tonify the Liver yang are Cinnamomi Cortex *(ròu guì)*, Zanthoxyli Pericarpium *(huā jiāo)*, and Cistanches Herba *(ròu cōng róng)*.

- Herbs to tonify the Liver qi are Gastrodiae Rhizoma *(tiān má)*, Atractylodis macrocephalae Rhizoma *(bái zhú)*, Chrysanthemi Flos *(jú huā)*, Zingiberis Rhizoma recens *(shēng jiāng)*, Asari Radix et Rhizoma *(xì xīn)*, Eucommiae Cortex *(dù zhòng)*, and sheep liver.

6. *Are the modifications listed for hernia only good for treating pain?*

All of the medicinals listed above for hernia are good for pain, but also have a healing effect by relaxing and strengthening the muscles. Thus they can also be used for patients that have an active hernia without pain.

5. Warm and Scatter the Exterior and Interior (温散表里 *wēn sàn biâo lǐ*)

[PRESENTATION] Pathogenic cold in both the interior and exterior; chills and a deep pulse

Prepared Ephedrae Herba *(zhì má huáng)*	2.4g
Glycyrrhizae Radix preparata *(zhì gān cǎo)*	1.5g
Aconiti Radix lateralis preparata *(zhì fù zǐ)*	4.5g
Perillae Folium *(zǐ sū yè)*	4.5g
Asari Radix et Rhizoma *(xì xīn)*	2.4g
Saposhnikoviae Radix *(fáng fēng)*	4.5g
Zingiberis Rhizoma recens *(shēng jiāng)*	2 slices

COMMENTARY

ADDITIONAL SIGNS AND SYMPTOMS

- Intense headache
- Tight, cold, and painful muscles and joints
- Sore and painful back and neck
- Chronic asthma, wheezing, or cough that worsens with cold
- Profuse phlegm
- Sore throat
- In addition to the chills, which may be quite severe, there is often a mild fever (elevated body temperature)
- The pulse is deep, tight, and thin
- The tongue is dark pale, swollen, with a wet and grey, white, or black coating

DISCUSSION

PATTERN AND ETIOLOGY: This pattern is approximately a 50% interior (root) and 50% exterior (branch). It consists of a constitutional Kidney yang deficiency with an invasion of a cold pathogen into the *tài yáng* and *shào yīn* channels. This external component is either wind-cold or wind-cold with dampness. This pattern is not very common and may be seen in peasants or those who have limited access to adequate shelter. It is especially appropriate if the patient looks very pale, has low blood pressure, and a weak pulse.

After taking the formula, the patient should stay warm to encourage a slight sweat. There is usually no need to take it for more than 1-2 weeks. Once the appetite returns and they do not feel cold, the formula can be discontinued or changed to a constitutional formula.

MEDICINAL ANALYSIS

- Aconiti Radix lateralis preparata *(zhì fù zǐ)*, Cinnamomi Ramulus *(guì zhī)*, and Zingiberis Rhizoma recens *(shēng jiāng)* support and aid the deficient yang qi and dispel internal cold.

- Aconiti Radix lateralis preparata *(zhì fù zǐ)* vitalizes the yang qi in the interior, and forces the pathogenic cold out. It can also secure the protective level. It should be pre-cooked for 45 minutes.

- Cinnamomi Ramulus *(guì zhī)* is acrid, slightly sweet, and warm. It unblocks the yang, releases the muscle layer, and warms the middle burner.

- Zingiberis Rhizoma recens *(shēng jiāng)* is acrid, dispersing, and warm. It expels cold and dampness from the interior and wind and cold from the exterior.

- Asari Radix et Rhizoma *(xì xīn)* unblocks and penetrates deep into the collaterals of the Kidney channel, assisting Aconiti Radix lateralis preparata *(zhì fù zǐ)*. It also assists the medicinals that focus more on the surface, such as prepared Ephedrae Herba *(zhì má huáng)*, in scattering cold from the exterior. It is very effective in reducing pain.

- Clear-prepared Glycyrrhizae Rhizoma preparata *(qīng zhì gān cǎo)* regulates and tonifies the Spleen.

- Saposhnikoviae Radix *(fáng fēng)*, prepared Ephedrae Herba *(zhì má huáng)*, and Cinnamomi Ramulus *(guì zhī)* promote sweating, thus one has to be careful to consider the possibility that their use can lead to devastated yang.

- Prepared Ephedrae Herba *(zhì má huáng)*, Perillae Folium *(zǐ sū yè)*, and Saposhnikoviae Radix *(fáng fēng)* scatter cold from the exterior.

- Prepared Ephedrae Herba *(zhì má huáng)* diffuses and disseminates the yang qi on the outer aspects of the body, and opens, discharges, and scatters cold.

- Perillae Folium *(zǐ sū yè)* is acrid. It diffuses the Lungs and scatters wind-cold and dampness on the exterior and scatters cold in the interior. It also has the ability to aromatically transform dampness and phlegm that may accumulate in the interior as a result of the cold.

Dr. Qin's formula is based on Ephedra, Asarum, and Aconite Accessory Root Decoction *(má huáng xì xīn fù zǐ tāng)*.

Ephedra, Asarum, and Aconite Accessory Root Decoction *(má huáng xì xīn fù zǐ tāng)*
SOURCE: *Discussion of Cold Damage* (c. 220)

Ephedrae Herba *(má huáng)* 6g
Aconiti Radix lateralis preparata *(zhì fù zǐ)* 9g
Asari Radix et Rhizoma *(xì xīn)* 6g

MODIFICATIONS OF DR. QIN'S FORMULA

More significant cold on the exterior aspect:

Schizonepetae Spica *(jīng jiè suì)* 4.5g

Headache (severe):

Ligustici Rhizoma *(gǎo běn)* 4.5g

More significant cold in the interior aspect:

Cinnamomi Cortex *(ròu guì)* 2g

***Tài yīn* cold** (stomachache, abdominal pain, and diarrhea):

Zingiberis Rhizoma *(gān jiāng)* 2-3g
Evodiae Fructus *(wú zhū yú)* 1g

▶ Remove Zingiberis Rhizoma recens *(shēng jiāng)*

8

Treatment Guidelines for

Summerheat 暑 (shǔ)

Summerheat is one of the six pernicious influences. While the five other pathogens can occur in any season, summerheat usually only occurs in the summer. Furthermore, summerheat occurs with dampness and this makes it different than warm-heat disease. Another difference is that a summerheat pathogen can have a direct attack which is different than damp-heat diseases.

The basic idea in the treatment is to first and foremost clear heat and facilitate resolution of dampness. Treatments, such as an ice bath, while necessary in severe cases, can trap dampness in the body and prolong recovery time.

> **PATTERNS**
>
> 1. Fever, sweating with wheezing, irritability, thirst, excessively wild talking,[i] fatigue, and shortness of breath; may have bleeding from the lower burner, jaundice, or eruption of maculae

This usually occurs in people with prior Spleen qi deficiency. The jaundice and eruption of maculae (which are usually just dimly visible) are seen when the pattern in severe. The fever is usually low and occurs in the afternoon. The sweating is usually sticky and not profuse. There may also be dizziness, stifling sensation in the chest, head distention, nausea/vomiting, loose stools, dark urine, a floating, soft, or soggy pulse, and a puffy tongue that is orange or dark. Apart from acute attacks, this pattern is also seen in chronic diseases and corresponds to the "dissipate heat and dispel summerheat" method described below.

2. Invasion of a pathogen into the Pericardium, which disperses through the blood vessels and enters the brain; there is muscle twitching in the extremities and loss of consciousness

This is called summerheat collapse, which first enters the Pericardium and then the Pericardium collaterals. The intense heat makes its way to all the body's collaterals, spreads throughout the blood, and then enters the brain. There is often a fire toxin component when it attacks the Heart and brain, which can manifest as loss of consciousness, convulsions, high fever, and bleeding. This requires immediate treatment or the situation can become critical.

However, one can have a less serious presentation of this pattern with no loss of consciousness but a sensation of intense heat, fever, nausea, and vomiting. Both of these are more serious than the previous pattern and correspond to the method "clear the Heart and flush away summerheat" described below.

PULSE

In cases of deficiency: Deficient, large, and lacks strength; or small and frail
In cases of excess: Flooding, overabundant, and fast

1. Dissipate Heat and Dispel Summerheat (宣热祛暑 *xuān rè qū shú*)

[PRESENTATION] Early stage contraction of a summerheat pathogen; physical fatigue, irritability, and thirst

Pogostemonis/Agastaches Herba *(huò xiāng)*[1] 6g
Forsythiae Fructus *(lián qiáo)* . . . . 4-6g[2]
Eupatorii Herba *(pèi lán)*[3] 6g
Trichosanthis Pericarpium *(guā lóu pí)* 9g
Six-to-One Powder *(liù yī sǎn)* 12g
Nelumbinis Plumula *(lián zǐ xīn)* 2.4g
Nelumbinis Folium *(hé yè)*[4] 6-9g

COMMENTARY

ADDITIONAL SIGNS AND SYMPTOMS

- Heavy sensation in the head, head distention, muddle-headed, or unclear thinking; not an actual headache

1. Pogostemonis/Agastaches Herba recens *(xiān huò xiāng)* 6g was originally used.

2. Forsythiae Pericarpium *(lián qiáo ké)* 9g was originally used. Here, Forsythiae Fructus *(lián qiáo)* is written because it is most commonly what one receives nowadays. The smaller dose reflects the need for a lighter action, which Forsythiae Pericarpium *(lián qiáo ké)* inherently has.

3. Eupatorii Herba recens *(xiān pèi lán)* 6g was originally used.

4. One piece of Nelumbinis Folium recens *(xiān hé yè)* was originally used, which weighs approximately 20-30g.

- Dizziness
- Grimy complexion (looks like the face has not been washed, slightly dark and oily)
- Tired, very lethargic, no desire to move
- Nausea, sometimes vomiting
- Loose stools
- Bloating and gas
- No appetite
- Low fever (37.5°C/99.5°F) that is higher in the afternoon
- Aversion to wind and drafts
- Achy joints/back pain
- Urine is dark and cloudy
- The tongue is slightly red on the tip, with a thin, wet and slightly yellow coating
- The pulse is floating, soft, and soggy (occasionally rapid); in severe cases it can be large and scattered

DISCUSSION

PATTERN AND ETIOLOGY: This is a summerheat pathogen (with aspects of dampness) that attacks the protective level and the Spleen. This looks like a mild heat stroke or a cold and usually occurs in the summer season when the outside temperature is high.

TREATMENT PRINCIPLE: Clear summerheat from the Lungs, Stomach, Spleen, Bladder, and brain.

MEDICINAL ANALYSIS

- Pogostemonis/Agastaches Herba *(huò xiāng)* is slightly warm and aromatically diffuses and vents the dampness from the upper burner and exterior. It also regulates qi in the middle, loosens up the chest, and transforms dampness. It is the number one choice for expelling summerheat, and is especially suitable for symptoms such as vertigo, dizziness, and headache.

- Eupatorii Herba *(pèi lán)* is similar to Pogostemonis/Agastaches Herba *(huò xiāng)*, however it works on a deeper level (muscular level and Spleen) while Pogostemonis/Agastaches Herba *(huò xiāng)* works more on the surface and Stomach. It also has the ability to promote movement to resolve dampness in the qi aspect.

- Forsythiae Fructus *(lián qiáo)* is bitter, cool, and mildly expels and clears heat from the Pericardium and Heart.[ii] Medicinals such as Mori Folium *(sāng yè)*, Chrysanthemi Flos *(jú huā)*, and Lonicerae Flos *(jīn yín huā)* are inappropriate for this function.[5]

- Trichosanthis Pericarpium *(guā lóu pí)* is cold, slippery, and can clear summerheat. The peel is more for expelling than is the entire fruit, but it also has some ability to open the bowels, although less so than the seeds.

---

5. Although these clear heat and evict the pathogen, they do not enter the Heart and Pericardium.

- Six-to-One Powder *(liù yī sǎn)* is a 6:1 powder of Talcum *(huá shí)* and Glycyrrhizae Radix *(gān cǎo)*. Talcum *(huá shí)* not only can expel dampness and heat through the urine but also has some ability to expel outward. Thus it can be used in treating early-stage problems. The diuretic component is an essential principle for this pattern. Glycyrrhizae Radix *(gān cǎo)* protects the Stomach from the cold nature of Talcum *(huá shí)*.

- Nelumbinis Plumula *(lián zǐ xīn)* clears summerheat from the collaterals of the Heart and helps prevent loss of consciousness.

- Nelumbinis Folium *(hé yè)* is sweet, slightly aromatic, and able to expel the wet and sticky aspects of summerheat from all regions of the body, particularly the deep collaterals.

Dr. Qin's formula is based on Patchouli/Agastache Powder to Rectify the Qi *(huò xiāng zhèng qì sǎn)*.

Patchouli/Agastache Powder to Rectify the Qi *(huò xiāng zhèng qì sǎn)*
SOURCE: *Formulary of the Pharmacy Service for Benefiting the People in the Taiping Era* (1107)

Pogostemonis/Agastaches Herba *(huò xiāng)* 12g
Magnoliae officinalis Cortex *(hòu pò)* 9g
Citri reticulatae Pericarpium *(chén pí)* 9g
Perillae Folium *(zǐ sū yè)* 6g
Angelicae dahuricae Radix *(bái zhǐ)* 6g
Pinelliae Rhizoma preparatum *(zhì bàn xià)* 9g
Arecae Pericarpium *(dà fù pí)* 9g
Atractylodis macrocephalae Rhizoma *(bái zhú)* 12g
Poria *(fú líng)* 9g
Platycodi Radix *(jié gěng)* 9g
Glycyrrhizae Radix preparata *(zhì gān cǎo)* 3g

---

MODIFICATIONS OF DR. QIN'S FORMULA

Nausea:

Bambusae Caulis in taeniam *(zhú rú)* 4.5g
Pinelliae Rhizoma preparatum *(zhì bàn xià)* 4.5g

Slightly burning and painful urination that is dark:

Tetrapanacis Medulla *(tōng cǎo)* 2g
Phragmitis Rhizoma *(lú gēn)* 6g

Stuffy chest, tight flanks, and overly emotional or depressed:

Aurantii Fructus *(zhǐ ké)* 4.5g
Curcumae Radix *(yù jīn)* 4.5g

2. Clear the Heart and Flush Away Summerheat (清心涤暑 qīng xīn dí shǔ)

[PRESENTATION] Summerheat pathogen accosts internally; fainting with fever

Coptidis Rhizoma *(huáng lián)*	1.5g
Forsythiae Fructus *(lián qiáo)*	9g
Artemisiae annuae Herba *(qīng hāo)*[6]	4.5g
Talcum *(huá shí)*[7]	12g
Black Gardeniae Fructus *(hēi zhī zǐ)*	4.5g
Nelumbinis Caulis *(lián gěng)*[8]	6-9g
Purple Snow *(zǐ xuě)*	0.9g (swallowed)

COMMENTARY

ADDITIONAL SIGNS AND SYMPTOMS

- Loss of consciousness
- Spasms
- Strong headache
- Red face, ears, and eyes
- Strong thirst
- May or may not sweat
- Dark urine accompanied by a painful, burning sensation
- Constipation
- Higher fever than in the previous method (e.g. 39-40°C/102.2-104°F)
- The pulse is soggy, floating, and rapid
- The tongue is bright red with yellow, sticky coating

DISCUSSION

Many times when people have a strong heat stroke they may try to cool themselves down with ice packs on the neck, etc. Sometimes this is necessary in critical situations because it can reduce the fever, however it can also lead to increased stagnation (e.g., congealed dampness), resulting in more lethargy, no appetite, a thicker, white, sticky tongue coating, and the patient may not recover for 1-3 weeks.

PATTERN: This is summerheat stroke that attacks the Heart and brain. There must usually be some underlying deficiency for this to occur.

---

6. Artemisiae annuae Caulis *(qīng hāo gěng)* 4.5g was originally used.

7. Flying Talcum *(fēi huá shí)* 12g was originally used.

8. A one-third meter length of Nelumbinis Caulis *(lián gêng)* was originally used. This is also called Nelumbinis Folium stalks *(hé yè gêng)*.

MEDICINAL ANALYSIS

- Gardeniae Fructus *(zhī zǐ)*, Forsythiae Fructus *(lián qiáo)*, and Coptidis Rhizoma *(huáng lián)* are all cold and bitter and clear heat (especially Heart fire) and flush away summerheat.

- Coptidis Rhizoma *(huáng lián)* also clears Stomach heat and dries dampness.

- Forsythiae Fructus *(lián qiáo)* is bitter, cool, and clears heat from the Heart.[iii]

- The shell of Gardeniae Fructus *(zhī zǐ)* is better at expelling than the seeds. One can therefore remove the seeds.

- Artemisiae annuae Herba *(qīng hāo)* and Nelumbinis Caulis *(lián gěng)* both resolve summerheat and have the ability to thrust the pathogen out from the deep layers of the body. Here this function pertains to taking the pathogen from the nutritive level of the Pericardium/Heart to the surface via first the qi level and then the protective level. Consequently, they can produce a mild sweat.

- Artemisiae annuae Herba *(qīng hāo)* is bitter, cold, acrid, aromatic, and can also clear deficiency heat.

- Nelumbinis Caulis *(lián gěng)* is sweet and slightly aromatic. It clears heat, promotes the resolution of dampness and removes it from the deep collaterals, and unblocks the orifices. If unavailable, one can substitute Nelumbinis Folium *(hé yè)*. However the stem of Nelumbinis Caulis *(lián gěng)* is like a tube or straw, which is thought to allow it to travel throughout the body, making it more effective at circulating the qi in the channels.

- Talcum *(huá shí)* clears heat and promotes the resolution of dampness. It prevents the pathogen from entering into the deeper regions of the body. Because of this, it can be used in either the early or late stages of disease. It should be wrapped and pre-cooked for 30 minutes. If available, Talcum in pieces *(huá shí kuài)* is preferred over the powdered form.

- Purple Snow *(zǐ xuě)* is a patent formula that should be added to the strained decoction. For example, take 0.45g with each dose (if twice a day). If unavailable, substitute Bovis Calculus *(niú huáng)* or Saigae tataricae Cornu *(líng yáng jiǎo)* 1g, as a fine powder, also added to the strained decoction.

MODIFICATIONS OF DR. QIN'S FORMULA

If there is damage to the yin and blood:

Lonicerae Flos *(jīn yín huā)* 4-6g

Moutan Cortex *(mǔ dān pí)* 4-6g

If the presentation is very serious, for example, loss of consciousness, stroke, or high fever, consider one of the three precious formulas:

Calm the Palace Pill with Cattle Gallstone *(ān gōng niú huáng wán)*

Purple Snow *(zǐ xuě)*

Greatest Treasure Special Pill *(zhì bǎo dān)*

QUESTIONS

1. *Why are Lonicerae Flos (jīn yín huā) and Moutan Cortex (mǔ dān pí) chosen as modifications for yin and blood damage?*

Severe heat can easily damage the yin and blood. At this stage, the way to protect the yin and blood is to expel the heat from the blood aspect. Tonics are inappropriate.

2. *Since there may be severe heat, could Gypsum fibrosum (shí gāo) or Scutellariae Radix (huáng qín) be used?*

Gypsum fibrosum *(shí gāo)* is inappropriate because it does not address the dampness. Scutellariae Radix *(huáng qín)* is also not the best choice because it mainly addresses the Lungs and Large Intestine. Here the Heart is the fundamental concern, thus Coptidis Rhizoma *(huáng lián)* is chosen.

9

Treatment Guidelines for

Dampness 湿 (shī)

NATURE

A heavy, turbid, substantial pathogen

Dampness is a yin pathogen that is very sticky and sluggish and does not transform easily. It has a tendency to sink down into the lower burner as well as into the minute collaterals. For these reasons, it can be difficult to eliminate.

ETIOLOGY

Externally-contracted: Mountain mist miasmic malarial disorder,[1] moisture and steaming of rain, making a long journey through water,[2] long-time residence in a damp location, or wearing clothes that have become damp from sweating

---

Damp weather or a damp environment may be major contributing factors, as may be actions such as not properly drying one's hair, which can cause such symptoms as headaches and migraines.

Internally-generated: Eating rich foods and having a fondness for roasted, raw, cold, or greasy foods may all result in the Spleen yang failing to transport.

---

1. 山岚瘴气 *(shān lán zhàng qì)*. A qi *(vapor)* given owff by putrescent matter in damp mountain forest areas and held to be one cause of malaria-like conditions.

2. This refers not only to traveling, but to working in water, for example, standing barefoot in water or dampness.

LOCATION
In the upper burner: Heavy head, yellowing of the eyes, nasal congestion, and a plugged-up sounding voice

The head may feel large, distended, swollen, or one may have a feeling of glue inside the head after shaking it. There may be dull or unclear thinking, dull headache, puffy face, swelling under eyes, lots of mucus in the throat, muffled voice, nasal discharge, tearing and eye discharge, loud tinnitus (like an airplane), blurry vision, or swollen hands and feet.

In the middle burner: Focal distention, a stifling sensation, and an uncomfortable feeling

There may also be nausea, plum pit qi, a sloshing sound upon palpation, or a feeling of water in the abdomen. The focal distention will be most obvious around the center of the epigastrium.

In the lower burner: Floating edema in the feet and lower legs

There may also be difficult urination, dribbling urination, cloudy urine, scanty urine, swollen legs (especially swelling of the instep), abdominal fullness, sticky or loose bowels that are difficult to fully void, hemorrhoids, or vaginal discharge.

Dampness in any of the three burners will present with a worsening of symptoms in the morning or after eating inappropriate foods (especially those mentioned above) and improvement after moving around. However, if dampness is mixed with heat, as in a damp-heat disorder (see method no. 6 below), then the symptoms will worsen in the afternoon and improve upon waking.

In the channels and collaterals: Late afternoon fever and aching pain in the sinews and bones

Apart from a low fever, there is a general sense of discomfort, weakness, soreness or heaviness of the limbs; fatigue, nausea, a stifling sensation in the chest, and very sore joints, which are more prevalent between 2–6 p.m. There may also be lower back pain or numbness and tingling in the sinews that make it difficult to move around.

In the muscles: Swelling and fullness that feels like mud when pressed.

This is pitting edema.

In the limb joints: Stiffness when bending or stretching.

Joints may also be sore and painful.

In the passages and pathways: Fixed and heavy with no movement

The passages and pathways (隧道 *suì dào*) are considered to be much deeper than the channels and collaterals. For example, the channels and collaterals refer to the superficial aspects of the muscles, joints, sinews, vessels, and bones. The passages and pathways refer to the deeper aspects of these same tissues. Both can present with soreness and pain. However, whole body soreness from conditions like the flu pertains to the channels and collaterals, whereas long-term sore conditions like ALS, MS, or rheumatoid arthritis pertain to the passages and pathways.

In the skin: Stubborn numbness and tingling

There may also be rashes with pustules/vesicles (e.g., some type of eczema). Numbness is more blood aspect, while tingling is more qi aspect.

In the qi and blood: Fatigue
In the Lungs: Wheezing, fullness, and cough

The mucus will be sticky or frothy.

In the Spleen: Phlegm-oral mucus with distention and swelling

There may also be profuse mucus in the throat, generalized body swelling, and abdominal bloating and gas.

In the Liver: Fullness in the flanks and bulging qi disorder

There may also be pain in the flanks.

In the Kidneys: Lower back pain and sweating around the genitals

There may also be a rash or dermatitis located over the perineum. The lower back pain can also present as heaviness that feels like one is carrying a heavy weight.

Enters the yang organs: Borborygmus, vomiting, painful urinary dribbling with turbidity, diarrhea with tenesmus; urination must be rough and yellow or red

Enters the yin organs: Stuporous and unable to be roused, fixed eyes, and soundlessly staring straight ahead

This can manifest as loss of consciousness, Tourette's syndrome, or petit-mal seizures. This is dampness attacking the deepest aspects, usually the Heart, Liver, and Kidneys.

TREATMENT
Use wind medicinals to prevail over dampness.

This idea is not only for external dampness but is also important for many internal damp conditions. For example, one often applies such medicinals in cases of leukorrhea instead of just binding,[3] as well as conditions such as Intestinal wind or vaginal bleeding. For example, Saposhnikoviae Radix *(fáng fēng)*, Schizonepetae Herba *(jīng jiè)*, and Notopterygii Rhizoma seu Radix *(qiāng huó)* are wind medicinals that expel and remove internal dampness by lifting. Using dry-fried or charred medicinals is best—dry-frying or charring allows the medicinals to enter a deeper layer of the body as well as making them "drier" so that they can better absorb dampness.

> Drain out urine to guide out dampness.

For example, consider Talcum *(huá shí)*, Benincasae Exocarpium *(dōng guā pí)*, Benincasae Semen *(dōng guā zǐ)*, or Alismatis Rhizoma *(zé xiè)*.

> Unblock the bowels to drive out dampness.

This is typically used for severe conditions such as ascites, in which eliminating dampness solely through the urine is not enough. It can also be used in less severe presentations when there is heat and dampness in the Large Intestine. In this situation, one can use formulas such as Unripe Bitter Orange Pill to Guide Out Stagnation *(zhǐ shí dǎo zhì wán)*, Aucklandia and Betel Nut Pill *(mù xiāng bīng láng wán)*, or Regulate the Middle and Reduce the Four [Stagnations] Pill *(tiáo zhōng sì xiāo wán)*.[4] This method, if applied correctly, should not produce watery diarrhea, but large and complete bowel movements, sometimes with sticky mucus. Charred Rhei Radix et Rhizoma *(dà huáng tàn)* is especially useful for damp-heat stagnation.

> Expectorate or vomit out phlegm-oral mucus to dispel dampness.

In an acute situation, where the patient has eaten some bad food or overeaten and has symptoms such as nausea, fever, and headache, they can drink 200cc of Gardenia and Prepared Soybean Decoction *(zhī zǐ chǐ tāng)* slowly.[5] Then, after 5-10 minutes, the patient can tickle the throat with a feather to induce vomiting. This method is not very common at present.

> If in the upper part of the body, it is appropriate to promote sweating.

For example, for slight vertigo, headache, profuse mucus, and nausea, one can use Patchouli/Agastache Powder to Rectify the Qi *(huò xiāng zhèng qì sǎn)*.[6]

> If in the lower upper part of the body, it is appropriate to leach out and drain [dampness].

---

3. For example, End Discharge Decoction *(wán dài tāng)*.

4. Ingredients for these three formulas can be found in the supplementary formulas section of Ch. 2 (pp. 53-54).

5. This is Sojae Semen preparatum *(dàn dòu chǐ)* and Gardeniae Fructus *(zhī zǐ)*. Sometimes this method can be used for epilepsy or asthma in children. Zhang Zi-He often used this method.

6. Ingredients can be found in Ch. 8 (p. 186).

For example, for edema and nephritis, one can use Five-Peel Drink *(wǔ pí yǐn)*.[7] For damp-heat in the lower burner, such as a urinary tract infections (dark and painful urination) with lower abdominal pain, one can use Eight-Herb Powder for Rectification *(bā zhèng sǎn)*.[8]

> **If there is interior deficiency, it is appropriate to bolster the Spleen.**

This is dampness in the middle burner and one should tonify to increase the transportation function of the Spleen.

> **If complicated with wind, it is appropriate to release the muscle layer.**

This is wind accompanied by dampness. For example, in cases of damp rashes or dermatitis, one should use medicinals such as Saposhnikoviae Radix *(fáng fēng)*, Cicadae Periostracum *(chán tuì)*, Dictamni Cortex *(bái xiān pí)*, Atractylodis Rhizoma *(cāng zhú)*, or Tribuli Fructus *(cì jí lí)*.

> **If there is yang deficiency then it is appropriate to tonify the fire.**

This is dampness accompanied by deficiency in the gate of vitality. For example, one can use Kidney Qi Pill from the *Golden Cabinet (jīn guì shèn qì wán)*.[9] This may present as a wide range of manifestations from chronic nephritis to easily catching colds. It may also present as edema, pale face, lower back pain, generalized sensation of cold, or frequent urination. In this situation, merely applying diuretics will make the situation worse.

> **If there is yin deficiency, it is appropriate to fortify the water.**

This is a difficult situation with many permutations. One must tonify the yin without generating more dampness, and this requires promoting urination. One definitely cannot simply nourish the yin. A reasonable starting place is Six-Ingredient Pill with Rehmannia *(liù wèi dì huáng wán)*.[10] It contains yin-tonifying medicinals with others that can help eliminate dampness. One can also add medicinals such as Benincasae Semen *(dōng guā zǐ)*, Plantaginis Semen *(chē qián zǐ)*, Polyporus *(zhū líng)*, Achyranthis bidentatae Radix *(niú xī)*, and Coicis Semen *(yì yǐ rén)* to guide the dampness down and out. Using a medicinal like Atractylodis macrocephalae Rhizoma *(bái zhú)* with the intention of strengthening the Spleen and transforming dampness is inappropriate. This is because it does not tonify the yin and does not sufficiently remove the water.

---

7. Mori Cortex *(sāng bái pí)*, Zingiberis Rhizomatis Cortex *(shēng jiāng pí)*, Poriae Cutis *(fú líng pí)*, Citri reticulatae Pericarpium *(chén pí)*, and Arecae Pericarpium *(dà fù pí)*.

8. Akebiae Caulis *(mù tōng)*, Talcum *(huá shí)*, Plantaginis Semen *(chē qián zǐ)*, Dianthi Herba *(qú mài)*, Polygoni avicularis Herba *(biān xù)*, Gardeniae Fructus *(zhī zǐ)*, wine-washed Rhei Radix et Rhizoma *(jiǔ xǐ dà huáng)*, Junci Medulla *(dēng xīn cǎo)*, and Glycyrrhizae Radix preparata *(zhì gān cǎo)*.

9. Rehmanniae Radix *(shēng dì huáng)*, Corni Fructus *(shān zhū yú)*, Dioscoreae Rhizoma *(shān yào)*, baked Aconiti Radix lateralis *(bāo fù zǐ)*, Cinnamomi Ramulus *(guì zhī)*, Alismatis Rhizoma *(zé xiè)*, Poria *(fú líng)*, and Moutan Cortex *(mǔ dān pí)*.

10. Rehmanniae Radix preparata *(shú dì huáng)*, Corni Fructus *(shān zhū yú)*, Dioscoreae Rhizoma *(shān yào)*, Poria *(fú líng)*, Moutan Cortex *(mǔ dān pí)*, and Alismatis Rhizoma *(zé xiè)*.

A useful clinical example of this pattern is seen in many cases of restless legs syndrome that occur in the elderly. They may also have tingling and numbness, or a heavy, swollen sensation. Many times, one must tonify the Kidney yin and essence and simultaneously remove the dampness. One may consider a base formula such as Rehmannia Drink *(dì huáng yǐn zi)*[11] to which is added light medicinals that eliminate dampness such as Chaenomelis Fructus *(mù guā)*, Bombycis Faeces *(cán shā)*, Arecae Semen *(bīng láng)*, Trachelospermi Caulis *(luò shí téng)*, Luffae Fructus Retinervus *(sī guā luò)*, and Tetrapanacis Medulla *(tōng cǎo)*.

> If there is heat with the dampness, it is appropriate to use a bitter and cold formula to dry it.

Heat plus dampness (in which heat predominates) usually requires bitter and cold medicinals such as Coptidis Rhizoma *(huáng lián)*, Scutellariae Radix *(huáng qín)*, Phellodendri Cortex *(huáng bǎi)*, and Rhei Radix et Rhizoma *(dà huáng)*.

> If there is cold with the dampness, it is appropriate to use an acrid and hot formula to eliminate it.

It is appropriate to use dry and warm medicinals such as Tsaoko Fructus *(cǎo guǒ)*, Atractylodis Rhizoma *(cāng zhú)*, Asari Radix et Rhizoma *(xì xīn)*, Eucommiae Cortex *(dù zhòng)*, Dipsaci Radix *(xù duàn)*, Angelicae pubescentis Radix *(dú huó)*, and Zingiberis Rhizoma preparata *(páo jiāng)*.

SUMMARY OF TREATMENT
Transform, dry, promote sweating, drive out, clear, and facilitate the resolution of dampness.

1. Aromatically Transform Dampness (芳香化湿 *fāng xiāng huà shī*)

[PRESENTATION] Damp-turbidity collects internally; disharmony of the Spleen and Stomach

Pogostemonis/Agastaches Caulis *(huò xiāng gěng)*	4.5g
Amomi Fructus rotundus *(bái dòu kòu)*	2.4g
Pinelliae Rhizoma preparatum *(zhì bàn xià)*	4.5g
Amomi Fructus *(shā rén)*	2.4g
Citri reticulatae Pericarpium *(chén pí)*	4.5g
dry-fried Coicis Semen *(chǎo yì yǐ rén)*	9g
Citri sarcodactylis Fructus *(fó shǒu)*	3g

---

11. Rehmanniae Radix preparata *(shú dì huáng)*, Corni Fructus *(shān zhū yú)*, Cistanches Herba *(ròu cōng róng)*, Morindae officinalis Radix *(bā jǐ tiān)*, Aconiti Radix lateralis preparata *(zhì fù zǐ)*, Cinnamomi Cortex *(ròu guì)*, Dendrobii Herba *(shí hú)*, Ophiopogonis Radix *(mài mén dōng)*, Acori tatarinowii Rhizoma *(shí chāng pú)*, Polygalae Radix *(yuǎn zhì)*, Poria *(fú líng)*, and Schisandrae Fructus *(wǔ wèi zǐ)*.

COMMENTARY

ADDITIONAL SIGNS AND SYMPTOMS

- Indigestion, lack of appetite, possibly a sensation of bloating
- Stifling sensation in the chest
- Epigastric focal distention
- Sticky and bland taste in the mouth
- Usually mild nausea, but if severe, vomiting
- Heavy head
- Swollen face
- The pulse is floating and soggy
- The tongue has a swollen and large body with a greasy white or grey coating or a slightly yellow and thick coating that can be scraped off

DISCUSSION

ETIOLOGY: This pattern is usually a result of external dampness (e.g., humid environment) invading and causing disharmony of the Spleen and Stomach. It can also come about from dietary irregularities and eating excessive raw and cold foods (such as melons and fruits) or food that is too rich.

DURATION: This method is used for the early stages of damp disorders, usually acute or subacute in nature (one day to a few weeks).

LOCATION: The upper and middle burners are most affected and the Stomach is usually more affected than the Spleen.

TREATMENT PRINCIPLE: Aromatically transform and vent out dampness and harmonize the Stomach qi. If the damp pathogen stagnates, causing constraint and stoppage of the qi dynamic, this will contribute further to the retention of the damp pathogen, and one should then aromatically regulate the qi and transform dampness.

MEDICINAL ANALYSIS

SUMMARY

- This formula is aromatic and should not be cooked for a long time. One can soak the medicinals for 20–30 minutes, then bring the formula to a boil and simmer for 10 minutes.
- All the medicinals are acrid and warm except for Coicis Semen *(yì yǐ rén)*.
- All the medicinals are aromatic except for Pinelliae Rhizoma preparatum *(zhì bàn xià)* and Coicis Semen *(yì yǐ rén)*.
- All the medicinals transform and eliminate dampness.

INDIVIDUAL CHARACTERISTICS

- Pogostemonis/Agastaches Caulis *(huò xiāng gěng)*—the stem—regulates the qi in the middle, loosens the chest, and transforms dampness. It is not overly drying or hot and is milder than the entire herb, Pogostemonis/Agastaches Herba *(huò xiāng)*, which has more of an effect on the upper and exterior. Both will aromatically diffuse and vent the damp pathogen. The leaf, Pogostemonis/Agastaches Folium *(huò xiāng yè)*, has a stronger tendency to disperse and resolve the exterior and can be used if there is more exterior involvement. The stem is usually preferred for this pattern.

- Amomi Fructus rotundus *(bái dòu kòu)*, Citri reticulatae Pericarpium *(chén pí)*, Citri sarcodactylis Fructus *(fó shǒu)*, Amomi Fructus *(shā rén)*, and Pinelliae Rhizoma preparatum *(zhì bàn xià)* all act on the middle to aromatically regulate the qi and transform dampness.

- Amomi Fructus rotundus *(bái dòu kòu)* and Amomi Fructus *(shā rén)* have similar properties of promoting the movement of qi and harmonizing the middle. Amomi Fructus *(shā rén)* is better at warming and opening the Stomach, increasing appetite, and alleviating vomiting. Amomi Fructus rotundus *(bái dòu kòu)* focuses more on the Spleen, increasing its circulation and aiding in the elimination of dampness. Together they open the Stomach and awaken the Spleen. They should be crushed and added during the final 3-5 minutes of cooking.

- Dry-fried Coicis Semen *(chǎo yì yǐ rén)* functions on the lower burner and is sweet and bland, able to leach out dampness, and strengthens the Spleen. It regulates, drains, and dries dampness without guiding the pathogen deeper into the body. The dry-fried preparation should be used when aromatic medicinals that dry dampness are also used. Dry-frying moderates its cold nature and improves its ability to strengthen the Spleen and harmonize the middle. Conversely, the raw form is better at opening the channels and collaterals, enabling it to treat painful obstruction, atrophy, expel pus, and reduce swelling.

Dr. Qin's formula is roughly based on Patchouli/Agastache Powder to Rectify the Qi *(huò xiāng zhèng qì sǎn)*.

Patchouli/Agastache Powder to Rectify the Qi *(huò xiāng zhèng qì sǎn)*
SOURCE: *Formulary of the Pharmacy Service for Benefiting the People in the Taiping Era* (1107)

Pogostemonis/Agastaches Herba *(huò xiāng)* 12g
Magnoliae officinalis Cortex *(hòu pò)* 9g
Citri reticulatae Pericarpium *(chén pí)* 9g
Perillae Folium *(zǐ sū yè)* 6g
Angelicae dahuricae Radix *(bái zhǐ)* 6g
Pinelliae Rhizoma preparatum *(zhì bàn xià)* 9g
Arecae Pericarpium *(dà fù pí)* 9g
Atractylodis macrocephalae Rhizoma *(bái zhú)* 12g
Poria *(fú líng)* 9g
Platycodi Radix *(jié gěng)* 9g
Glycyrrhizae Radix preparata *(zhì gān cǎo)* 3g

---

MODIFICATIONS OF DR. QIN'S FORMULA

Mucus in throat:

 Eupatorii Herba *(pèi lán)* 4.5g

**Slight aversion to wind, or with the etiology of consumption
of excessively cold and damp foods:**

 Perillae Folium *(zǐ sū yè)* 4.5g

Simultaneous external dampness and cold:

 Perillae Folium *(zǐ sū yè)* 4.5g

 Saposhnikoviae Radix *(fáng fēng)* 6g

 Notopterygii Rhizoma seu Radix *(qiāng huó)* 4.5g

Spleen deficiency:

 Poria *(fú líng)* 9g

Fullness and bloating:

 Magnoliae officinalis Cortex *(hòu pò)* 4.5g
  (for epigastric fullness)

 Aucklandiae Radix *(mù xiāng)* 4.5g
  (for lower abdominal fullness)

History of poor digestion:

 scorched Massa medicata fermentata *(jiāo shén qū)* 9g

Sticky stools with yellow, sticky coating:

 Dry-fried Coptidis Rhizoma *(chǎo huáng lián)* 3g

 Dry-fried Massa medicata fermentata *(chǎo shén qū)* 9g

QUESTIONS

1. *Why does Dr. Qin include Citri sarcodactylis Fructus (fó shǒu) in this prescription?*

   Citri sarcodactylis Fructus *(fó shǒu)* is included because of its light, aromatic, out-thrusting nature. Furthermore, it works together with Pogostemonis/Agastaches Herba *(huò xiāng)* to lightly thrust out and transform dampness. Citri sarcodactylis Fructus *(fó shǒu)* is not chosen because of its ability to regulate the Liver qi.

2. *What does "transform dampness" mean?*

   The strategy of transforming dampness is one of three primary methods used in the treatment of dampness. The other two are facilitating the resolution of dampness and expelling dampness.

    However, transforming dampness is a general term that can encompass three additional treatment principles:

   a. Aromatically transform dampness is used in mild patterns, as above.

b. Bitter, warm and dry dampness method is used when the dampness is relatively more severe (see treatment method no. 2 below).

c. Clear and transform damp-heat (often shortened to clear dampness) involves one aspect of clearing heat and another of transforming dampness, although transforming dampness should be emphasized in such a pattern. Method no. 6 below demonstrates this approach.

3. *What are some concerns when using the method of transforming dampness?*

Medicinals that transform dampness can easily damage the fluids and it is important to discontinue them before this occurs. However, the nature of dampness is congealing and stagnating, and eliminating it can sometimes be relatively slow. Thus if one uses an excessive amount of aromatic and dry medicinals, frequently the dampness will not be reduced and transformed, but it will begin to damage the fluids, and an impasse will develop that is very difficult to treat.

4. *Why does Dr. Qin only use one medicinal (Coicis Semen [yì yǐ rén]) that leaches out/ facilitates resolution of dampness?*

This is a relatively superficial and light damp pathogen and one does not need to overly facilitate resolution (or dry out) dampness to accomplish one's goal.

5. *What do the terms "leach out dampness" and "facilitate resolution of dampness" mean?*

Facilitate resolution of dampness (利湿 *lì shī*) is a general treatment strategy that eliminates dampness through the urine. It can be divided into 'blandly leach out and eliminate dampness' (淡渗除湿, *dàn shèn chú shī*) and 'unblock and promote urination' (通利小便, *tōng lì xiǎo biàn*). Commonly, one or two medicinals that blandly leach out dampness (such as Coicis Semen *(yì yǐ rén)*, Tetrapanacis Medulla *(tōng cǎo)*, Poria *(fú líng)*, Poria rubra *(chì fú líng)*, or Benincasae Exocarpium *(dōng guā pí)*) are added to formulas that aromatically transform dampness. Medicinals that promote urination are different and are used when dampness leads to urinary symptoms such as scanty, short, yellow, dark, and inhibited urination. This is described below under the method "move downward and facilitate the resolution of dampness" (p. 207).

6. *What is the relationship between this method (aromatically transform dampness) and the following one (warm and dry damp-turbidity), and how does one differentiate the symptomology?*

This method is for more superficial/acute/Stomach-related problems while the "warm and dry damp-turbidity" method is for deeper/more chronic/Spleen-related problems. Thus the former uses lighter medicinals.

As one might suspect, the key differentiating feature for the "warm and dry damp-turbidity" method is related more to Spleen symptoms such as slow digestion and loose and sticky stools, hence the addition of "warming (the Spleen)" into the method's name. However, in practice, one might combine the two, emphasizing the treatment principles that are most closely linked to the presenting symptoms.

7. *Which symptoms indicate that the damp pathogen is more serious and how does this relate to the following method, "warm and dry damp-turbidity"?*

The pathogen is more severe (and deeper) when one starts to see focal distention and a stifling sensation in the chest and epigastrium, heavy body and fatigue, reduced food intake with vomiting and nausea, and a thick and greasy tongue coating. For these symptoms, one might modify the treatment strategy to a more 'drying' approach and consider including Magnoliae officinalis Cortex *(hòu pò)* and Atractylodis Rhizoma *(cāng zhú)*, while deemphasizing the lighter medicinals. This makes it closer to the following method.

However, if these symptoms are not present and one just sees, for example, reduced food intake, a bland taste in the mouth, and an upward flow into the throat that is just short of vomiting with a white, greasy tongue coating, then one may emphasize the lighter medicinals and possibly use Amomi Pericarpium rotundum *(bái dòu ké)*, Amomi Pericarpium *(shā rén ké)*, and Magnoliae officinalis Flos *(hòu pò huā)*, while at the same time removing the heavier medicinals such as Coicis Semen *(yì yǐ rén)* and Pinelliae Rhizoma preparatum *(zhì bàn xià)*. As with many of Dr. Qin's formulas, this is right in the middle of a pattern, allowing for flexible treatment through modifications.

OTHER TIPS

- If there is blockage/tightness at the center of the epigastrium—or just lack of appetite—one can chew Amomi Fructus *(shā rén)* or Amomi Fructus rotundus *(bái dòu kòu)* seeds (no shells) 2-3 times a day.
- One can eat Massa Fortunellae Fructus *(jīn jú bǐng)* (2 pieces) after meals to help Spleen circulation.
- After meals, the patient can perform self massage down the Conception vessel, starting at CV-14 *(jù què)*.

2. Warm and Dry Damp-Turbidity (温燥湿浊 *wēn zào shī zhuó*)

[PRESENTATION] Entrenched damp-turbidity; greasy tongue and a stifling sensation in the chest and upper abdomen

Atractylodis Rhizoma *(cāng zhú)* / Atractylodis macrocephalae Rhizoma *(bái zhú)*	4.5g (each)
Magnoliae officinalis Cortex *(hòu pò)*	4.5g
Amomi Fructus rotundus *(bái dòu kòu)*	2.4g
Dry-fried Aurantii Fructus *(chǎo zhǐ ké)*	4.5g
Acori tatarinowii Rhizoma *(shí chāng pú)*	2.4g
Citri reticulatae viride Pericarpium *(qīng pí)* / Citri reticulatae Pericarpium *(chén pí)*	2.4g (each)
Massa medicata fermentata *(shén qū)*	9g

COMMENTARY

ADDITIONAL SIGNS AND SYMPTOMS

- Focal distention and fullness in the central abdomen
- Abdominal distention with tenderness or water-splash sounds on percussion at the center of the epigastrium
- Lack of desire to eat
- Slow digestion
- Loose or sticky stools
- Nausea, and if severe, vomiting (induced by strong smells)
- Profuse and sticky saliva
- Fatigue
- Swollen face, legs, or hands
- Vaginal discharge
- Frequent but scanty urination with dribbling
- Cloudy or dark urine
- Flatulence
- The tongue is swollen with teeth marks, a tight (close to the body) white or grey, greasy or slippery coating. The coating is not especially thick or yellow.
- The pulse is very soggy and soft, not floating. The right middle position is deeper than others.

DISCUSSION

LOCATION: Primarily the middle burner, particularly the Spleen

PATTERN AND PATHODYNAMIC: This method is suitable for cold-damp-turbidity entrenched in the middle burner, impairing the ability of the Spleen to transport.

ETIOLOGY: This is a result of external dampness (e.g., a humid environment) invading and causing a disharmony of the Spleen and Stomach. This may also come about from dietary irregularities or eating excessively raw and cold foods, melons and fruits, or food that is too rich. This pattern can result from the improper resolution of the previous pattern, after which the Stomach dampness migrates into the Spleen.

DIFFERENTIATION AND TREATMENT PRINCIPLES: The previous pattern primarily affects the Stomach, while this pattern primarily affects the Spleen. Although dampness of the Stomach and Spleen have similar etiologies, there are key points of distinction based on their differing natures. Stomach dampness often occurs in the early stages of damp-turbidity obstruction, as seen in the method "aromatically transform dampness" described earlier in this chapter. Thus the treatment is to aromatically transform dampness and diffuse and unblock the stagnation. This pattern—entrenched damp-turbidity in the Spleen—is more serious and has more dampness. Consequently, the use of an expelling method alone is not enough. One must also warm and dry the damp-turbidity, while paying attention to Spleen yang (see below).

MEDICINAL ANALYSIS

SUMMARY

- All the medicinals have the ability to transform dampness.

- All the medicinals are warm and treat cold-damp pathogens.

- All the medicinals except Atractylodis macrocephalae Rhizoma *(bái zhú)* are acrid.

- All the medicinals except Atractylodis Rhizoma *(cāng zhú)*, Atractylodis macrocephalae Rhizoma *(bái zhú)*, and Acori tatarinowii Rhizoma *(shí chāng pǔ)* regulate the qi and direct it downward.

- All the medicinals except Atractylodis macrocephalae Rhizoma *(bái zhú)*, dry-fried Aurantii Fructus *(chǎo zhǐ ké)*, Citri reticulatae viride Pericarpium *(qīng pí)*, and Massa medicata fermentata *(shén qū)* are aromatic.

Medicinal	Warm	Acrid	Directs Qi Down	Aromatic	Regulates qi
Atractylodis Rhizoma *(cāng zhú)*	X	X		X	
Atractylodis macrocephalae Rhizoma *(bái zhú)*	X				
Magnoliae officinalis Cortex *(hòu pò)*	X	X	X	X	X
Amomi Fructus rotundus *(bái dòu kòu)*	X	X	X	X	X
Aurantii Fructus *(zhǐ ké)*		X	X		X
Acori tatarinowii Rhizoma *(shí chāng pǔ)*	X	X		X	
Citri reticulatae viride Pericarpium *(qīng pí)*	X	X	X		X
Citri reticulatae Pericarpium *(chén pí)*	X	X	X	X	X
Massa medicata fermentata *(shén qū)*	X	X	X		X

INDIVIDUAL CHARACTERISTICS

- Atractylodis Rhizoma *(cāng zhú)* is acrid, bitter, and very strongly dries dampness, especially when a damp pathogen has encroached on the Spleen. By contrast, Atractylodis macrocephalae Rhizoma *(bái zhú)* primarily builds up the Spleen. Together they are able to dry dampness and strengthen the Spleen, as Atractylodis Rhizoma *(cāng zhú)* raises the yang and Atractylodis macrocephalae Rhizoma *(bái zhú)* supplements and augments the Spleen qi and yang. They should be used when the transportation and transformation functions of the Spleen are impaired.

- Dry-fried Aurantii Fructus *(chǎo zhǐ ké)* is acrid and promotes the movement of qi and resolves dampness to eliminate the stifling sensation in the chest. It also works specifically to strengthen the Spleen's circulation (regulating and harmonizing the Spleen and Stomach qi), which helps transform and move dampness.

- Magnoliae officinalis Cortex *(hòu pò)* aromatically dries dampness and regulates the qi, eliminating the stifling sensation and fullness in the chest. Its strength in drying dampness is not as great as that of Atractylodis Rhizoma *(cāng zhú)*, but it is much better at eliminating fullness.

- Amomi Fructus rotundus *(bái dòu kòu)* is acrid, aromatic, and promotes the movement of qi and dampness (making it less sticky), as well as drying dampness and warming and harmonizing the middle. It is especially good for slow digestion, fatigue, and a sensation of heaviness. Crush it and add to the decoction during the last 3-5 minutes of cooking.

- Citri reticulatae Pericarpium *(chén pí)* aromatically regulates the qi and is drying in order to assist in transforming dampness. Citri reticulatae viride Pericarpium *(qīng pí)* is acrid, breaks up qi stagnation, dredges and regulates the Liver qi, and should be used when there are Liver channel signs such as hypochondriac and flank distention and fullness. It is inappropriate to use this in the absence of such signs or if the patient is clearly deficient. Citri reticulatae Pericarpium *(chén pí)* is better for digestion, while Citri reticulatae viride Pericarpium *(qīng pí)* is better for the Liver. However, using both of these medicinals together synergistically improves their ability to move the qi.

- Acori tatarinowii Rhizoma *(shí chāng pǔ)* is acrid and aromatic. It awakens the Spleen and moves and "cleans up" any damp-turbidity that is encumbering the Spleen, which manifests as a poor appetite, sticky and greasy mouth, focal distention, and stifling sensation in the central abdomen.

- Massa medicata fermentata *(shén qū)* is an excellent medicinal for building up the Spleen and Stomach, eliminating stagnation, and transforming accumulations. Consider using a filter when cooking it.

Dr. Qin's formula is based on Calm the Stomach Powder *(píng wèi sǎn)* and Unripe Bitter Orange and Atractylodes Pill *(zhǐ zhú wán)*.

Calm the Stomach Powder *(píng wèi sǎn)*

SOURCE: *Formulary of the Bureau of Medicines of the Taiping Era* (1078)

Atractylodis Rhizoma *(cāng zhú)* 12–15g
Magnoliae officinalis Cortex *(hòu pò)* 9–12g
Citri reticulatae Pericarpium *(chén pí)*. 9–12g
Glycyrrhizae Radix preparata *(zhì gān cǎo)*. 3–6g
    (taken as a draft with Zingiberis Rhizoma recens [*shēng jiāng*] and Jujubae Fructus [*dà zǎo*])

Unripe Bitter Orange and Atractylodes Pill (zhǐ zhú wán)

SOURCE: *Clarifying Doubts about Damage from Internal and External Causes* (1247)

Aurantii Fructus immaturus (zhǐ shí). 12-18g
Atractylodis macrocephalae Rhizoma (bái zhú) 6-9g
  (made into pills with rice fried in Nelumbinis Folium [hé yè])

MODIFICATIONS OF DR. QIN'S FORMULA

Chronic Spleen deficiency:

Poria *(fú líng)* 9g

Loose stools (several times per day):

Roasted Puerariae Radix *(wēi gé gēn)* 6g

Heaviness in the head, clouded thinking, muddled hearing, and cloudy vision:

Pogostemonis/Agastaches Herba *(huò xiāng)* 4.5g

Eupatorii Herba *(pèi lán)* 4.5g

Cloudy urine or difficult or dribbling urination:

Coicis Semen *(yì yǐ rén)* 9g

Alismatis Rhizoma *(zé xiè)* 6g

Damp-heat:

Coptidis Rhizoma *(huáng lián)* 3-5g

Phellodendri Cortex *(huáng bǎi)* 3-5g

QUESTIONS

1. *What are the important preparation methods to consider for these herbs?*

   Many of these medicinals, such as Atractylodis Rhizoma *(cāng zhú)*, Atractylodis macrocephalae Rhizoma *(bái zhú)*, Aurantii Fructus *(zhǐ ké)*, Citri reticulatae Pericarpium *(chén pí)*, Citri reticulatae viride Pericarpium *(qīng pí)*, and Massa medicata fermentata *(shén qū)*, can be dry-fried, which improves their ability to dry dampness and to remove dampness by increasing the Spleen's circulation. In addition, dry-frying these medicinals can moderate certain aspects of their properties, for example, making them easier to digest, which can be important when digestion is already compromised. For example, raw Atractylodis Rhizoma *(cāng zhú)* can bring about headaches and sore throat, and mostly works on the surface. It can create a sweat and is used to eliminate wind, cold, and dampness. Dry-frying it moderates its moving and dispersing qualities and enables it to work more on the middle burner.

2. *Why does Dr. Qin include Acori tatarinowii Rhizoma (shí chāng pǔ) in this prescription?*

   Long-term dampness encumbering the Spleen has a tendency to reduce its function by "covering the Spleen" and making it "sleepy." Acori tatarinowii Rhizoma *(shí chāng pǔ)* can awaken the Spleen, as well as the Heart or mind, which may have become cloudy as a result of the dampness. It should be noted that Acori tatarinowii Rhizoma *(shí chāng pǔ)* is not chosen for its ability to aromatically open the orifices. It has the important function of being able to open up and separate the dampness. If one just dries dampness, the outside (of the dampness) may become dry, but the inside remains damp. It also guides other herbs up and outward, increasing their ability to expel dampness, and is especially useful when there are symptoms such as heaviness in the head or a cloudy mind. Without this, the action of the formula will be confined to the middle.

Furthermore, medicinals such as Pogostemonis/Agastaches Herba *(huò xiāng)* and Eupatorii Herba *(pèi lán)* are too mild for this action, as they cannot penetrate its sticky dampness.

3. *Could one use Pogostemonis/Agastaches Herba (huò xiāng) or Eupatorii Herba (pèi lán)?*

Generally speaking, these medicinals are best reserved for acute or subacute conditions. However, because of their releasing and dispersing nature, they can be used if there is symptomology that affects the head (see Modifications above).

4. *What if the Large Intestine also needs awakening?*

Often, dampness will also affect the Large Intestine, having a similar dampening effect to that which it has on the Spleen. This will manifest as bloating, gas, and bowel movements that are difficult to move and fully void. Allii macrostemi Bulbus *(xiè bái)* is an important herb that can be added for this situation.

5. *Dr. Qin chooses to use Citri reticulatae viride Pericarpium (qīng pí) in this prescription and Citri sarcodactylis Fructus (fó shǒu) in the previous one. Why?*

The reason lies in the difference between the treatment methods. This method (no. 2) utilizes a more warming and drying strategy than the aromatic approach in method no. 1. Since dampness is more entrenched in this pattern, a stronger, more forceful approach is needed. Thus the fierce and strong nature of Citri reticulatae viride Pericarpium *(qīng pí)* can penetrate deeply into the organs and uproot the entrenched dampness. On the other hand, Citri sarcodactylis Fructus *(fó shǒu)* has a lighter, more aromatic, out-thrusting quality. Citri sarcodactylis Fructus *(fó shǒu)* is best used in situations in which there is some damp-turbidity in the upper burner or even exterior of the body, such as in method no. 1, "aromatically transform dampness."

6. *Is there a difference between moving qi and moving dampness?*

A fundamental principle for eliminating dampness is promoting the movement of qi. However, certain herbs also have the ability to move dampness, which breaks up dampness and makes it less sticky. This is different from drying dampness. For example, Citri reticulatae viride Pericarpium *(qīng pí)*, Cyperi Rhizoma *(xiāng fù)*, and Aurantii Fructus *(zhǐ ké)* are able to move the qi and can assist in the removal of dampness, but do not directly move dampness. Medicinals such as dry-fried Aurantii Fructus *(chǎo zhǐ ké)* and Amomi Fructus rotundus *(bái dòu kòu)* are able to move the dampness.

7. *If Aurantii Fructus immaturus (zhǐ shí) is originally used in Unripe Bitter Orange and Atractylodes Pill (zhǐ zhú wán), why does Dr. Qin use the dry-fried preparation?*

   This situation primarily manifests in the upper abdomen. Aurantii Fructus immaturus *(zhǐ shí)* is best used for fullness in the lower abdomen, while the dry-fried preparation is best for the epigastrium.

8. *In the differentiation and treatment principles sections for this method, it says to "pay attention to Spleen yang." What does this mean?*

   Spleen dampness is mostly from middle yang deficiency, which is unable to fortify (build up) its transportation and transformation functions. Although Spleen dampness has a tendency toward cold, the warming in the title of this treatment principle not only has the literal meaning of warming (to remove cold), but also the meaning of increasing the Spleen yang. Even if there is only a temporary constraint of Spleen yang, it is also important to look after the root by strengthening the Spleen's ability to transform dampness. Thus one may consider taking this method a step further and use Cinnamomi Ramulus *(guì zhī)*, making it an "acrid, warm [bitter] drying" method.

---

3. Move Downward and Facilitate the Resolution of Dampness
(下行利湿 *xià xíng lì shī*)

[PRESENTATION] Damp-turbidity in the lower burner; rough urination and swelling of the feet

Poriae Cutis *(fú líng pí)*	12g
Plantaginis Semen *(chē qián zǐ)*	9g
Arecae Pericarpium *(dà fù pí)*	9g
Alismatis Rhizoma *(zé xiè)*	9g
Phaseoli Semen *(chì xiǎo dòu)*	9g
Stephaniae tetrandrae Radix *(hàn fáng jǐ)*	4.5g
Benincasae Exocarpium *(dōng guā pí)*	9g

COMMENTARY

ADDITIONAL SIGNS AND SYMPTOMS

- Scanty, difficult, red, rough, and/or dribbling urination
- Floating edema in the lower limbs
- Fatigue
- Lower back is painful, encumbered, and/or heavy
- Lower abdominal bloating
- Diarrhea or alternating constipation and diarrhea[12]

---

12. Alternating constipation and diarrhea is not a typical symptom for this pattern, but may occur. If it does, it indicates that the Spleen is deficient and not transporting; appropriate adjustments to the treatment should be made

- The pulse is soggy and weak in the proximal positions
- The tongue is swollen, pale, wet, and teeth-marked

DISCUSSION

This is water-dampness collecting in the lower burner. Edema is an important symptom for this pattern, and this method can be used for almost any type of edema (e.g., menopausal edema), especially if there is no major pathology affecting the Heart and Kidneys. It may also be used for some urinary tract infections or even some patients with the diagnosis of nephritis or glomerulonephritis.

ETIOLOGY AND PATHODYNAMIC: This pattern is usually a result of invasion of external dampness (e.g., humid environment) causing disharmony of the Spleen and Stomach, or from dietary irregularities such as excessive raw and cold foods, melons and fruits, or food that is too rich. There is usually some underlying Spleen and Kidney yang deficiency, which may be constitutional or caused by the above dietary irregularities. However, the essential idea is that there is stagnation because of damp-turbidity collecting in the lower burner.

TREATMENT PRINCIPLE: Facilitate resolution of dampness (by bland percolation and opening and promoting urination),[13] strengthen the Spleen, and promote the movement of qi.

COMPARISON: The previous two methods address damp-turbidity collecting in the middle burner. This method addresses water-dampness in the lower burner by means of promoting urination. This method mainly refers to the *Inner Classic's* treatment method of "if it is in the lower [burner], guide it out and expel it."

Location	Method
Middle burner (Stomach)	Aromatically transform (disperse outward)
Middle burner (Spleen)	Warm, dry, and move qi
Lower burner	Promote urination

MEDICINAL ANALYSIS

SUMMARY

The ingredients in this formula can be separated into two groups:

Facilitate resolution of dampness by blandly leaching it out and opening and promoting urination	Plantaginis Semen *(chē qián zǐ)*, Alismatis Rhizoma *(zé xiè)*, Stephaniae tetrandrae Radix *(hàn fáng jǐ)*, Benincasae Exocarpium *(dōng guā pí)*
Strengthen the Spleen, promote the movement of qi, and assist in the elimination of dampness	Poriae Cutis *(fú líng pí)*, Phaseoli Semen *(chì xiǎo dòu)*, Arecae Pericarpium *(dà fù pí)*

accordingly, such as adding Atractylodis macrocephalae Rhizoma *(bái zhú)*.

13. See the question section under the method "aromatically transform dampness" (p. 199).

INDIVIDUAL CHARACTERISTICS

- Poriae Cutis *(fú líng pí)* is sweet and neutral. It enters the collaterals and is principally a diuretic that drains dampness from the muscles and skin. Its tonifying ability is slight.

- Plantaginis Semen *(chē qián zǐ)* is slightly bitter, sweet, and cool. It is best for chronic edema.

- Arecae Pericarpium *(dà fù pí)* is bitter, acrid, and warm. It is able to promote the movement of qi and water downward (promoting urination/facilitating resolution of dampness), as well as promoting bowel movements. It is especially good for bloating and gas. It has no tonifying qualities.

- Alismatis Rhizoma *(zé xiè)* is sweet, bland, and cold. It leaches out dampness and is commonly used to promote urination (move water).

- Phaseoli Semen *(chì xiǎo dòu)* is sweet and slightly cold. It promotes urination, primarily by moving dampness in the blood aspect, but also by moving water in the qi aspect. Although it is relatively mild, it also moves blood stasis and cools the blood.

- Stephaniae tetrandrae Radix *(hàn fáng jǐ)* is bitter and cold. It promotes urination and facilitates the resolution of dampness, enabling it to clear damp-heat accumulation from the lower burner, especially when there is swelling. If it is unavailable, one can substitute Dianthi Herba *(qú mài)* 6g.[14]

- Benincasae Exocarpium *(dōng guā pí)* is sweet, cold, gentle, and harmonious. It promotes urination, clears heat and dampness, and is especially good for edema in the muscles and skin.

Dr. Qin's formula is based on Five-Peel Powder *(wǔ pí sǎn)* with Cheng Guo-Peng's modifications for dampness in the lower burner.

Five-Peel Powder *(wǔ pí sǎn)*

SOURCE: *Treasury Classic* (4th century)

Poriae Cutis *(fú líng pí)* 15g
Arecae Pericarpium *(dà fù pí)* 15g
Zingiberis Rhizomatis Cortex *(shēng jiāng pí)* 6g
Citri reticulatae Pericarpium *(chén pí)* 9g
Mori Cortex *(sāng bái pí)* 15g

Cheng Guo-Peng's modifications:

Phaseoli Semen *(chì xiǎo dòu)*
Poria rubra *(chì fú líng)*
Alismatis Rhizoma *(zé xiè)*
Plantaginis Semen *(chē qián zǐ)*
Dioscoreae hypoglaucae Rhizoma *(bì xiè)*
Stephaniae tetrandrae Radix *(hàn fáng jǐ)*
   (dosages not given)

---

14. Indicated especially if there is slight pain with urination.

MODIFICATIONS OF DR. QIN'S FORMULA

Fever or heat from yin deficiency:

Polyporus *(zhū líng)* 4.5g

Difficult urination:

Talcum *(huá shí)* 9g

Cloudy urination:

Dioscoreae hypoglaucae Rhizoma *(bì xiè)* 4.5g

Burning sensation during urination, with occasional blood in the urine:

Cirsii Herba *(xiǎo jì)* 6g

Burning sensation during urination and difficulty passing urine:

Polygoni avicularis Herba *(biǎn xù)* 6g

Burning sensation during urination with internal heat
(e.g., sore throat, fever, red tip, and yellow coating):

Plantaginis Herba *(chē qián cǎo)* 6g

(forming a strong synergistic herbal pair with Plantaginis Semen
[chē qián zǐ], in which case its dosage may be reduced to 6g)

Lower abdominal bloating:

Dry-fried Pharbitidis Semen *(chǎo qiān niú zǐ)* 6g

Frequently feeling cold, and a pale face:

Cinnamomi Ramulus *(guì zhī)* 3g

Zingiberis Rhizomatis Cortex *(shēng jiāng pí)* 6g

▶ These two medicinals strengthen Kidney yang to help
facilitate the elimination of dampness.

Renal or urinary tract stones:

Lysimachiae Herba *(jīn qián cǎo)* 9g

Lygodii Spora *(hǎi jīn shā)* 6g

Unprepared Gigeriae galli Endothelium corneum *(shēng jī nèi jīn)* 4-6g

QUESTIONS

1. Why is Phaseoli Semen (chì xiǎo dòu) included in this formula?

Qin Bo-Wei noticed that many nephritis patients have blood in their urine as well as swelling. Phaseoli Semen *(chì xiǎo dòu)* addresses this by moving blood stasis and cooling the blood. It can also ease the bowels without causing diarrhea.

2. Since the majority of medicinals in this formula are cool, is there a heat component?

Often, stagnation can turn to heat. However, this formula is only slightly cool and therefore can only address a small accumulation of heat. If there is an overwhelming amount of heat, the formula should be modified. If there are simultaneous yang deficiency signs with cold, then warmer medicinals can be added (see question below).

3. *Since this condition is caused by an underlying deficiency, wouldn't one want to add some tonifying herbs?*

Even though this condition is primarily due to a Spleen and Kidney yang deficiency, it is important for this method to strongly promote urination and eliminate the edema. Thus if there is small amount of deficiency, it is unnecessary to tonify at this time. However, if the deficiency is prominent, one can add medicinals such as Aconiti Radix lateralis preparata *(zhì fù zǐ)*, bland Zingiberis Rhizoma *(dàn gān jiāng)*, or others to tonify the appropriate deficiency (Spleen and/or Kidney). For example, if one sees floating edema with physical cold, fear of cold, a deep and thin pulse, an especially faint proximal position, and a pale white tongue body, then some supplementation is appropriate. As with all treatments, one must gauge how much deficiency, excess, cold, and heat are present. If there is an overwhelming amount of Spleen and Kidney yang deficiency, then of course this method may not be appropriate. One may consider using a method from the deficiency or cold chapters of this book, or some combination of the three.

4. *How long can this method be used?*

There are no time restrictions on this method. Generally speaking, this is not a harsh formula and can be taken for many years if needed. However, this is usually an acute condition and long-term use is probably not warranted. When the swelling is eliminated, one may change to addressing the underlying cause.

5. *How does this formula differ from Five-Peel Powder (wǔ pí sǎn)?*

Although this formula is rooted in Five-Peel Powder *(wǔ pí sǎn)*, its focus is different. Five-Peel Powder *(wǔ pí sǎn)* primarily treats a pattern of edema that derives from vigorous dampness and qi stagnation with Spleen deficiency. Qin Bo-Wei's formula adds medicinals to direct its action more to the lower burner.

---

4. Drive Out Dampness and Move Water (逐湿利水 *zhú shī lì shuǐ*)

[PRESENTATION] Water-dampness buildup and accumulation; swelling, distention, and urinary blockage

Pharbitidis Semen *(qiān niú zǐ)*	2.4g
Arecae Semen *(bīng láng)*	4.5g
Lepidii/Descurainiae Semen *(tíng lì zǐ)*	4.5g
Phytolaccae Radix *(shāng lù)*	2.4g
Processed Kansui Radix *(zhì gān suì)*	1.5g
Stephaniae tetrandrae Radix *(hàn fáng jǐ)*	4.5g
Gyllulus *(xī shuài)* /Gryllotalpa *(lóu gū)* [15]	4 pieces each

---

15. These are two types of crickets (males preferred). See commentary for substitutions.

COMMENTARY

ADDITIONAL SIGNS AND SYMPTOMS

- The swelling and distention (mentioned above) occurs on the arms, legs, or abdomen.

- There will usually be swelling in other parts of the body (e.g., legs, hips, head, and feet).

- Scanty, sometimes brown, urine with a volume of usually less than 200cc per day, or even no urination for 24 hours

- Difficulty breathing when lying down

- Bloating, gas, and constipation, with possible fecal blockage

- The pulse is soft, big, hollow, and floating, or dry-drumskin and rapid.

- The tongue is (dark) purple red, swollen, wet, with a white or grey coating

DISCUSSION

This is an excess presentation and must be treated as such. An attacking approach is the only way to drive out the water. Although there is certainly some deficiency underneath this pattern, it should not be the focus of treatment.

This is mostly for ascites or pleurisy, in which there is water under the ribs or between the lungs and ribs. The water is not in the organs (e.g., bladder) but in between the tissues. This is difficult to remove. It requires a strong treatment, more so than the previous methods.

This formula purges water out through the urine and bowels. After taking the formula, it is normal to hear abdominal gurgling and then to expel watery diarrhea.

Note: This is a very strong formula. One should use it for only 1-2 days because of its potential damaging effects.

MEDICINAL ANALYSIS

- Pharbitidis Semen *(qiān niú zǐ)* and Lepidii/ Descurainiae Semen *(tíng lì zǐ)* very strongly promote urination. Pharbitidis Semen *(qiān niú zǐ)* is bitter and cool and can break up qi stagnation, promote the movement of water, and unblock and drain the bowels (specifically of dampness and heat). The unprocessed form is much stronger than dry-fried, and one will often experience gurgling intestines and then watery stool after consuming 9-12g. Lepidii/ Descurainiae Semen *(tíng lì zǐ)* is bitter and cold, forcefully descends and drains, moves water, dampness, and phlegm downward and out. It also has some ability to loosen the stool. However, most pharmacies carry a processed version (often dry-fried), which moderate its effect.

- Kansui Radix *(gān suì)* and Phytolaccae Radix *(shāng lù)* fiercely drive out water. Because both of these are toxic, they need to be used with caution. If Phytolaccae Radix *(shāng lù)* is unavailable, one can substitute Euphorbiae pekinensis Radix *(jīng dà jǐ)* 2.4g.

- Stephaniae tetrandrae Radix *(hàn fáng jǐ)* is bitter and cold and promotes urination, enabling it to clear damp-heat accumulation from the lower burner, especially when there is swelling. If unavailable, one can substitute Dianthi Herba *(qú mài)*[16] 6g or Alismatis Rhizoma *(zé xiè)* 6g.

- Gyllulus *(xī shuài)*/Gryllotalpa *(lóu gū)* can open and free water-dampness from the deep collaterals. If unavailable, one can substitute Pheretima *(dì lóng)* 4.5g and Benincasae Exocarpium *(dōng guā pí)* 9g.

- Arecae Semen *(bīng láng)* assists the other medicinals by moving the qi, promoting urination, and reducing swelling. It is able to unblock the bowels, guide everything out, pass gas, and move downward.

Dr. Qin's formula is based on Vessel and Vehicle Pill *(zhōu chē wán)* and Dredging and Chiseling Drink *(shū záo yǐn zi)*

Vessel and Vehicle Pill *(zhōu chē wán)*

SOURCE: *Formulas from Benevolent Sages Compiled during the Taiping Era*

Kansui Radix *(gān suì)*	30g
vinegar Genkwa Flos *(cù yuán huā)*	30g
vinegar Euphorbiae pekinensis Radix *(cù dà jǐ)*	30g
Pharbitidis Semen *(qiān niú zǐ)*	120g
Rhei Radix et Rhizoma *(dà huáng)*	60g
Citri reticulatae viride Pericarpium *(qīng pí)*	15g
Citri reticulatae Pericarpium *(chén pí)*	5g
Arecae Semen *(bīng láng)*	15g
Aucklandiae Radix *(mù xiāng)*	15g
Calomelas *(qīng fěn)*	3g

Dredging and Chiseling Drink *(shū záo yǐn zi)*

SOURCE: *Formulas to Aid the Living* (1253)

Alismatis Rhizoma *(zé xiè)*
Phytolaccae Radix *(shāng lù)*
Phaseoli Semen *(chì xiǎo dòu)* (dry-fried)
Notopterygii Rhizoma seu Radix *(qiāng huó)* (nodes removed)
Arecae Pericarpium *(dà fù pí)*
Zanthoxyli Semen *(jiāo mù)*
Akebiae Caulis *(mù tōng)*
Gentianae macrophyllae Radix *(qín jiāo)* (reed removed)
Poriae Cutis *(fú líng pí)*
Arecae Semen *(bīng láng)*
    (all equal parts)

MODIFICATIONS OF DR. QIN'S FORMULA

This method is more effective with the addition of some qi-moving medicinals, especially if there has been no urination for eight hours. Consider the following:

Aucklandiae Radix *(mù xiāng)*	4.5g
Cinnamomi Ramulus *(guì zhī)*	4.5g

---

16. Indicated especially if there is slight pain during urination.

Scanty urination (need to increase the volume):

Plantaginis Semen *(chē qián zǐ)*. 9g

Leonuri Herba *(yì mǔ cǎo)*. 6g

Alismatis Rhizoma *(zé xiè)*. 6g

Bloating:

Aurantii Fructus immaturus *(zhǐ shí)* 6g

Arecae Pericarpium *(dà fù pí)*. 6g

Linderae Radix *(wū yào)*. 6g

▶ These all move and guide the qi downward, to assist in guiding out the water.

One can also use Ten-Jujube Decoction *(shí zǎo tāng)* from the *Discussion of Cold Damage.* Boil all the herbs with Jujubae Fructus *(dà zǎo)* for one hour. Then eat the Jujubae Fructus *(dà zǎo)* throughout the day. For example, take three in the morning, four in the afternoon, and four in the evening. Do not drink the decoction, as it can cause severe nausea, vomiting, and diarrhea. Although eating the Jujubae Fructus *(dà zǎo)* from this cooked formula will still cause diarrhea, it will be moderated, as this medicinal also helps tonify the Spleen.

External treatment:

Combine 3-4 small to medium size cloves of garlic with Moschus *(shè xiāng)* 0.1g or Caryophylli Flos *(dīng xiāng)* 0.5g into a paste. Put this paste on CV-8 *(shén què)* for two hours. This promotes urination. This can be used with the above herbs or by itself. One can use a tissue as a buffer if the patient's skin is sensitive.

QUESTIONS

1. *Is there a method by which one can use this formula for longer than just two days?*

   One strategy that will allow the use of this formula to be extended to a treatment period of up to two weeks is to alternate it with a tonifying formula. For example, give this formula for one day, then tonify the Spleen for 1-3 days (e.g., Six-Gentleman Decoction *(liù jūn zǐ tāng)*), depending on how severe the condition is.

2. *Can this formula be given in conjunction with aspiration of the fluid?*

   These patients will most likely be under hospital care, during which they are likely to have their fluids drained. Following this procedure, one can administer the formula the next day, because the fluid is likely to return. If they aspirate too much fluid too quickly, the patient can become weak, experience a decline in blood pressure, and even fall into a coma. These patients must have a diet of good, simple, light, and nutritious food. For example, rice congee is beneficial, and high protein foods like steamed egg are essential, because the extracted fluid is rich in protein and many nutrients.

5. Promote Sweating and Dispel Dampness (发汗祛湿 *fā hàn qū shī*)

[PRESENTATION] Dampness spreading into the muscles and skin and wind-water overflowing thin mucus

Spirodelae Herba *(fú píng)* 2.4g

prepared Ephedrae Herba *(zhì má huáng)* 2.4g

Notopterygii Rhizoma seu Radix *(qiāng huó)*/
    Angelicae pubescentis Radix *(dú huó)* . . . . 2.4g (each)

Atractylodis Rhizoma *(cāng zhú)*[17] 2.4g

Saposhnikoviae Radix *(fáng fēng)* 4.5g

Alismatis Rhizoma *(zé xiè)* 9g

Zingiberis Rhizomatis Cortex *(shēng jiāng pí)* 2.4g

COMMENTARY

ADDITIONAL SIGNS AND SYMPTOMS

- Fever (may be high) and chills
- Aversion to wind and drafts
- Absence of sweating
- Whole body floating edema
- Scanty urine
- Constipation

There may also be:

- Headache with a strong distending quality, but should not be severely painful
- Cough (which is not too loud)
- Heavy body
- Fatigue
- Swollen or painful joints or muscles (e.g., neck and back)
- On biomedical examination there may be white or red blood cells and/or protein in the urine.
- The pulse is floating
- The tongue has a thin, white, and greasy coating

Note: This pattern many times correlates with a biomedical diagnosis of an acute form of nephritis and is usually serious.

DISCUSSION

PATTERNS: The key feature is an *external contraction* that is accompanied by pernicious dampness (water swelling) in the muscle layer and skin. Wind-water is the most likely

---

17. The original text prescribed Atractylodis Rhizomatis Cortex *(cāng zhú pí)* 2.4g.

classical disease name for this pattern. However, it can also treat patterns of wind edema, overflowing thin mucus, and some conditions of skin edema (see question no. 3 below).

ETIOLOGY AND PATHODYNAMIC: The wind in wind-water refers to wind-cold. This cold pathogen contends with the protective qi and fetters the Lungs, which inhibits the normal circulation of Lung qi and results in swelling, mostly in the upper part of the body. There is usually no deficiency addressed by this method; however, there may be underlying deficiency.

This pattern often occurs after swimming or exposure to rain, which consequently leads to an exterior pattern. Although there is always an external component to this pattern, there are basically three possibilities:

1. External contraction of a wind-cold pathogen
2. External contraction of a damp pathogen that invades the *tài yáng*
3. Chronic edema with the further contraction of exterior wind-cold

TREATMENT PRINCIPLE: First and foremost, one should follow the *Inner Classic*'s direction, "Open the ghost gates, and completely cleanse the yang organs." Opening the ghost gates, about 80% of this formula, refers to promoting sweat by opening the pores, which will disperse the pathogen and vent the dampness. This is necessary because the pathogen resides in the exterior levels. Completely cleansing the yang organs refers to opening the bladder.

One should also abide by the adage, "Lift the pot and remove the lid." This refers to opening and diffusing the Lungs to free the lower orifices and promote urination. It is incorrect to solely use a drain-dampness method. Proper treatment can prevent the development of chronic nephritis.

PATIENT RECOMMENDATIONS

1. The patient should keep warm, especially the area around the kidneys, trying to actively prevent any potential for catching a cold, which can easily trigger a relapse.

   These patients need a diet low in salt and sweets, as well as good quality, easily absorbable protein. Their digestives systems are usually already impaired (Spleen qi deficiency). Consider the following two ideas.

   • **Tofu skin recipe:** Bring soy milk to a boil, cool, and use a stick to remove the layer that forms on top. Fresh is best. It has lots of protein and is very easy to digest

   • **Egg and meat pudding:** One can also grind up some small pieces of fish or meat and mix with one egg and some water. Steam all of this together for 20 minutes. Flavor to one's liking (e.g., soy sauce). This is also very easy to digest.

2. After treatment, the patient should not perform strenuous exercise for 3-6 months.

MEDICINAL ANALYSIS

Note: This formula should not be taken for a long period of time.

- Prepared Ephedrae Herba *(zhì má huáng)* (processed by water frying), Spirodelae Herba *(fú píng)*, and Zingiberis Rhizomatis Cortex *(shēng jiāng pí)* are acrid and warm and promote sweating, dissipate dampness, promote urination, and reduce swelling.

- Spirodelae Herba *(fú píng)* is very effective at removing dampness on the surface by promoting a sweat. It unblocks the waterways to promote urination and reduce swelling.

- Saposhnikoviae Radix *(fáng fēng)*, Notopterygii Rhizoma seu Radix *(qiāng huó)*, and Angelicae pubescentis Radix *(dú huó)* eliminate wind and prevail over dampness.

- Zingiberis Rhizomatis Cortex *(shēng jiāng pí)* is used because the peel promotes movement and eliminates water-dampness from the skin.

- Atractylodis Rhizoma *(cāng zhú)* is acrid, warm, and expels wind, cold, and dampness.

Dr. Qin's formula is based on Notopterygium Decoction to Overcome Dampness *(qiāng huó shèng shī tāng)* and Wondrous Atractylodes Decoction *(shén zhú tāng)*

Notopterygium Decoction to Overcome Dampness *(qiāng huó shèng shī tāng)*

SOURCE: *Clarifying Doubts about Damage from Internal and External Causes* (1247)

Notopterygii Rhizoma seu Radix *(qiāng huó)*	3g
Angelicae pubescentis Radix *(dú huó)*	3g
Ligustici Rhizoma *(gǎo běn)*	1.5g
Saposhnikoviae Radix *(fáng fēng)*	1.5g
Chuanxiong Rhizoma *(chuān xiōng)*	1.5g
Viticis Fructus *(màn jīng zǐ)*	0.9g
Glycyrrhizae Radix preparata *(zhì gān cǎo)*	1.5g

---

Wondrous Atractylodes Decoction *(shén zhú tāng)*

SOURCE: *Concise Cases of Yin Patterns* (1236)

Atractylodis Rhizoma *(cāng zhú)*	6g
Saposhnikoviae Radix *(fáng fēng)*	6g
Dry-fried Glycyrrhizae Radix *(chǎo gān cǎo)*	3g

---

MODIFICATIONS OF DR. QIN'S FORMULA

Severe headache:

Ligustici Rhizoma *(gǎo běn)*	4-6g
Viticis Fructus *(màn jīng zǐ)*	4-6g

Very obvious floating edema:

Benincasae Exocarpium *(dōng guā pí)*	6-9g
Plantaginis Semen *(chē qián zǐ)*	6-9g

Water-dampness in the interior:

Plantaginis Semen *(chē qián zǐ)*	4-6g
Stephaniae tetrandrae Radix *(hàn fáng jǐ)*	4-6g

QUESTIONS

1. *If this treatment method is only for external contraction (an excess pathogen), then how could it be appropriate for a chronic edema pattern with a wind-cold invasion?*

   Chronic edema patterns usually have some underlying deficiency and hence are not excessive. This method is not indicated for patterns of deficiency. It is primarily indicated for externally-contracted patterns of excess, and thus the herbs are all reducing and dispersing. However, sometimes a long-term problem caused by deficiency may need a short-term formula to evict a newly incoming pathogen. Of course, if the patient is obviously deficient, this strategy may be too strong. For this reason, the strategy should not be used for a long period of time in patients who have chronic edema.

2. *If there is only an external pattern, why does Dr. Qin include Alismatis Rhizoma (zé xiè)?*

   In this pattern, one will often see inhibited urination. This can be because of the Lungs' relationship to the Bladder, or because of a preexisting condition of dampness. Therefore, Alismatis Rhizoma *(zé xiè)* is used to drain fluid via the urine. However, if there is an external presentation with just edema and no inhibited urination, one may decide not to include Alismatis Rhizoma *(zé xiè)*. One should note that even with the removal of Alismatis Rhizoma *(zé xiè)*, many of the medicinals will have some ability to open the bladder and enable dampness to drain through the urine.

3. *I thought that skin edema and overflowing thin mucus are internal problems. How can this formula treat them?*

   Both of these disease categories can arise from internal deficiency. For example, skin edema can have its root cause in Spleen deficiency or Kidney yang deficiency. This strategy would therefore be inappropriate for these types. However, skin edema can also come about from the above-discussed etiologies. For example, for this formula to be appropriate there must be an external component. If wind-cold fetters the Lungs and causes edema, this method may be used regardless of whether there is a preexisting condition (e.g., deficiency); however, if the deficiency is severe, then short-term use or even a different strategy may be appropriate. With qi deficiency, one may decide to add Astragali Radix *(huáng qí)*. One cannot use this medicinal by itself because its ability to promote urination is mild. However, one may also include Poriae Cutis *(fú líng pí)* and Benincasae Exocarpium *(dōng guā pí)* to assist. These are all mild and do not damage the qi, and still utilize the idea of treating the skin with peels.

4. *If this is essentially an excess external wind-cold condition, then why would you use prepared Ephedrae Herba (zhì má huáng) instead of Ephedrae Herba (má huáng)?*

   If this were a simple wind-cold pathogen (excess presentation), then unprepared Ephedrae Herba *(má huáng)* would of course be appropriate. However, in this situation there are the complications of edema and dampness. If one releases the exterior too quickly, the dampness will be left behind. The appropriate method needs to be a bit more moderate and slow; therefore, Dr. Qin chooses to use prepared Ephedrae Herba *(zhì má huáng)*, whose diaphoretic properties are tempered by the processing.

---

6. Clear and Transform Damp-Heat (清化湿热 *qīng huà shī rè*)

[PRESENTATION] Dampness and heat intertwining and stagnating with each other, damp-heat [disorders] with dark urination

Armeniacae Semen *(xìng rén)*	9g
Pinelliae Rhizoma preparatum *(zhì bàn xià)*	4.5g
Amomi Fructus rotundus *(bái dòu kòu)*	2.4g
Talcum *(huá shí)*	9g
Coicis Semen *(yì yǐ rén)*	9g
Lophatheri Herba *(dàn zhú yè)*[18]	4.5g
Poria rubra *(chì fú líng)* / Polyporus *(zhū líng)*	9g each

COMMENTARY

ADDITIONAL SIGNS AND SYMPTOMS

This type of pattern has a wide range of presentations; however, here are three key aspects:

1. The condition has been ongoing for a long period of time.
2. The condition is not very serious and waxes and wanes. It is worse with humid weather and after the consumption of food and drink that generate dampness.
3. The pulse is soggy and the tongue is wet.

SECONDARY DIAGNOSTIC CLUES

- Cold hands and feet, however the central abdomen is warm.
- The palmar surface of the forearm is cold and sticky to the touch, but changes to being warm and sticky if pressure is maintained for a couple minutes (this is a sign of unsurfaced or contained fever). This area may also be moist.

THE FOLLOWING SYMPTOMS MAY OR MAY NOT BE PRESENT

- Fever that is usually chronic, low-grade, unsurfaced, generalized, and worse in the afternoons or summertime. There may be no fever in the evening, night, or morning.
- Complexion is usually dark, grey, and lacking luster. It looks dirty, as if the face had not been washed.
- Sweating does not resolve the condition and generally leaves the patient feeling fatigued. The sweat will be sticky.
- Skin is usually moist and slightly sticky.
- Fatigue may be extreme.

---

18. The original text prescribed fresh Lophateri Herba *(xiān zhú yè)* 4.5g.

- Generalized body heaviness (not severe) or pain
- Difficulty moving the limbs (due to a feeling of tightness or lack of desire)
- Numbness on the back
- Often feels like one is catching a cold.

HEAD

- Discharge from the eyes, unclear vision
- Tinnitus
- Loss of smell, congested sinuses
- Frequent but unproductive clearing of the throat
- Sticky or dry sensation in the mouth with a slightly bitter or sweet taste. Saliva may be sticky, thick, and/or profuse. Drinking may make the dryness worse, or patients may have no desire to drink.
- Dizziness or vertigo

IF THE DAMP-HEAT AFFECTS THE SPLEEN AND STOMACH, THE FOLLOWING WILL BE SEEN

- Poor digestion
- Chest and abdominal fullness, especially after eating
- Abdominal bloating and gas
- Nausea
- Poor appetite
- Frequent, loose, malodorous, sticky stools that are difficult to fully void and which may contain mucus

ADDITIONAL LOWER BURNER SYMPTOMS

- Hemorrhoids
- Difficult and dribbling urination with occasional burning
- Genital itching or discharge that is yellow and sticky
- Cloudy urination

Note: many of these symptoms—not just the fever—may become worse in the afternoon.

- The pulse is soggy, sticky, and rapid (especially if there is a fever). It may be floating and soft.
- The tongue has a pale, dark, swollen body with teeth marks and a dirty, sticky or wet, yellow, and greasy coating.

DISCUSSION

This common condition can manifest in a wide range of presentations. Although not serious, its manifestation can sometimes seem quite complex. Dampness and heat are the pathogens that result in the pattern called damp-heat. However, this method can also treat patterns that are not technically damp-heat. The formula associated with this method addresses equal amounts of dampness and heat.

Note: If the patient does not have dark urine, the main symptom listed above by Dr. Qin, it does not preclude the use of this formula. What we describe here is a larger presentation that more closely matches a broader-based Three-Seed Decoction *(sān rén tāng)* presentation. This differs from the other chapters where the chief symptom is usually essential for the pattern. Present or not, the chief symptom does tell us something significant about the pattern.

Although this formula is excellent for urinary conditions (e.g., infections and prostatitis), if there are no symptoms related to urination it would be best to remove or reduce the dosage of Poria rubra *(chì fú líng)* and Polyporus *(zhū líng)*. However, as one will recall, medicinals that drain dampness are an integral part of Three-Seed Decoction *(sān rén tāng)* and one may decide to use the lighter Tetrapanacis Medulla *(tōng cǎo)*.

DURATION: This is usually a chronic presentation that progresses slowly and is thus slow and difficult to cure. However, this method may be used for some acute presentations.

LOCATION: The damp-heat is primarily in both the superficial and deep collaterals at the qi aspect of the organs and limbs. It can also be conceptualized as located throughout the entire body (e.g. all three burners, channels and collaterals, and interstices of the flesh), or lodged in the *shào yáng*.

ETIOLOGY: Environment, diet, and constitutional Spleen deficiency. All factors can occur at the same time.

PATHODYNAMIC: Dampness is a yin pathogen and heat is a yang pathogen. When they intertwine and stagnate together, they block the qi dynamic and thus restrict the normal flow of yang.

TREATMENT PRINCIPLE: Besides clearing and transforming damp-heat, one should:

1. Diffuse and open the qi dynamic and qi transformation, which transforms dampness.
2. Lightly clear and facilitate the resolution of damp-heat.

Depending on which pathogen is more prevalent, one should either emphasize clearing (of heat) or transforming (of dampness). One should not use overly-drying medicinals for dampness that is accompanied by heat.

One should start out by taking one bag a day, then switch to one bag every two days. Finally, one can switch over to drafts. The treatment should last at least 2-4 weeks, during which time gradual improvement should be seen.

MEDICINAL ANALYSIS

CHIEF HERBS

Upper burner: Armeniacae Semen *(xìng rén)* is acrid and opens and circulates the Lung qi in order to dissipate dampness. Armeniacae Semen amarum *(kǔ xìng rén)* is best for this purpose.

Middle burner: Amomi Fructus rotundus *(bái dòu kòu)* is warm, awakens the Spleen, and increases circulation in order to transform dampness. It should be crushed and added in the last 3-5 minutes of cooking.

Lower burner: Coicis Semen *(yì yǐ rén)* is cool and promotes urination in order to facilitate the resolution of dampness. It not only enters the organs, but can also guide the effects of the formula into the collaterals and minute channels.

Together, these three medicinals promote circulation in all three burners, increasing the body's ability to eliminate dampness.

ASSISTANTS

- Lophatheri Herba *(dàn zhú yè)* is light, clears heat, and vents dampness. It also enters the collaterals, guiding the chief herbs through all the channels and collaterals.

- Pinelliae Rhizoma preparatum *(zhì bàn xià)* is bitter, enabling it to descend. It is acrid and warm, enabling it to disperse, open, and expel. It mildly dries dampness and works on the organ level (versus the channels and collaterals).

- Talcum *(huá shí)* is sweet, bland, and cool, leaching out dampness and cooling heat. It is slippery and thus especially good for difficult urination with heat (e.g., cloudy, burning).

- Poria rubra *(chì fú líng)* clears heat and dampness from the blood aspect and minute channels via urination. There is no need to use Poria *(fú líng)* or Poriae Cutis *(fú líng pí)* because there is no need to tonify.

- Polyporus *(zhū líng)* clears heat and dampness through the urine. This is a strong diuretic.

- This is a very flexible formula that can be adjusted according to which burner is most affected, as well as the ratio of heat to dampness. This may be as simple as changing the dosages or modifying the formula (see below). Usually, all three burners are affected, as well as the deep channels and collaterals.

Dr. Qin's formula is based on Three-Seed Decoction *(sān rén tāng)* and Polyporus Decoction *(zhū líng tāng)*. It is very mild and light. It contains no herbs that promote sweating, directly clear heat, or overly dry dampness.

Three-Seed Decoction *(sān rén tāng)*

SOURCE: *Systematic Differentiation of Warm Pathogen* (1798)

Armeniacae Semen *(xìng rén)* 15g
Amomi Fructus rotundus *(bái dòu kòu)*. 6g
Magnoliae officinalis Cortex *(hòu pò)* 6g
Pinelliae Rhizoma preparatum *(zhì bàn xià)* 9g
Coicis Semen *(yì yǐ rén)* 18g
Tetrapanacis Medulla *(tōng cǎo)* 6g
Lophatheri Herba *(dàn zhú yè)* 6g
Talcum *(huá shí)* 18g

Polyporus Powder (*zhū líng sān*)

SOURCE: *Essentials from the Golden Cabinet* (c. 220)

Polyporus (*zhū líng*)
Poria (*fú líng*)
Atractylodis macrocephalae Rhizoma (*bái zhú*)
  (equal amounts)

MODIFICATIONS OF DR. QIN'S FORMULA

Nausea:

Ginger-prepared Bambusae Caulis in taeniam (*jiāng zhú rú*) 4.5g

Bloating and gas in the epigastrium:

Magnoliae officinalis Cortex (*hòu pò*) 4.5g

Arecae Pericarpium (*dà fù pí*) 6g

Upper burner involvement/exterior condition (such as fever, chills/aversion to wind):

Sojae Semen germinatum (*dà dòu juǎn*) 9g

Sojae Semen preparatum (*dàn dòu chǐ*) 9g

▶ Do not use medicinals such as Schizonepetae Herba (*jīng jiè*)
  because they are too dispersing

▶ Eupatorii Herba (*pèi lán*) or Pogostemonis/Agastaches Herba (*huò xiāng*) can also be considered (see question no. 3 below).

Difficult urination:

Tetrapanacis Medulla (*tōng cǎo*) 3g

Downcast and dispirited, stifled and depressed mood, and muddleheadedness:

Acori tatarinowii Rhizoma (*shí chāng pǔ*) 4.5g

Curcumae Radix (*yù jīn*) 4.5g

Frequently feels hot with a bitter taste and sticky sensation in the mouth:

Arisaema cum Bile (*dǎn nán xīng*) 4.5g

QUESTIONS

1. *What is the difference between this formula and Three-Seed Decoction (sān rén tāng) and why does Dr. Qin remove Magnoliae officinalis Cortex (hòu pò) and Tetrapanacis Medulla (tōng cǎo)?*

   Three-Seed Decoction *(sān rén tāng)* treats a damp-heat pattern that is more dampness than heat. This pattern, though, has equal degrees of dampness and heat. Thus Magnoliae officinalis Cortex *(hòu pò)* is removed because it is too warm and Tetrapanacis Medulla *(tōng cǎo)* is removed because it is too light. Both may be added back into the formula if needed (see modifications for this formula above). However, as with any modification, one should be aware of how it changes the overall formula. For example, knowing that

Dr. Qin removed Magnoliae officinalis Cortex *(hòu pò)* because of its warmth demonstrates how it will affect the formula if added back in for the modification "bloating and gas in the epigastrium." Therefore, to preserve the thermal nature of the formula, one may decide to add an additional cooling medicinal.

2. *Why is dark urine listed as a main symptom when Three-Seed Decoction (sān rén tāng) can be used for a large array of systemic symptoms?*

Dr. Qin uses this key symptom to draw attention to the two key aspects, heat and the lower burner. Although this formula is based on Three-Seed Decoction *(sān rén tāng)*, Dr. Qin's changes (the addition of Poria rubra *(chì fú líng)* and Polyporus *(zhū líng)*) direct the focus of the formula to the lower burner. Thus the pattern is more likely to have some urinary problems. There is also more heat in this pattern than for the Three-Seed Decoction *(sān rén tāng)* pattern. Regardless, this formula may be used to treat a wide variety of symptoms.

3. *What is the rationale behind the above modifications for external involvement?*

When there is dampness with an external pathogen, one must be careful not to release the exterior too quickly, otherwise the dampness will linger behind. Thus stronger medicinals such as Schizonepetae Herba *(jīng jiè)* are contraindicated. By contrast, Sojae Semen germinatum *(dà dòu juǎn)* is very light and mild, with only a minor ability to induce a sweat. Sojae Semen preparatum *(dàn dòu chǐ)* is also mild and has a tonifying quality and can be used when there is underlying Spleen qi deficiency. One can use both of these together.

Eupatorii Herba *(pèi lán)* and Pogostemonis/Agastaches Herba *(huò xiāng)* are also possible modifications. They enter the Spleen and Stomach and are able to expel dampness upward and outward, especially in the upper burner. However, because long-term dampness usually enters the Spleen collaterals, the soybeans are preferred because they are able to enter the deep collaterals. By contrast, Eupatorii Herba *(pèi lán)* and Pogostemonis/Agastaches Herba *(huò xiāng)* enter the superficial collaterals.

4. *What seemingly appropriate approaches are contraindicated for this pattern?*

- Acrid, warm, release the exterior medicinals will cause a rising up and counterflow steaming, which can impair consciousness.

- If there is a concurrent external presentation and one uses formulas such as Honeysuckle and Forsythia Powder *(yín qiáo sǎn)* or Mulberry Leaf and Chrysanthemum Drink *(sāng jú yǐn)*, they can make the dampness stickier as they are overly cold and acrid. Not only will the fever not come down and other exterior symptoms increase, but the nausea and vomiting will become more severe, the head will become heavy and painful, and the digestion will get worse.

- Patchouli/Agastache Powder to Rectify the Qi *(huò xiāng zhèng qì sǎn)* can cause a temporary reduction in a fever by producing a mild sweat; however, the fever will return (sometimes higher) the next day. This formula works too superficially to be appropriate for this pattern.

- Strong descending (or purging) medicinals can cause the Spleen qi to sink and lead to diarrhea.

- If one uses an enriching, cooling formula to treat symptoms mistakenly attributed to yin deficiency, the pathogen will become more solidified and tangled up and therefore more difficult to unravel.

- If one merely uses cooling medicinals, the dampness will not be transformed.

- Hot medicinals, such as Cinnamomi Ramulus *(guì zhī)* or Ephedrae Herba *(má huáng)*, can give rise to fire-toxin and lead to loss of consciousness.

5. *If this is a heat-based pattern, why does it include cold hands and feet and a craving for warm beverages?*

The cold hands and feet are from dampness blocking the qi dynamic, preventing the yang qi from reaching outward. Oftentimes, there is a subjective sense of internal heat, or an objective feeling of heat upon palpation. This is not unlike a Frigid Extremities Powder *(sì nì sǎn)* pattern. Damp-heat patients often crave warm beverages because the warmth disperses the dampness and brings some relief, whereas cold beverages will produce further congealing.

6. *Why does Dr. Qin use Coicis Semen (yì yǐ rén) instead of dry-fried Coicis Semen (chǎo yì yǐ rén)?*

In previous methods, where there is dampness, dry-fried Coicis Semen *(chǎo yì yǐ rén)* is used because it is better at drying dampness and strengthening the Spleen. However, in this case one wants to facilitate the resolution of dampness, and promote movement in the channels and collaterals, and not tonify. In addition, Coicis Semen *(yì yǐ rén)* is cooler than dry-fried Coicis Semen *(chǎo yì yǐ rén)*, making it more suitable for conditions that have both dampness and heat.

10

Treatment Guidelines for

Dryness 燥 *(zào)*

NATURE

The yin aspect is parched and consumed.

The yin aspect includes body fluids, blood, and yin. Both deep and superficial patterns can belong to the yin aspect, including patterns of Spleen yin deficiency, Stomach fluid deficiency, or just loss of fluids due to excessive sweating.

PATHODYNAMIC

The Lungs contract scorching fire, yang fluids are expended in the upper burner and are unable to irrigate the body and unable to supply nourishment to the hundred bones; the complexion is dry and without moisture or luster.

Both internal and external influences can lead to Lung heat or fire. This, in turn, can damage the Lung's yin, fluids, and qi. The Lungs lose their ability to transport and this leads to systemic dryness (e.g., organs, hair, and skin).

A serious disease that takes too great a toll, inappropriate administration of drying and tonifying yang formulas, or excessive ingestion of alcohol, meat, or spicy-hot foods, especially contribute to pathogenic fire. This damages the true yin and simmers, such that the blood and fluids become debilitated and consumed.

This "serious disease" is usually a warm disease or *yáng míng* type disease that has excessive heat/fire. There may be bleeding or high fever, etc. Furthermore, apart from the above-mentioned foods, lifestyle choices such as smoking cigarettes or marijuana can all increase heat and damage the fluids.

LOCATION

Exterior: Chapped or cracked skin
Upper: Dry throat and nose

The mouth may also be affected (e.g., lack of saliva).

Middle: Water and yin fluids are sapped and sparse with irritability and thirst.

There may also be hunger and increased urination.

Lower: Gastrointestinal fluids are withered and dried up with difficult bowel movements.

There may also be bloating and gas. While any type of constipation can be accompanied by focal distention and fullness, excess patterns are marked by focal distention, fullness, and dry, hard, painful stools. Since this is a case of deficiency stagnation, the pain, hardness, and severe stool dryness will be missing. Similarly, this pattern should not have burning anus or strongly malodorous stools.

Lungs: Dry cough with clumped phlegm
Womb: Melancholy with a desire to cry

This can occur in perimenopausal syndrome or restless organ disorder.

Hands and feet: Weathered, frail, and weak

There may be heaviness or atrophy. This can occur is such serious conditions as multiple sclerosis.

Vessels: Thin, rough, and faint pulse

If there is dryness in the vessels, one can feel it in the pulse. This may manifest like other dryness patterns and have typical symptoms like dryness of the skin and hair, and thirst. However, there may also be manifestations such as numbness (e.g., carpal tunnel) or pain in the vessels themselves.

TREATMENT METHOD

Sweet and cold medicinals moisten these problems. The main types of medicinals to use are those that clear, moisten, are sweet, and cold.

To nourish the yin fluids of the Lungs and Stomach, one's first choice is to use sweet and cold flavors. Furthermore, in order to enrich the essence of the Liver and Kidneys, one should use salty and cold medicinals. Acrid-hot, bitter-cold, bland-percolating, and aromatic medicinals are generally used to drain excess and should not be used for dryness.

This chapter not only addresses yin deficiency but also fluid deficiency, which is a common scenario in modern clinical situations. For example, if one sees back ache and weak joints with a thin, weak, and *hard* pulse, consider dryness, not just painful obstruction (wind-cold-dampness). Restless leg syndrome (RLS) is also a common complaint that often has an aspect of dryness. Dryness, however, can occur with other pathogens and one must consider the ratios appropriately.

For example, heat commonly occurs with dryness or yin deficiency. In such situations, one should refrain from using strong heat-clearing medicinals such as Coptidis Rhizoma *(huáng lián)*, Scutellariae Radix *(huáng qín)*, and Phellodendri Cortex *(huáng bǎi)*. These are too dry and will further damage the yin. However, there are always exceptions when one can use these medicinals, especially if the heat is severe. In general, though, one should focus on sweet, cool, and moist medicinals. It is also not uncommon for dampness or phlegm to accompany dryness. This is a complex pattern where methods from this chapter should be combined with others in the book.

1. Moisten the Upper and Clear Dryness (润上清燥 *rùn shàng qīng zào*)

[PRESENTATION] Heart and Lungs contract dryness; dry cough, irritability, and thirst

Glehniae Radix *(běi shā shēn)*	4.5g
Armeniacae Semen dulce *(tián xìng rén)*	9g
Ophiopogonis Radix *(mài mén dōng)*	6g
Fritillariae cirrhosae Bulbus *(chuān bèi mǔ)*	6g
Mume Fructus *(wū méi)*	3 pieces
Trichosanthis Radix *(tiān huā fěn)*	9g
Fresh Pyri Exocarpium *(lí pí)*	9g

COMMENTARY

ADDITIONAL SIGNS AND SYMPTOMS

- In addition to a dry cough there may also be dried phlegm that is difficult to expectorate.
- Loss of voice, low voice, or hoarse voice
- Cracked lips
- Bitter taste
- Palpitations
- Insomnia
- Restlessness
- Shortness of breath
- Overall sensation of warmth
- There may also be symptoms that manifest in the other burners, for example, scanty urination, dry constipation, and a constant sense of hunger with an inability to eat much.
- The pulse is thin, slightly choppy, slightly rapid, and dry. The distal pulse is more choppy, thin, and dry.

- The tongue has a dry and red body with cracks (sometimes on the tip) with a scanty coating.

DISCUSSION

ETIOLOGY: This presentation can occur from dry environmental or climatic influences (especially common in the autumn), or from internally-generated dryness such as from the excessive consumption of spicy and fried foods.

TREATMENT PRINCIPLE: Moisten the upper burner, tonify the Lung yin, clear dryness, and stop the coughing.

MEDICINAL ANALYSIS

- Glehniae/Adenophorae Radix *(shā shēn)*, Ophiopogonis Radix *(mài mén dōng)*, and Trichosanthis Radix *(tiān huā fěn)* all generate yang fluids, nourish yin fluids, and clear yin-fluid deficient heat from the upper burner.

- Armeniacae Semen dulce *(tián xìng rén)* moistens the Lungs and Large Intestine, stops coughing, and is suitable for deficiency cough. If unavailable, one can substitute raw Pruni Amygdali Semen *(bā dàn xìng rén)* 9g (American almond),[1] which is more moistening than Armeniacae Semen dulce *(tián xìng rén)*.

- Fritillariae cirrhosae Bulbus *(chuān bèi mǔ)* is sweet and cool. It strongly moistens dryness, tonifies Lung yin, and stops coughing. It lightly clears the Lung heat. Three grams of powdered Fritillariae cirrhosae Bulbus *(chuān bèi mǔ)* dissolved into the strained decoction can be used instead of the 6g noted above.

- Mume Fructus *(wū méi)* is excellent at generating yang fluids and is suitable for upper, middle, and lower dryness patterns.

- Fresh Pyri Exocarpium *(xiān lí pí)* is sweet and cold. It clears and moistens dryness and generates yang fluids. The skin from one Asian pear should be washed and boiled with the other medicinals and then the pear should be eaten.

Dr. Qin's formula is based on Mulberry Leaf and Apricot Kernel Decoction *(sāng xìng tāng)* and Glehnia and Ophiopogonis Decoction *(shā shēn mài mén dōng tāng)*

Mulberry Leaf and Apricot Kernel Decoction *(sāng xìng tāng)*
SOURCE: *Systematic Differentiation of Warm Pathogen Diseases* (1798)

Mori Folium *(sāng yè)*	3g
Gardeniae Fructus *(zhī zǐ)*	3g
Sojae Semen preparatum *(dàn dòu chǐ)*	3g
Armeniacae Semen *(xìng rén)*	4.5g
Fritillariae thunbergii Bulbus *(zhè bèi mǔ)*	3g
Glehniae/Adenophorae Radix *(shā shēn)*	6g
Pyri Exocarpium *(lí pí)*	3g

---

1. It is sweet and balanced, moistens the Lungs, stops coughing, transforms phlegm, and causes the qi to descend.

Glehnia and Ophiopogonis Decoction (*shā shēn mài mén dōng tāng*)

SOURCE: *Systematic Differentiation of Warm Pathogen Diseases* (1798)

Glehniae/Adenophorae Radix (*shā shēn*) 9g
Ophiopogonis Radix (*mài mén dōng*) 9g
Polygonati odorati Rhizoma (*yù zhú*) 6g
Mori Folium (*sāng yè*) 4.5g
Trichosanthis Radix (*tiān huā fěn*) 4.5g
Lablab Semen album (*biǎn dòu*) 4.5g
Glycyrrhizae Radix (*gān cǎo*) 3g

MODIFICATIONS OF DR. QIN'S FORMULA

In general, one may choose to add Lophatheri Herba (*dàn zhú yè*) and Imperatae Rhizoma (*bái máo gēn*), which are sweet and cold and able to clear heat and generate yang fluids. However, even though there may be heat, one should not use bitter, cold medicinals because these can induce the formation of more dryness and forcefully remove the yang fluids.

Burning, dark, or scanty urine:

Imperatae Rhizoma *(bái máo gēn)* 6g
Phragmitis Rhizoma *(lú gēn)* 6g
Lophatheri Herba *(dàn zhú yè)* 4.5g

Dry and hoarse voice:

Chebulae Fructus *(hē zǐ)* . . . . 4.5g (chronic)
Galli Membrana Ovi *(fèng huáng yī)*[2] 1.5g

A feeling of phlegm stuck in the throat (with or without
actual phlegm), and scratchy throat:

Bambusae Concretio silicea *(tiān zhú huáng)* 4.5g
Lilii Bulbus *(bǎi hé)* 6g

Voice easily lost or hoarse:

Sterculiae lychnophorae Semen *(pàng dà hǎi)* 3p
Glycyrrhizae Radix *(gān cǎo)* 3g

Menopause with dry mouth, thirst, insomnia, and dry tongue:

Tritici Fructus *(xiǎo mài)* 9g
Ligustri lucidi Fructus *(nǚ zhēn zǐ)* 6g

FOOD THERAPY

1. Five-Juice Drink (*wǔ zhī yǐn*)

   Nelumbinis Nodus Succus *(ǒu zhī)*, Eleocharitis Succus *(bí qi zhī)*,[3] Phragmitis Rhizomatis Succus *(lú gēn zhī)*, Pyri Succus *(lí zhī)*, and Ophiopogonis Succus *(mài mén dōng zhī)*.

---

2. See Ch. 1, p. 12, n. 7 for more details.

3. Patients can make this water chestnut, Eleocharitis Rhizoma *(bí qi)*, juice for themselves. Remove the tops, clean, cut into small pieces, and grind into liquid. It does not have to be peeled.

Use 50g of each, and as much as 200g, then combine with 50% water.

This is from *Systematic Differentiation of Warm Pathogen Diseases* and was originally indicated for the aftermath of high fever with severe dryness.

If these ingredients are unavailable, one can make a drink based on other juices, such as watermelon juice, tomato juice, daikon juice, cucumber juice, and celery juice. Take about eight ingredients and make a juice. However, do not use orange, pineapple, or mango juices because they are too warm. If desired, some grapefruit juice could be added for taste because it is cool. Note that apple and carrot juices are neutral; cherry, grape, raspberry, and strawberry juices are slightly warm. Also consider adding medicinals such as Menthae haplocalycis Herba recens *(xiān bò hé)* or two pieces of Mume Fructus *(wū méi)* (dried or soaked in water with the pulp cut off).

2. Fritillariae and Pear *(chuan bèi lí)* (see Ch. 5, p. 119, for preparation instructions).

QUESTIONS

1. If this is dryness in the upper burner, why do quite a few of the listed symptoms belong to the lower burner?

The presence of dryness in a specific burner does not mean that the other burners are unaffected. It means that the principal manifestation occurs in that burner. However, dryness is usually systemic, therefore it is not uncommon for there also to be dryness in the lower burner when the upper burner is mainly affected. One can explain this in many ways. For example, Lung dryness can transfer to Large Intestine dryness. When one sees obvious involvement of different areas of the body, one can add medicinals to address each of the areas. For example, with dryness in the Large Intestine, one may add Trichosanthis Semen *(guā lóu rén)* or Cannabis Semen *(huǒ má rén)*.

2. What is the difference between Lung fluid deficiency and Lung yin deficiency?

Both patterns are similar and can be hard to differentiate, although they require slightly different treatment strategies and have a different prognosis. Simply speaking, Lung fluid deficiency is milder and more superficial than Lung yin deficiency. The former manifests as dry mouth, thirst, and dry cough. It often occurs as part of an acute presentation, for example, after a high fever, heavy sweat, intense exercise, or working in a hot environment. It is easy to rebuild.

The more severe Lung yin deficiency incorporates Lung fluid deficiency. It will have more systemic symptoms such as afternoon or night fevers, night sweating, steaming bone syndrome, and heat in the five centers. There is also usually difficulty digesting food and drink. It typically does not appear suddenly, but comes about from a chronic disease or a long-term disorder. If yin deficiency becomes too severe, yin tonics alone will not suffice (see also question no. 6 below, the discussion of Sjögren's syndrome).

Dry mouth is a common distinguishing symptom. In Lung yin deficiency the mouth is drier at night but one is unable to drink much.[4] By contrast, in a pattern of fluid defi-

---

4. This is because in yin deficiency it is difficult to nourish the body with water; the body simply cannot absorb the

ciency the mouth will be dry all day and one will be able to drink much more. It should be remembered that many 'dry' symptoms can occur secondarily to other patterns. For example, dampness may cause signs of dryness, such as thirst. One must consider the whole picture before starting to nourish the fluids.

Three common causes of dry mouth:

Fluid deficiency: can drink large amounts of water; may also have dry tongue with cracks

Yin deficiency: cannot drink too much; worse at night

Internal dampness ('false dryness'): the mouth will feel dry, yet the tongue may be wet and/or sticky [5]

---

3. *There seem to be heat signs mentioned above. What is the pathodynamic of this heat?*

Dr. Qin mentions irritability and thirst as chief symptoms. In addition, one may have restlessness, insomnia, sore throat, as well as dry eyes and mouth. This all suggest the involvement of heat. However, this is not excess heat or a heat pathogen that must be removed by strong medicinals such as Coptidis Rhizoma *(huáng lián)* or Scutellariae Radix *(huáng qín)*. Such medicinals will exacerbate the problem, as this heat is from dryness. For example, as dryness reduces the fluids, the fluids are unable to cool the body; this, in turn, leads to a relatively hot presentation. Thus, in general, the medicinals in Dr. Qin's formula are cooling (clearing heat) and moistening. Apart from patterns of cool dryness, dryness will almost always lead to some relative heat signs.

4. *Why is Chebulae Fructus (hē zǐ) recommended for dry and hoarse voice instead of other typical herbs such as Schisandrae Fructus (wǔ wèi zǐ) or Oroxyli Semen (mù hú dié)?*

Chebulae Fructus *(hē zǐ)* is best used for chronic cough and has the ability to hold in liquids, which helps the dry and hoarse voice. Oroxyli Semen *(mù hú dié)* works too superficially for this type of pattern, but could be used for an acute pattern. Schisandrae Fructus *(wǔ wèi zǐ)* can work synergistically with Ophiopogonis Radix *(mài mén dōng)*, and can be used if there is also Heart yin deficiency (e.g., palpitations).

5. *Can one use Armeniacae Semen amarum (kǔ xìng rén) instead of Armeniacae Semen dulce (tián xìng rén)?*

Armeniacae Semen amarum *(kǔ xìng rén)* is slightly bitter, slightly sweet, warm, and diffuses, scatters, and directs the Lung qi downward. It is also somewhat toxic and is inappropriate in this situation. Armeniacae Semen dulce *(tián xìng rén)* is superior because it has no scattering/diffusing nature.

---

liquid.

5. Many times this corresponds to a pattern of internal dampness with external dryness. For example, there may be dry skin, finger or feet cracking and bleeding. This is dampness in the channels, which blocks the movement of qi and fluids.

6. Can this method treat the autoimmune disorder Sjörgen's syndrome?

Sjögren's syndrome is a condition with the hallmark signs of dryness, such as dry mouth and dry eyes. The dryness can be very severe, where eating one piece of bread might require two cups of water. However, even such a severe dry pattern can arise from either *real dryness* or *false dryness*, and must be differentiated. Damp-heat is one possibility of false dryness and can manifest like severe dryness. However, it will have differentiating signs such as a bitter taste, burning tongue and gums, yellow, dry tongue coating, dark urine, constipation, and a soggy and rapid pulse.

A true dryness pattern is one with actual fluid and yin deficiency. Although it may seem similar to the signs and symptoms that are appropriate to this method, one must be careful when dryness becomes extreme. Even though the dryness looks very severe, one cannot be overly aggressive and use sticky and heavy medicinals such as Rehmanniae Radix *(shēng dì huáng)*, Rehmanniae Radix preparata *(shú dì huáng)*, Testudinis Plastrum *(guī bǎn)*, and Polygoni multiflori Radix *(hé shǒu wū)*. This will damage the qi mechanism, which is already compromised. This lack of function prevents fluids from being properly distributed throughout the body. Even using Qin's Moisten the Upper and Clear Dryness formula (above) may be too much when the dryness is severe.

Therefore, in such a case, one should only lightly tonify the body fluids, using mild medicinals to assist the qi mechanism combined with moistening medicinals. For example, consider Lophatheri Herba *(dàn zhú yè)* 4.5g, Lablab Testa *(biǎn dòu yī)* 3g, Tetrapanacis Medulla *(tōng cǎo)* 1g, Eupatorii Folium *(pèi lán yè)* 4.5g, Lycopi Herba *(zé lán)* 3g, Nelumbinis Folium *(hé yè)* 4.5g, Mori Folium *(sāng yè)* 6g, Pseudostellariae Radix *(tài zǐ shēn)* 6g, Ecliptae Herba *(mò hàn lián)* 4.5g, Glehniae/Adenophorae Radix *(shā shēn)* 6g, Dendrobii Herba *(shí hú)* 6g, Phragmitis Rhizoma *(lú gēn)* 9g, Trichosanthis Radix *(tiān huā fěn)* 6g, Scrophulariae Radix *(xuán shēn)* 4.5g—1 bag per day. Boil for 10-15 minutes in 2 liters of water and drink all day. Such a pattern usually has only a slightly red, tender tongue (like a baby's tongue), but with cracks and the presence of an insipid taste. The pulse is thin, soft, and weak.

---

2. Moisten the Middle and Clear Dryness (润中清燥 *rùn zhōng qīng zào*)

[PRESENTATION] Spleen and Stomach contract dryness; wasting and thirsting disorder accompanied by being easily hungry

Rehmanniae Radix *(shēng dì huáng)*[6]	9g
Anemarrhenae Rhizoma *(zhī mǔ)*	9g
Dendrobii Herba *(shí hú)*[7]	9g
Trichosanthis Radix *(tiān huā fěn)*	9g
Polygonati odorati Rhizoma *(yù zhú)*	9g

---

6. The original text prescribed Rehmanniae Radix recens *(xiān dì huáng)* 9g.

7. The original text prescribed Dendrobii Herba recens *(xiān shí hú)* 9g.

Phragmitis Rhizoma *(lú gēn)*[8] 9g
Sacchari Caulis Succus (sugar cane juice) *(gān zhè zhī)* . . . . 1 cup

COMMENTARY

ADDITIONAL SIGNS AND SYMPTOMS

- Thirst and dry mouth
- Fever
- Restlessness
- Unclear or poor vision
- Vertigo or dizziness
- Burping, hiccough, reflux
- Frequent urination
- Constipation
- The pulse is thin, choppy, with a deeper right middle position. The pulse may also be jumpy and rapid.
- The tongue has a dry, cracked, red body with a dry, yellow coating and possibly patches without any coating.

MEDICINAL ANALYSIS

- Rehmanniae Radix *(shēng dì huáng)* is sweet, bitter, and cold, enriches and moistens the yin and fluids, and clears Stomach heat in order to moisten dryness.

- Anemarrhenae Rhizoma *(zhī mǔ)* and Phragmitis Rhizoma *(lú gēn)* are sweet, moist, and cool to cold, and are able to generate fluids.

- Anemarrhenae Rhizoma *(zhī mǔ)* is also bitter and enters the Stomach and Kidney. It enriches the yin, directs fire downward, moistens dryness, and lubricates the Intestines. It is usually used when there is more severe heat.

- Phragmitis Rhizoma *(lú gēn)* is mild, not cloying, generates fluids, and does not have the disadvantage of constraining the pathogen. It clears heat on the qi level and works more superficially than Dendrobii Herba *(shí hú)*.

- Dendrobii Herba *(shí hú)*, Trichosanthis Radix *(tiān huā fěn)*, and Polygonati odorati Rhizoma *(yù zhú)* are excellent medicinals for generating yang fluids.

- Dendrobii Herba *(shí hú)* nourishes the Stomach, alleviates thirst, and moistens dryness. It is best for chronic or late-stage illnesses. If unavailable, one can substitute Glehniae Radix *(běi shā shēn)*.

- Polygonati odorati Rhizoma *(yù zhú)* is sweet, neutral, and slightly cool, and is especially important for cases of swift digestion accompanied by being easily hungry and dry mouth and thirst. It is not very cloying.

---

8. The original text prescribed Phragmitis Rhizoma recens *(xiān lú gēn)* 30g.

- Trichosanthis Radix *(tiān huā fěn)* is bitter, cool, moist, and clears heat.

- Sacchari Caulis Succus *(gān zhè zhī)* is able to promote the flow in the Large Intestine and drain heat; it should be added to the boiled herbs. If unavailable, one can substitute Eleocharitis Rhizoma *(bí qí)* 9 pieces. One can also use 5 pieces of canned water chestnuts. Wash the water chestnuts well, removing and discarding all the juice from the can, then grind into a liquid and add to the boiled herbs.

MODIFICATIONS OF DR. QIN'S FORMULA

High fever, sensation of burning heat, prone to sweating, with a floating and forceful pulse and a red tongue with a yellow coating:

Gypsum fibrosum *(shí gāo)* 9g

Glauberitum *(hán shuǐ shí)* 9g

▶ One will usually give 1-2 bags of this formula to reduce heat, even with very deficient patients, such as those with HIV or leukemia.

Strong appetite accompanied by being easily hungry, red tongue, dry yellow coating, and constipation:

Bubali Cornu *(shuǐ niú jiǎo)* 15-30g

Steamed Rhei Radix et Rhizoma *(shú dà huáng)* 4-6g
 (if constipation is severe)

FOOD THERAPY

- Beancurd or soybean milk[9]
- Jellied beancurd *(dòu fǔ huā):* best eaten at slightly higher than body temperature, which allows for better absorption
- Herba Dendrobii Officinalis *(tiě pí shí hú)* and/or Panacis quinquefolii Radix *(xī yáng shēn):* no more than 2g/day

---

3. Moisten the Lower and Clear Dryness (润下清燥 *rùn xià qīng zào*)

[PRESENTATION] Liver, Kidneys, and Large Intestine contract dryness; frail, withered, and weak legs and clumping of the stool

Rehmanniae Radix *(shēng dì huáng)*[10] 9g

Asparagi Radix *(tiān mén dōng)* 9g

Scrophulariae Radix *(xuán shēn)* 9g

Paeoniae Radix alba *(bái sháo)* 9g

Cistanches Herba *(ròu cōng róng)* 6g

Cannabis Semen *(huǒ má rén)* 6g

Trichosanthis Fructus *(quán guā lóu)* 9g

---

9. Note that while cow's milk is warm, soymilk is cool and moistening.

10. The original text prescribed Rehmanniae Radix recens *(xiān dì huáng)* 9g.

COMMENTARY

ADDITIONAL SIGNS AND SYMPTOMS

- Overall dryness (e.g., hair, eyes, and skin, which may be so severe as to resemble tree bark)
- Skin that lacks luster
- Emaciated body and general body weakness (especially lower limb weakness and atrophy)
- Poor appetite and digestion
- Sore gums and loose teeth
- Insomnia
- Restlessness
- Night sweats
- Tinnitus, dizziness, and tremors (see questions below)
- Burning pain on the sole of the foot
- Lower back pain
- Scanty menstrual period
- Constipation (often 3-7 days without a bowel movement)
- Frequent and scanty urination
- The pulse is thin, rapid, and lacks strength; especially weak in the proximal positions.
- The tongue is dark red with cracks and has only a scanty amount of fluids.

DISCUSSION

LOCATION AND PATTERN: Apart from the above-mentioned organs, the Bladder may also be affected. This is essentially a Liver and Kidney fluid, yin, and sometimes essence deficiency that affects the Large Intestine and Bladder.

ETIOLOGY AND DURATION: This usually follows from a long-term illness or sometimes more quickly from events such as chemotherapy or radiation treatment.

TREATMENT PRINCIPLE: Tonify the fluids, yin, and essence and moisten the Large Intestine. The latter aspect is often said to "increase the water to sail the boat" (refloat a grounded ship) because "without water, the boat stops."

MEDICINAL ANALYSIS

- All of the medicinals are tonifying as well as draining.
- Both Scrophulariae Radix *(xuán shēn)* and Rehmanniae Radix *(shēng dì huáng)* enrich the yin (especially of the Kidneys), generate fluids, moisten dryness, and clear heat. Scrophulariae Radix *(xuán shēn)* is salty, cold, and most important for this treatment principle. Rehmanniae Radix *(shēng dì huáng)* and Paeoniae Radix alba *(bái sháo)* cool, calm, and nourish the blood.
- Rehmanniae Radix *(shēng dì huáng)* is sweet, bitter, and cold. Paeoniae Radix alba *(bái*

sháo) is sour and nourishes and preserves (restrains) the yin.

- Cannabis Semen *(huǒ má rén)* is sweet, cool, moistens the lower burner and Intestines, and unblocks the bowels.

- Trichosanthis Fructus *(quán guā lóu)* is sweet, cool, moistens the Lungs and the Large Intestine, causes the Lung qi to descend, and unblocks the bowels.

- Cistanches Herba *(ròu cōng róng)* is salty, warm, tonifies the Kidneys, descends, and moistens the Intestines in order to unblock the bowels.

Dr. Qin's formula is based on Generate the Pulse Powder *(shēng mài sǎn)* plus Hemp Seed Pill *(má zǐ rén wán)*

Generate the Pulse Powder *(shēng mài sǎn)*

SOURCE: *Expounding on the Origins of Medicine* (Yuan)

Ginseng Radix *(rén shēn)*	9-15g
Ophiopogonis Radix *(mài mén dōng)*	9-12g
Schisandrae Fructus *(wǔ wèi zǐ)*	3-6g

---

Hemp Seed Pill *(má zǐ rén wán)*

SOURCE: *Discussion of Cold Damage* (c. 220)

Cannabis Semen *(huǒ má rén)*	500-600g
Armeniacae Semen *(xìng rén)*	150-250g
Paeoniae Radix *(sháo yào)*	150-250g
Aurantii Fructus immaturus *(zhǐ shí)*	150-250g
Magnoliae officinalis Cortex *(hòu pò)*	150-250g
Rhei Radix et Rhizoma *(dà huáng)*	300-500g

---

MODIFICATIONS OF DR. QIN'S FORMULA

If severe Kidney yin deficiency:

Testudinis Plastrum *(guī bǎn)*	9g
or Testudinis Plastri Colla *(guī bǎn jiāo)*	9g
Anemarrhenae Rhizoma *(zhī mǔ)*	6-9g
Lycii Cortex *(dì gǔ pí)*	6-9g
Pearls of Asini Corii Colla *(ē jiāo zhū)*	4-6g

Fevers at night:

Trionycis Carapax *(biē jiǎ)*	6-9g

EDIBLE PASTE INSTRUCTIONS (膏 *gāo*)

This type of formula can be made into an edible paste. For example, boil three packs of herbs with a small amount of water for 3-4 hours, then add crushed Testudinis Plastri Colla *(guī bǎn jiāo)* 50g and Asini Corii Colla *(ē jiāo)* 100g and soak overnight. This will yield a jelly-like decoction, which then should be double-boiled for one hour. After that, one can add some honey, raw sugar, cashews, or walnuts for taste. Take one teaspoon to one tablespoon daily, finishing the three bags in a week. This is excellent for tonifying the Liver and Kidney yin-essence. It is unsuitable for patients with a thick tongue coating.

FOOD THERAPY

Grind 10g of raw Pini Semen *(sōng zǐ rén)* together with some wild rice, soymilk, Juglandis Semen *(hé táo rén)*, Sesami Semen nigrum *(hēi zhī má)*, and Glycinis Semen *(hēi dòu)*. One can then consume in soup, power shakes, on cereal, etc.

QUESTIONS

1. *Why are there symptoms of tinnitus, dizziness, and tremors mentioned above; and if these are present, does this change the treatment strategy?*

   Tinnitus, dizziness, and tremors are definitely not typical but may occur is this pattern. This indicates a more extreme condition where wind manifests from yin deficiency. Consequently, one would adjust the formula by adding medicinals such as prepared Testudinis Plastrum *(zhì guī bǎn)*, Anemarrhenae Rhizoma *(zhī mǔ)*, and Achyranthis bidentatae Radix *(niú xī)*. If there is tinnitus, one can add Magnetitum *(cí shí)* and Anemarrhenae Rhizoma *(zhī mǔ)*. Although these two are often combined with Phellodendri Cortex *(huáng bǎi)*, here that medicinal is inappropriate because it can be too bitter and drying. *Note:* Yin-deficient patterns of dryness with accompanying sensation of heat, vertigo, dizziness, possible loss of consciousness, and paralysis of a large part of the body or just the face requires careful discrimination because this may be a wind attack (stroke).

2. *What is the difference between this method and "enrich the yin and replenish the water" from Ch. 5 on deficiency?*

   These are similar methods with a fair amount of overlap. This method can be viewed as a milder version of the "enrich the yin and replenish the water" method. Depending on the relative intensity of the dryness versus the deficiency, these two patterns can be viewed as a continuum. For example, if this pattern is one's starting point and there is more signs of deficiency, such as weak knees and lower back, then one should use more medicinals such as Testudinis Plastrum *(guī bǎn)*, Ligustri lucidi Fructus *(nǚ zhēn zǐ)*, and Rehmanniae Radix preparata *(shú dì huáng)*. This then brings the formula closer to the "enrich the yin and replenish the water" method. In general, this method focuses on the liquid and yin aspect, while the "enrich the yin and replenish the water" method (p. 132) focuses on the Kidney yin and essence. Furthermore, in this pattern the chief complaint is constipation; the focus is accordingly on medicinals that moisten and open the bowels. If constipation is not present, one may still use the formula, but probably in a modified form.

11

Treatment Guidelines for

Fire 火 *(huǒ)*

NATURE

Fire is the essential core of heat and heat is the manifestation and function of fire.

This was a phrase that Dr. Qin was fond of using, which differentiates between fire and heat. Fire is pathological and is the foundation of the pathodynamic that causes heat. This may come about from an external pathogen or be internally generated, such as from the excessive buildup of yang qi. Heat is the physical manifestation of this process and appears in such symptoms as red face, fever, dry mouth, burning urine, thirst, sweating, or constipation. To put it simply, first there is fire, which you cannot see or feel until it becomes heat.

It should be noted that clinically, fire is often used to describe patterns of intense heat that primarily ascend. That is, the term fire can mean three different, if related, things: a physiological phenomenon that drives metabolism, the foundation of a pathodynamic, and an extreme manifestation of that pathodynamic. This is one of the many terms in Chinese medicine that has overlapping layers of meaning and requires context to understand more specifically.

PHYSIOLOGY

If fire is anchored and stored, it can warm and nourish the hundred bones and secure longevity.

PATHOLOGY

If fire is stimulated and stirred up, it stews the thin and thick fluids, and damages and robs the primal qi.

Fire can be physiological (e.g., fire at the gate of vitality or sovereign fire) or pathological. This chapter fundamentally deals with the latter, which can damage the blood, fluids, and yin.

CAUSES OF DISEASE

- With qi constraint, fire arises in the Lungs.

This is not a reference to Liver qi constraint, but to a blockage of Lung qi, such as caused by catching a cold.

- With becoming enraged, fire arises in the Liver.
- With drunkenness or overeating, fire arises in the Spleen.
- With excessive thinking and deliberation, fire arises in the Heart.
- With excessive bedroom activity, fire arises in the Kidneys.

The five yin organs govern the five emotions. Thus, any excess of the five emotions can transform into fire.

LOCATION

Stomach fire: Toothache, bleeding, ulcerated or swollen gums, and swollen cheeks and jowls

This area may also feel hot and manifest with something like a carbuncle or mumps and similar conditions.

Gallbladder fire: Yellowing of the eyes, bitter taste in the mouth, and inability to calmly sit or lie down

There may also be red eyes.

Large Intestine fire: Thick tongue coating and swollen and sore throat, constipation that may be severe

The thick tongue coating will be yellow, brown, or black. There may also be hard stools with a strong odor, as well as a dry throat.

Small Intestine fire: Urinary blockage, dribbling urination, red, white, and turbid vaginal discharge

There may also be burning, cloudy, or dark urine.

Bladder fire: Painful lower abdomen, with difficult urination

There may also be blood in the urine. Both Small Intestine fire and Bladder fire can lead to urinary symptoms. Proper differentiation is important for proper treatment. Bladder fire is usually burning, painful, and sometimes contains blood. Small Intestine fire usually results in urine that is cloudy, dark, and viscous.[i] This is because the Small Intestine governs the separation of the clear from the turbid. Small Intestine fire is usually accompanied by other Heart fire symptoms such as insomnia, restlessness, and a red-tipped tongue with cracks. With Bladder fire the tongue has a thicker yellow coating on the root with a bitter or salty taste in the mouth.

> *Triple Burner fire*: Dizziness, physical fatigue, heat in the palms and soles

There may also be a hot or cloudy sensation in the head, slight vertigo, heavy sensation in the body, bloating and gas, and a feeling of warmth in the palmar surface of the forearm, chest, palms and feet.

> **TRANSFORMATION OF SYMPTOMS**
>
> *Constrained fire in the middle burner*: Chills and shivering, the six pulses are hidden and small, and there is heat forming with cold

This is a severe heat and a severe inversion pattern. There is excessive and constrained heat that leads to an obstruction of yang qi and creates signs of cold. This is true heat and false cold and is very serious. The patient may have a high thermal temperature. The tongue and the temperature of the palmar surface of the forearm and epigastrium area will show the true situation. Another possible interpretation is that there is intense cold causing constraint and leading to fire. This would render the last part of the above phrase "heat that has been transformed from cold."

> *Heat clumping in the Stomach*: Coughing and vomiting up of clumped phlegm, with a slippery and excessive radial pulse

This is excess Stomach heat that affects the Lungs, resulting in phlegm-heat. There are often dietary factors leading to food and phlegm stagnation in the Stomach that contributes to the initial heat. There may also be some chills on the back, frequent phlegm in the throat, epigastric pain, and a floating pulse, especially in the distal and proximal positions.

> *Heat lodged in the lower burner*: Turbid painful urinary dribbling disorder, and a flooding and slippery pulse at the proximal position

The pulse at the proximal position will also be more forceful or edgy. This corresponds to heat, dampness, and stagnation in the lower burner.

> The two conditions above both have fire and heat confined with damp turbidity.

TREATMENT

- If there is excess fire, drain it.
- If there is deficiency fire, tonify it.
- If there is fire from constraint, discharge it.
- If there is yang fire, directly break it up.

Differentiating yang fire and excess fire: Although yang fire is a fire of excess, there are differences in its manifestation and treatment. For example, symptoms of yang fire include red face, red eyes, manic agitation, ongoing sensation of heat, easily sweating, loud voice, and a forceful and rapid pulse. Dr. Qin instructs us to use the treatment method of "directly break it up." One might choose a formula such as Clear Epidemics and Overcome Toxicity Drink *(qīng wēn bài dú yǐn)*,[1] Five-Ingredient Drink to Eliminate Toxin *(wǔ wèi xiāo dú yǐn)*,[2] or Rhinoceros Horn and Rehmannia Decoction *(xī jiǎo dì huáng tāng)*.[3]

On the other hand, excess fire corresponds more with excess heat in the organs resulting in an Order the Qi Decoction *(chéng qì tāng)* pattern. For example, symptoms include bad temper, very active, always feeling hot, easily sweating, dark urine, constipation, loud voice, forceful and rapid pulse, and a bright red tongue with yellow coating. One therefore "drains it" with formulas such as Major Order the Qi Decoction *(dà chéng qì tāng)*.[4]

- If there is yin fire, warm and guide it.

Yin fire is a fire of deficiency. This refers to Li Dong-Yuan's method for treating yin fire. In our modern society, it is not so common clinically. See Ch. 3, p. 75, for a more complete discussion of yin fire.

SUMMARY
Clear and direct downward.

Fire's nature is to ascend. Clinically, we refer to intense heat that rises as fire. If it is internal and does not effuse, then it is heat. Thus, for the treatment of heat one uses a clearing method and for fire a descending method. In short, there is only excess and deficiency. Excess fire must be cleared, directed downward, and drained, and deficiency fire must be anchored, nourished, and grasped (i.e., by the Kidneys).

---

1. See Ch. 12, p. 271.

2. Lonicerae Flos *(jīn yín huā)*, Taraxaci Herba *(pú gōng yīng)*, Violae Herba *(zǐ huā dì dīng)*, Chrysanthemi indici Flos *(yê jú huā)*, Semiaquilegiae Radix *(tiān kuí zǐ)*.

3. See medicinal analysis under method no 1 in this chapter for ingredients.

4. See Ch. 2, p. 45.

1. Calm and Quiet the Sovereign Fire (宁静君火 *níng jìng jūn huô*)

[PRESENTATION] Hyperactive Heart fire; irritability, restlessness, and crimson tongue

Saigae tataricae Cornu *(líng yáng jiǎo)*[5]	1g
Rehmanniae Radix *(shēng dì huáng)*	9g
Coptidis Rhizoma *(huáng lián)*	1.5g
Lophatheri Herba *(dàn zhú yè)*	4.5g
Forsythiae Fructus *(lián qiáo)*	9g
Gardeniae Fructus *(zhī zǐ)*	4.5g
Junci Medulla *(dēng xīn cǎo)*	4 bundles (1g)

COMMENTARY

ADDITIONAL SIGNS AND SYMPTOMS

- Palpitations
- Insomnia (awaken easily, cannot sleep for very long, sometimes only for a few minutes at a time)
- Fever
- Manic agitation
- Heat in the palms
- A mind that races and cannot be turned off
- Rough, dark, burning, or scanty urination
- Red rashes under eyes or skin, visible blood vessels in the sclera
- The pulse is rapid (100-120 bpm), floating, and edgy (especially in the left distal position)
- The tongue has a fresh red tip that is sometimes painful or burning; there may also be cracks/erosion or a swollen protrusion under the tongue, which is a serious sign

DISCUSSION

PATTERN: This is an acute excess presentation that is a manifestation of hyperactive Heart fire or Heart heat spreading to the Small Intestine. There may be some consequential minor damage to the yin.

MEDICINAL ANALYSIS

- Dr. Qin originally called for Rhinocerotis Cornu *(xī jiǎo)*, which enters the Heart, cools the blood, clears fire toxin, and open the orifices. This is the best medicinal for emergency situations, as it can prevent loss of consciousness. However, it is harvested from an endangered species and thus we need to look for substitutes. Bubali Cornu *(shuǐ niú jiǎo)* 15-20g (ground or small pieces that are precooked for 1 hour) can be used if the situation is mild. Saigae tataricae Cornu *(líng yáng jiǎo)* 1g is used for more severe

---

5. The original text prescribed Rhinocerotis Cornu *(xī jiâo)* 0.6g.

presentations, especially if there is wind with spasms. If these are unavailable, one can use Nelumbinis Plumula *(lián zǐ xīn)* 1.5g or Isatidis Folium *(dà qīng yè)* 4.5g. Another option is Glauberitum *(hán shuǐ shí)* 9-12g, especially if the patient presents with red eyes, red face, strong sensation of heat, and migraines. All of these cool Heart fire.

- Rehmanniae Radix *(shēng dì huáng)* is sweet, bitter, and cold. It enters the Heart, clears heat, and cools the blood. It also enters the Kidneys, nourishes the yin, and generates fluids. If the Kidney water is sufficient, the Heart fire is able to descend. It is especially suitable when there is Heart channel heat with damage to the fluids that is not that severe.

- Lophatheri Herba *(dàn zhú yè)* and Junci Medulla *(dēng xīn cǎo)* are sweet, bland, and cold. They clear the Heart, eliminate irritability, and guide heat downward, eliminating it through the urine.

- Coptidis Rhizoma *(huáng lián)*, Forsythiae Fructus *(lián qiáo)*, and Gardeniae Fructus *(zhī zǐ)* are all bitter and cold and are able to clear the Heart and drain fire. Gardeniae Fructus *(zhī zǐ)* is especially good for Heart agitation and anguish.

Dr. Qin's formula is based on Rhinoceros Horn and Rehmannia Decoction *(xī jiǎo dì huáng tāng)*.

Rhinoceros Horn and Rehmannia Decoction *(xī jiǎo dì huáng tāng)*

SOURCE: *Important Formulas Worth a Thousand Gold Pieces [for any Emergency]* (7th century)

Rhinocerotis Cornu *(xī jiǎo)* 3g
Rehmanniae Radix *(shēng dì huáng)* 24g
Paeoniae Radix *(sháo yào)* 9g
Moutan Cortex *(mǔ dān pí)* 6g

MODIFICATIONS OF DR. QIN'S FORMULA

Restlessness (unable to keep quiet):

Fossilia Dentis Mastodi *(lóng chǐ)* 9g

▶ If unavailable, use Fossilia Ossis Mastodi *(lóng gǔ)* or
Ostreae Concha *(mǔ lì)*

Sweats easily:

Tritici Fructus levis *(fú xiǎo mài)* 9g
Nelumbinis Plumula *(lián zǐ xīn)* 3g

Insomnia:

Ziziphi spinosae Semen *(suān zǎo rén)* 9g
Platycladi Semen *(bǎi zǐ rén)* 6g

Visible phlegm, unclear mind, and a sticky, yellow tongue coating:

Polygalae Radix *(yuǎn zhì)* 4.5g
Acori tatarinowii Rhizoma *(shí chāng pú)* 6g

Fever and blisters on tongue:

Lonicerae Flos *(jīn yín huā)* 6g

Scutellariae Radix *(huáng qín)* 4.5g

Red eyes with discharge:

Zaocydis Vesica Fellea *(wū shé dǎn)*[6] 0.3g
(powder and mix into decoction)

Bleeding from heat stirring the blood and forcing the blood to move chaotically:

Moutan Cortex *(mǔ dān pí)* 4-6g

High fever, loss of consciousness or delirium:

Bovis Calculus *(niú huáng)* 0.5g

Impaired consciousness with incoherent speech:

Purple Snow Special Pill *(zǐ xuě dān)*

QUESTIONS

1. *Is this pattern more serious than the pattern treated by the method "clear and cool the blood" in Ch. 4 (see p. 85)?*

   This pattern, described in Ch. 4, is due to a buildup of heat in the blood aspect. It is essentially bleeding with many of the same 'heat' symptoms presented above (insomnia, restlessness, irritability). However, compared to the bleeding pattern, the pattern here is deeper and more severe. Thus, the irritability and restlessness noted above is quite severe and acute, much more so than in the bleeding pattern. The treatment here also reflects the urgency, with the inclusion of Saigae tataricae Cornu *(líng yáng jiǎo)*. Therefore, this formula is not just for Heart fire in the patient with run-of-the-mill insomnia. However, if heat is the main factor in such a patient, this formula can be tempered and used in such cases by removing Saigae tataricae Cornu *(líng yáng jiǎo)*.

---

2. Use Bitter Medicinals to Drain Ministerial Fire
(苦泄相火 *kŭ xiè xiāng huŏ*)

[PRESENTATION] Liver and Gallbladder exuberant fire; deafness and wet dreams

Gentianae Radix *(lóng dǎn cǎo)*	2.4g
Rehmanniae Radix *(shēng dì huáng)*	9g
Phellodendri Cortex *(huáng bǎi)*	2.4g
Paeoniae Radix rubra *(chì sháo)*	4.5g
Scutellariae Radix *(huáng qín)*	4.5g
Clematidis armandii Caulis *(chuān mù tōng)*	4.5g
Prunellae Spica *(xià kū cǎo)*	4.5g

---

6. Zaocydis Vesica Fellea *(wū shé dǎn)* is cold, bitter, slightly sweet, and non-toxic. It dispels wind, clears heat, transforms phlegm, and clears the eyes. Other snake's bile (蛇胆 *shé dǎn*) can be used, such as Agkistrodonis Halydis Vesica Fellea (蝮蛇胆, *fù shé dǎn*), if it is dried. The current marketplace derives snake bile from a wide variety of snakes.

COMMENTARY

ADDITIONAL SIGNS AND SYMPTOMS

- Headache
- Easily angered (which may trigger or exacerbate any of the other symptoms)
- Red face, ears, eyes, or neck
- Bloody nose, especially after emotional upset or consumption of alcohol
- Eye infections (e.g., conjunctivitis)
- Bitter taste
- Dry mouth and throat
- Insomnia or profuse dreams and difficulty entering into deep sleep
- Sensation of pressure in the head or headache
- Pain or pus inside of ears
- Tinnitus
- Chest and flank fullness and pain
- Oral herpes simplex or herpes zoster
- Turbid painful urinary dribbling
- Constipation
- Persistent erection
- Irregular periods, PMS, or midcycle bleeding
- The pulse is wiry, rapid, and hard
- The tongue is fresh red or pink on sides, red prickles, dry yellow coating, or possibly a black and dry coating at the root

DISCUSSION

PATTERN: This method is suitable for ascending ministerial fire of the Liver and Gallbladder, or for Liver channel damp-heat that pours downward.

MEDICINAL ANALYSIS

SUMMARY

Enters the blood aspect: Paeoniae Radix rubra *(chì sháo)*, Rehmanniae Radix *(shēng dì huáng)*, and to some extent, Scutellariae Radix *(huáng qín)*.

Enters the qi aspect: Prunellae Spica *(xià kū cǎo)*, Gentianae Radix *(lóng dǎn cǎo)*, Scutellariae Radix *(huáng qín)*, Phellodendri Cortex *(huáng bǎi)*, and Akebiae Caulis *(mù tōng)*

INDIVIDUAL CHARACTERISTICS

- Gentianae Radix *(lóng dǎn cǎo)* is very bitter, very cold, drains excess fire from the Liver and Gallbladder, and eliminates damp-heat from the lower burner.

- Scutellariae Radix *(huáng qín)*, Prunellae Spica *(xià kū cǎo)*, and Phellodendri Cortex *(huáng bǎi)* are bitter and cold and are able to drain the excess heat in the Liver and

248

Gallbladder channels. Scutellariae Radix *(huáng qín)* and Prunellae Spica *(xià kū cǎo)* clear the *shào yáng* above, for extreme rebellion of Liver fire.

- Prunellae Spica *(xià kū cǎo)* cools Liver fire, discharges constrained heat, and opens up areas of clumped qi through its acrid (dispersing) and bitter nature.

- Scutellariae Radix *(huáng qín)* is bitter, balanced, clears heat and drains fire (especially from the Gallbladder), and dries dampness.

- Phellodendri Cortex *(huáng bǎi)* is bitter and cool, clears damp-heat in the lower burner, and drains damp-heat in the *jué yīn*.

- Rehmanniae Radix *(shēng dì huáng)* and Paeoniae Radix rubra *(chì sháo)* nourish the blood, augment the yin, cool and soften the Liver. They protect the yin from the medicinals that are bitter, drying, and leech out dampness, as well as augment the yin, helping it recover from the damage that may have occurred from the excess fire.

- Clematidis armandii Caulis *(chuān mù tōng)* is bitter and cold and guides damp-heat and fire out through the Kidneys and Bladder. In general, it is best for excess presentations, because its cold nature can damage the Spleen and Stomach as well as the Kidney yang. One should not use more than 5g. If unavailable, substitute Tetrapanacis Medulla *(tōng cǎo)* 2g or consider Alismatis Rhizoma *(zé xiè)* or Plantaginis Semen *(chē qián zǐ)*.

Dr. Qin's formula is based on Gentian Decoction to Drain the Liver *(lóng dǎn xiè gān tāng)*.

Gentian Decoction to Drain the Liver *(lóng dǎn xiè gān tāng)*

SOURCE: *Medical Formulas Collected and Analyzed* (1682)

Gentianae Radix *(lóng dǎn cǎo)*	3-9g
Scutellariae Radix *(huáng qín)*	6-12g
Gardeniae Fructus *(zhī zǐ)*	6-12g
Akebiae Caulis *(mù tōng)*	3-6g
Plantaginis Semen *(chē qián zǐ)*	9-15g
Alismatis Rhizoma *(zé xiè)*	6-12g
Bupleuri Radix *(chái hú)*	3-9g
Rehmanniae Radix *(shēng dì huáng)*	9-12g
Angelicae sinensis Radix *(dāng guī)*	6-12g
Glycyrrhizae Radix *(gān cǎo)*	3-6g

MODIFICATIONS OF DR. QIN'S FORMULA

Yin deficiency (e.g., insomnia and night sweats):

Anemarrhenae Rhizoma *(zhī mǔ)*	6g
Lycii Cortex *(dì gǔ pí)*	6g
Stellariae Radix *(yín chái hú)*	4g

Burning, dark urination:

Plantaginis Herba *(chē qián cǎo)* or Plantaginis Semen *(chē qián zǐ)* 6g

    ▶ If there are severe urinary problems, use Plantaginis Semen *(chē qián zǐ)*, which goes more to the organs. If there is more heat with fire rising in the channels, use Plantaginis Herba *(chē qián cǎo)*, which goes more to the channels.

Polyporus *(zhū líng)* 6g

Phragmitis Rhizoma *(lú gēn)* 6g

Six-to-One Powder *(liù yī sǎn)*[7] 6g

Throat pain:

Sophorae tonkinensis Radix *(shān dòu gēn)* 3g

Tinosporae Radix *(jīn guǒ lǎn)*[8] 6g

Dry mouth with intake of fluids:

Dendrobii Herba *(shí hú)* 6g

Scrophulariae Radix *(xuán shēn)* 6g

FOOD THERAPY

Tender Ilicis latifoliae Folium *(nèn kǔ dīng chá)* 3g; take as a tea. One can reuse the leaves for 2-3 cups (6g total a day). The young green leaves are the best. The older, larger leaves (black ones) are too bitter and can damage the yin and Stomach, resulting in reduced appetite.

QUESTIONS

1. *Why does Dr. Qin not use Angelicae sinensis Radix (dāng guī), as in the original Gentian Decoction to Drain the Liver (lóng dǎn xiè gān tāng)?*

    Quite simply, Angelicae sinensis Radix *(dāng guī)* is too warm for this pattern of Liver and Gallbladder exuberant fire. However, the usage of Angelicae sinensis Radix *(dāng guī)* in Gentian Decoction to Drain the Liver *(lóng dǎn xiè gān tāng)* is important to understand as it serves a couple of purposes. First, by tonifying and moving the blood, it prevents the ministerial fire from entering the blood aspect. Second, it balances the formula so that it is not too cold. Third, many of these patients have underlying yin and blood deficiency that Angelicae sinensis Radix *(dāng guī)* and Rehmanniae Radix *(shēng dì huáng)* can address. In the above presentation, there is too much fire and Angelicae sinensis Radix *(dāng guī)* can exacerbate the condition, so other medicinals are used to perform its function.

    However, if the fire is not that severe and one understands the three points above, one can choose to include dry-fried Angelicae sinensis Radix *(chǎo dāng guī)* or earth-fried Angelicae sinensis Radix *(tǔ chǎo dāng guī)*. Unprocessed Angelicae sinensis Radix *(dāng guī)* is too acrid and ascending. Other herbs to consider, if there is yin and blood deficiency, are Ligustri lucidi Fructus *(nǔ zhēn zǐ)*, Mori Fructus *(sāng shèn)*, Polygoni

---

7. This is a six-to-one ratio of Talcum *(huá shí)* and Glycyrrhizae Radix *(gān cǎo)* in powder form.

8. Tinosporae Radix (金果榄 *jīn guô lǎn*) is bitter and cold and enters the Lungs and Large Intestine. It clears heat, resolves toxicity, benefits the throat, and stops pain.

multiflori Radix *(hé shǒu wū)*, Scrophulariae Radix *(xuán shēn)*, Asparagi Radix *(tiān mén dōng)*, and Paeoniae Radix alba *(bái sháo)*.

2. *Why does Dr. Qin include Paeoniae Radix rubra (chì sháo)?*

Paeoniae Radix rubra *(chì sháo)* here moves the blood to help prevent the development of blood stasis from the use of so many cold, stagnating herbs. In this way, it substitutes for one aspect of the usage of Angelicae sinensis Radix *(dāng guī)* in Gentian Decoction to Drain the Liver *(lóng dǎn xiè gān tāng)*.

3. *Why does Dr. Qin also remove Bupleuri Radix (chái hú) from the original Gentian Decoction to Drain the Liver (lóng dǎn xiè gān tāng)?*

Some would say that Bupleuri Radix *(chái hú)* is an important component in the treatment of Liver and Gallbladder patterns, especially in Gentian Decoction to Drain the Liver *(lóng dǎn xiè gān tāng)*. With its ability, in concert with Scutellariae Radix *(huáng qín)*, to clear *shào yáng* heat, one must ask why did Dr. Qin remove it. Qin Bo-Wei follows in the footsteps of Ding Gan-Ren (one of his teachers) and Ye Tian-Shi, who believed that the long-term use of Bupleuri Radix *(chái hú)*, which is rising and expelling, can forcefully remove the yin from the Liver and is quite simply malpractice. Therefore, in such situations, whenever possible, Dr. Qin avoided its use. This is especially true because many of these patients are already at risk of depleting their yin and blood. This is because of the excess fire or a constitutional tendency. The more moderate Prunellae Spica *(xià kū cǎo)* takes the place of Bupleuri Radix *(chái hú)* in this formula, gently circulating the Liver qi with its acrid and scattering function, which differs from the ascending and scattering nature of Bupleuri Radix *(chái hú)*.

4. *Why did Dr. Qin reduce the amount of medicinals that promote urination as compared to Gentian Decoction to Drain the Liver (lóng dǎn xiè gān tāng)?*

Gentian Decoction to Drain the Liver *(lóng dǎn xiè gān tāng)* contains a few medicinals that promote urination, including Alismatis Rhizoma *(zé xiè)*, Plantaginis Semen *(chē qián zǐ)*, Akebiae Caulis *(mù tōng)*, and, to a lesser extent, Gardeniae Fructus *(zhī zǐ)*. Dr. Qin reduced the emphasis on this strategy because Liver and Gallbladder fire can easily damage the yin and promoting urination can damage the fluids. Dr. Qin often paid extreme attention to the body fluids and yin and therefore did not include such a strong approach when dealing with Liver and Gallbladder fire.

Of course, if there are strong signs of damp-heat in the lower burner these medicinals can be added. However, ministerial fire patients often have Kidney and Liver yin deficiency, and this is the point of these changes. Consequently, Qin's formula is milder and is able to be used for a longer period of time than its predecessor, Gentian Decoction to Drain the Liver *(lóng dǎn xiè gān tāng)*.

3. Order and Restrain Excess Fire (承制实火 *chéng zhì shí huǒ*)

[PRESENTATION] Excess fire in the Intestines and Stomach heat; abdominal pain, Stomach heat,[9] and hard, clumped stools

Rhei Radix et Rhizoma (*dà huáng*)	9g
Glycyrrhizae Radix (*gān cǎo*)	2.4g
Aurantii Fructus immaturus (*zhǐ shí*)	4.5g
Trichosanthis Fructus (*quán guā lóu*)	9g
Alumen (*míng fán*)	9g
Lonicerae Flos (*jīn yín huā*)	9g
Scorched Gardeniae Fructus (*jiāo zhī zǐ*)	4.5g

COMMENTARY

ADDITIONAL SIGNS AND SYMPTOMS

- Abdominal fullness, distention, and cramping
- Bloating and gas
- Constipation with no bowel movement for 3-5 days, or heat clumping with circumfluence[10]
- Fever
- Bitter taste
- Dry mouth
- If severe, there is irritability, restlessness, and delirious speech

PALPATION:

- Abdomen is hard and feels like a stone
- The area around the umbilicus is painful and feels hot

- The pulse is rapid, forceful, and slippery
- The tongue has a red body with a yellow, thick, and greasy coating

DISCUSSION

This is essentially a *yáng míng* bowel pattern from the *Discussion of Cold Damage*, where five key indicators are present:

> Focal distention (痞 *pǐ*)
> Fullness (满 *mǎn*)
> Dryness (燥 *zào*)

---

9. This key symptom of Stomach heat may or may not correspond to an actual sensation of heat in the Stomach. More importantly, it corresponds to the additional signs and symptoms that are typically known to accompany Stomach heat, such as bitter taste, etc.

10. This is hard stool in the intestines, allowing looser stool to pass around it. This manifests as constipation followed by extremely foul-smelling diarrhea.

Hardness (坚 *jiān*)

Excess (实 *shí*)

Although the patient may present with all of these symptoms, it is unnecessary to see every one of them to use this method.

The most important clinical features for this pattern are:

• Constipation
• Forceful pulse
• A yellow and greasy tongue coat
• Tenderness/pain with pressure at or around the umbilicus

For the acute stage, one bag is usually enough. After taking the formula, the stools may become dark, black, or red. This is a good sign and indicates that the fever will be reduced.

DURATION: This method is usually only for acute or sub-acute patterns. However, see question no. 3 below.

TREATMENT STRATEGY: Excess fire must be removed through the stool to prevent damage to the qi and yin.

MEDICINAL ANALYSIS

• Rhei Radix et Rhizoma *(dà huáng)* is very bitter and very cold. It drains heat, opens the bowels, flushes away excessive clumping, invigorates the blood, and moves stagnation. Use Rhei Radix et Rhizoma *(dà huáng)* without any further processing, as its effect is stronger and quicker.

• Glycyrrhizae Radix *(gān cǎo)* clears heat, drains fire, and harmonizes the other medicinals.

• Aurantii Fructus immaturus *(zhǐ shí)* directs qi downward, diminishes focal distention, and assists in the downward removal of accumulation and stagnation.

• Trichosanthis Fructus *(quán guā lóu)* moistens the Large Intestine and removes heat and fire.

• Natrii Sulfas siccatus *(xuán míng fěn)* is salty and cold, draws fluids into the intestines, lubricating the stools, increases yin fluids, drains heat, softens what is hard, and moistens what is dry. One can use Natrii Sulfas *(máng xiāo)* if Natrii Sulfas siccatus *(xuán míng fěn)* is not available, but it should be ground into powder and added into the strained decoction.

• Lonicerae Flos *(jīn yín huā)* is moist and clears qi-level heat. It is able to clear and facilitate the functions of the Large Intestine, and resolve toxicity. However, it primarily works on the upper burner.

• Scorched Gardeniae Fructus *(jiāo zhī zǐ)*, or dry-fried Gardeniae Fructus *(chǎo zhī zǐ)*, is bitter, cold, moist, and able to clear heat from the three burners by directly cooling as well as promoting urination. Unprocessed Gardeniae Fructus *(zhī zǐ)* may be unsuitable, especially in a patient with a tendency toward deficiency, because its cold and damp nature can damage the Spleen, Stomach, and Intestines.

Dr. Qin's formula is based on Regulate the Stomach and Order the Qi Decoction *(tiáo wèi chéng qì tāng)* and Major Order the Qi Decoction *(dà chéng qì tāng)*.

Regulate the Stomach and Order the Qi Decoction *(tiáo wèi chéng qì tāng)*

SOURCE: *Discussion of Cold Damage* (c. 220)

Rhei Radix et Rhizoma *(dà huáng)* 12g
Glycyrrhizae Radix *(gān cǎo)* 6g
Natrii Sulfas *(máng xiāo)* 9-12g

Major Order the Qi Decoction *(dà chéng qì tāng)*

SOURCE: *Discussion of Cold Damage* (c. 220)

Rhei Radix et Rhizoma *(dà huáng)* 12g
Natrii Sulfas *(máng xiāo)* 9-12g
Aurantii Fructus immaturus *(zhǐ shí)* 12-15g
Magnoliae officinalis Cortex *(hòu pò)* 24g

---

MODIFICATIONS OF DR. QIN'S FORMULA

Acne or rashes:

Patriniae Herba *(bài jiàng cǎo)* 6g
Taraxaci Herba *(pú gōng yīng)* 6g

Heat in the blood (such as very purple red lips or nosebleeds):

Violae Herba *(zǐ huā dì dīng)* 6g
Chrysanthemi indici Flos *(yě jú huā)* 5g
Cirsii japonici Herba sive Radix *(dà jì)* 4-6g

Enduring *yáng míng* heat with carbuncles:

Paridis Rhizoma *(chóng lóu)* 9g
Rhapontici Radix *(lòu lú)* 9g
   (use before or after pus has come out)

Laxative use with chronic constipation (this formula may not be strong enough):

Aloe *(lú huì)* 2g
Persicae Semen *(táo rén)* 9g

QUESTIONS

1. Why does Dr. Qin include Trichosanthis Fructus (quán guā lóu)?

There are many medicinals that moisten the intestines, but Trichosanthis Fructus *(quán guā lóu)* also has the ability to enter the Lungs and loosen up the chest. This makes use of the Lung and Large Intestine connection to assist in moving the bowels. Trichosanthis Semen *(guā lóu rén)* moistens the intestines more than Trichosanthis Fructus *(quán guā lóu)*, however it is not as appropriate because there is fire in all three burners and Trichosanthis Fructus *(quán guā lóu)* plays an important role for the upper burner symptoms such as dry throat, bitter taste, dry cough, burning nose, and nosebleeds.

2. *Why does Dr. Qin include Lonicerae Flos (jīn yín huā)?*

Lonicerae Flos *(jīn yín huā)* is sweet, enabling it to moisten, and cold, enabling it to clear heat. It is an excellent medicinal to clear qi-level heat but can also be used to treat any stage (protective, qi, nutritive, and blood) of a warm pathogen disease. Essentially, the proper treatment for a *yáng míng* pattern is to purge the heat out through the bowels and Lonicerae Flos *(jīn yín huā)* helps things move downward. Furthermore, Lonicerae Flos *(jīn yín huā)* can vent heat outward through the layers (not merely downward purging). This warm disease idea provides an additional avenue for heat to be evicted and is similar to its use in Clear the Nutritive Level Decoction *(qīng yíng tāng)*.

3. *Can this formula be used to treat a chronic presentation? In other words, can it be used for an extended period of time?*

This strategy may be used for acute, subacute, or even chronic stages. If symptoms are less severe (e.g., not a high fever) with something like food stagnation, one may consider a modification of this method. One must reduce the force of the purging as well as safeguard the body's resources. Therefore one may use charred Rhei Radix et Rhizoma *(dà huáng tàn)* and reduce Natrii Sulfas siccatus *(xuán míng fěn)* to 3-5g. One may also consider adding Cannabis Semen *(huǒ má rén)* 6g, Armeniacae Semen *(xìng rén)* 9g, and Paeoniae Radix alba *(bái sháo)* 6g.

---

4. Diffuse and Discharge Constrained Fire (宣发郁火 *xuān fā yù huǒ*)

[PRESENTATION] Internal clumping of wind and fire; toothache and insomnia

COMMENTARY: Toothache is just emblematic for any number of symptoms that can occur in the head with this pattern. This relates to the pathodynamic, which is fire from constraint located in the Liver channel leading to ascending Stomach fire. Actually, this may result in any number of symptoms in the head, for example, swollen gums, ulcerated gums, ringing in ears, tinnitus, poor hearing, nose bleeding, or even bleeding or discharge from the ears.

Bupleuri Radix *(chái hú)*	2.4g
Mori Folium *(sāng yè)*	2.4g
Dry-fried Menthae haplocalycis Herba *(chǎo bò hé)*	2.4g
Chrysanthemi Flos *(jú huā)*	4.5g
Uncariae Ramulus cum Uncis *(gōu téng)*	9g
Scutellariae Radix *(huáng qín)*	4.5g
Ilicis latifoliae Folium *(kǔ dīng chá)*	4.5g

COMMENTARY

ADDITIONAL SIGNS AND SYMPTOMS

EMOTIONAL:

- Melancholy or very sad and depressed
- Irritable, restless, and anxious
- Easily lose one's patience or become angry, although anger may be difficult to express (and fully resolve), which may result in headaches (or other physical symptoms listed below)
- Emotionally the patient may present as being very calm, but a trigger can lead to an eruption of symptoms.

HEAD:

- Headache (head feels blocked, distended, and painful) or migraines
- Bleeding or red gums, or gums that are swollen and painful
- Scanty nosebleeds
- Bitter taste
- Throat is dry, hot, and/or has a sensation of being blocked
- Sinus blockage
- Blurry vision with discharge or pain

BODY:

- Overall sensation of heat or dryness
- Chest and flank irritability and fullness

OTHER:

- Insomnia (either difficulty falling asleep or staying asleep)
- Profuse dreams of fire or heat (such as falling into a hot pot, shoes that are burning, etc.)
- Menstrual period is difficult to start, with many dark clots
- Difficulty sweating
- Urination is difficult or burning
- Constipation
- Red and painful skin lesions such as acne or carbuncles
- It is also common for symptoms to worsen during or prior to menstruation, during menopause, or during periods of increased stress.

THE PULSE AND TONGUE SIGNS ARE IMPORTANT
INDICATORS FOR THIS PATTERN:

- The pulse is choppy, stagnant, or wiry, and especially forceful in the middle position. There may also be a soggy quality if there is also dampness or phlegm present.
- The tongue is dark pale, dark red, deep red, or pale, rose-colored. It should not be fresh red. The sides may be especially dark red. The coating is usually thin, tight, and sticky; the color can be white or yellowish. It is not thick and remains intact with scraping.

DISCUSSION

LOCATION AND PATHOGEN: This is wind-heat in the *shào yáng* channels (half-interior and half-exterior). This is mostly a heat pathogen with a secondary wind component. It can also be understood as wind and heat located in the qi and blood aspects of the Liver and Gallbladder.

DURATION: This is usually a chronic presentation (from around 6 months to one year or longer).

PATHODYNAMIC: This pattern usually begins as Liver qi constraint that becomes Liver heat and then fire. Because the fire is constrained, it is trapped internally and unable to be expressed. One must open it up and expel it.

KEY IDEA AND CLUES FOR DIFFERENTIAL DIAGNOSIS:

The key idea in understanding this pattern is that there are symptoms that are unable to fully manifest or be expressed. For example, acne or carbuncles are unable to fully erupt (just residing under the skin); blood or sweat does not easily flow out; or there is difficulty in fully expressing emotions. This is because, due to the constraint, the heat is unable to be fully discharged. This is helpful in differentiating between more typical patterns of Liver fire.

It can also be differentiated from standard Liver qi stagnation in that there is some obvious component of fire, such as red eyes and red lips and symptoms that come and go. This coming and going is related directly to *shào yáng* disorders and further helps in the differentiation from other fire patterns. (See questions below.)

MEDICINAL ANALYSIS

SUMMARY

The treatment method is to use acrid and cool, dispersing and draining medicinals.

- Bupleuri Radix *(chái hú)* and Scutellariae Radix *(huáng qín)* work together to expel fire from the *shào yáng*. Bupleuri Radix *(chái hú)* is acrid, balanced, and slightly cold. Scutellariae Radix *(huáng qín)* is bitter, cold, and dry.

- Mori Folium *(sāng yè)*, Chrysanthemi Flos *(jú huā)*, and dry-fried Menthae haplocalycis Herba *(chǎo bò hé)* all disperse wind and heat outward from the blood aspect of the Liver channel.

INDIVIDUAL CHARACTERISTICS

- Mori Folium *(sāng yè)* is acrid, bitter, and cold, enabling it to treat constrained Liver fire. It is also sweet, which helps moisten and protect the fluids.

- Chrysanthemi Flos *(jú huā)* is bitter, slightly cold, clears the Liver fire and circulates the Liver qi. However, it primarily focuses on clearing the head and eyes (e.g., headache, head distention, dizziness, and vertigo). White Chrysanthemi Flos *(bái jú huā)* is the best. Mori Folium *(sāng yè)* also has this ability, but it is much better at expelling when compared to Chrysanthemi Flos *(jú huā)*, which is better at cooling. Both have the ability to settle the Liver and Chrysanthemi Flos *(jú huā)* is best for Liver yang rising.

- Dry-fried Menthae haplocalycis Herba *(chǎo bò hé)* is acrid and cool, dredges the Liver qi, and resolves constraint. It can disperse and expel heat from the blood aspect of the Liver. One can also use Menthae haplocalycis Herba *(bò hé tàn)*. The unprocessed Menthae haplocalycis Herba *(bò hé)* does not enter the blood aspect and so is not used here. These three medicinals should only be cooked for 10 minutes.

- Uncariae Ramulus cum Uncis *(gōu téng)* is light, circulates the Liver qi, expels fire outward, and is able to eliminate wind-heat from the interior of the body.

- Ilicis latifoliae Folium (*kǔ dīng chá*) is bitter, cool, enters and promotes circulation in the collaterals, promotes urination, expels Liver fire, and clears Liver and Gallbladder heat and dampness. It is more bitter than green tea.[11] If unavailable, one can use oolong or pu'er tea.

- Although all of these medicinals are cooling, this is not a cooling method, but an out-thrusting one. If cold medicinals are used without this out-thrusting aspect, it can make the problem worse. Thus do not use medicinals such as Rhei Radix et Rhizoma *(dà huáng)*, which is too cold and can cause further congealing, or Gypsum fibrosum *(shí gāo)*, which is best used for pathogens in the *yang míng*.

Dr. Qin's formula is based on Raise the Yang and Disperse Fire Decoction *(shēng yáng sàn huǒ tāng)* and Minor Bupleurum Decoction *(xiǎo chái hú tāng)*.

Raise the Yang and Disperse Fire Decoction *(shēng yáng sàn huǒ tāng)*

SOURCE: *Clarifying Doubts about Damage from Internal and External Causes* (1247)

Bupleuri Radix *(chái hú)*. 9g
Saposhnikoviae Radix *(fáng fēng)* 7.5g
Puerariae Radix *(gé gēn)*. 15g
Cimicifugae Rhizoma *(shēng má)* 15g
Notopterygii Rhizoma seu Radix *(qiāng huó)* 15g
Angelicae pubescentis Radix *(dú huó)*. 15g
Ginseng Radix *(rén shēn)* 15g
Paeoniae Radix alba *(bái sháo)* 15g
Glycyrrhizae Radix *(gān cǎo)*. 6g

Minor Bupleurum Decoction *(xiǎo chái hú tāng)*

SOURCE: *Discussion of Cold Damage* (c. 220)

Bupleuri Radix *(chái hú)*. 24g
Scutellariae Radix *(huáng qín)* 9g
Pinelliae Rhizoma preparatum *(zhì bàn xià)* 24g
Zingiberis Rhizoma recens *(shēng jiāng)*. 9g

---

11. There are three types of Ilicis latifoliae Folium *(kǔ dīng chá)*. The ones that are suitable for this pattern are the larger leaves sliced into small pieces and lie somewhere between the smaller *(tender)* leaves and longer rolled sticks that one finds in the modern tea stores. One can use the latter varieties, however they are milder and if the problem is severe, one should purchase the leaves from a reputable herb store.

Ginseng Radix (*rén shēn*) 9g
Glycyrrhizae Radix preparata (*zhì gān cǎo*) 9g
Jujubae Fructus (*dà zǎo*) 12p

MODIFICATIONS OF DR. QIN'S FORMULA

Painful throat with possible phlegm that is not easily expectorated:

Lasiosphaera/Calvatia *(mǎ bó)* 2g

Cicadae Periostracum *(chán tuì)* 3g

Bombyx batryticatus *(bái jiāng cán)* 5g

Painful and bleeding gums:

Isatidis Folium *(dà qīng yè)* 6-9g

Imperatae Rhizoma *(bái máo gēn)* 9g

Nelumbinis Nodus rhizomatis *(ǒu jié)* 9g

Red face and swollen gums:

Indigo naturalis *(qīng dài)* 2g

Gypsum fibrosum *(shí gāo)* 9g

Splitting headache:

Viticis Fructus *(màn jīng zǐ)* 9g

Glycinis Testa *(lǜ dòu yī)*[12] 3g

QUESTIONS

1. *Why does Dr. Qin include so many wind medicinals?*

This prescription contains five medicinals that have the ability to treat exterior wind conditions: Bupleuri Radix *(chái hú)*, Mori Folium *(sāng yè)*, Menthae haplocalycis Herba *(bò hé)*, Chrysanthemi Flos *(jú huā)*, and Uncariae Ramulus cum Uncis *(gōu téng)*. This strategy follows the admonition in the *Inner Classic*, "For fire [due to] constraint, discharge it." Ye Tian-Shi was also very fond of this method. Essentially, wind medicinals are used to vent fire that is locked in the interior of the body from constraint. Since this pattern occurs in the Liver, the medicinals all enter the Liver channel.

However, one should avoid at all costs using acrid, warm, ascending, and discharging medicinals that are used for wind-cold patterns. One should only use cool or neutral ones.

2. *Are there other ways to eliminate fire from constraint?*

In general, when there is fire from constraint there are three primary avenues of exit: sweat, tears, or sneezing; urine; and stool. In this case, however, the surface (sweat, tears, or sneezing) is the only appropriate avenue for elimination. This is because of the location of the pathogen, which here is the *shào yáng* channels. By contrast, for

---

12. Glycinis Testa (*lǜ dòu yī*) is able to cool the head by expelling fire outward from the superficial collateral channels, as well as nourish and protect the yin.

example, to eliminate via the stool, the pathogen must be located in the Large Intestine or Stomach. In Dr. Qin's pattern there may actually be some mild constipation; however, since this is from constraint, and not from a pathogen in the *yáng míng*, one would not add medicinals like Rhei Radix et Rhizoma *(dà huáng)* and Natrii Sulfas *(máng xiāo)*.

Thus, the exterior-releasing medicinals in Dr. Qin's formula vent the pathogen outward while at the same time opening the exterior to allow for their exit. One can also use the analogy of a teapot: If the teapot is closed, the heat and steam just stagnate internally; however, providing a small opening on the surface will allow the steam to escape.

One can see this strategy in other common formulas. For example, Drain the Yellow Powder *(xiè huáng sǎn)* is indicated for constrained fire (smoldering fire) in the Spleen and uses Pogostemonis/Agastaches Herba *(huò xiāng)* and Saposhnikoviae Radix *(fáng fēng)* to disperse it.

3. *Why does Dr. Qin include Bupleuri Radix (chái hú) in this pattern? Does he not worry about damaging the yin, as in the method "drain ministerial fire with bitterness" above?*

In this pattern there in no substitute for the ability of Bupleuri Radix *(chái hú)* to expel and break up the constraint in the Liver. One of course must still pay attention to patients who have yin deficiency.

4. *After giving this formula, would one expect anything in particular to happen?*

Since this is a pattern of constraint with symptoms related to inhibited flow, after giving the formula one should expect the expulsion of stagnation. This can manifest in a wide range of possibilities. For example, one might see bleeding with possible clots that were not present before, or a dark red nosebleed that is followed by the resolution of symptoms. This bleeding is a release of the heat, an idea that was first discussed in the *Discussion of Cold Damage*.

In addition, physical symptoms related to constraint, like pressure on the chest, may suddenly be replaced with the ability to take in deep breaths. Acne that previously lingered below the surface of the skin may manifest as a red dot and then resolve. Slightly inhibited urination might become more frequent, darker, and have a stronger odor than normal. The bowels may open, with possible sticky stools, where previously there might have been some mild constipation. This all occurs after opening up the qi dynamic, and not from medicinals that promote urination or open the bowels directly.

The above changes should only last about 2-3 days. In general, one should not expect to see an exacerbation of symptoms (emotional or physical) just because the "flood gates" have been opened up. If this occurs, the treatment is incorrect or too strong for the individual.

5. *The pathogen (wind-heat) is said to be located half-interior and half-exterior; what does this mean?*

Another way of understanding this pattern is a wind-heat pathogen that is lodged in the half-interior and half-exterior of the body. This location is often related to the *shào yáng.*

Thus one may see typical *shào yáng* symptoms such as alternating fever and chills, bitter taste, dry throat, dizzy head and vision, melancholy, etc. While most of the time there are no fluctuations in temperature, such as alternating fever and chills, there will usually be signs related to wind. Wind in this usage refers to symptoms that have an on-again off-again presentation. For example, red ears will come and go. This may occur with a wide variety of complaints such as migraines, red eyes, tinnitus, or toothache. Similarly, the patient's emotional state will be labile and their appetite variable.

---

5. Anchor and Nourish Deficiency Fire (潛養虛火 *qián yâng xū huô*)

[PRESENTATION] Yin aspect insufficiency; fire floats and thrusts upward

Rehmanniae Radix *(shēng dì huáng)*[13]	9g
prepared Testudinis Plastrum *(zhì guī bǎn)*	15g
Paeoniae Radix alba *(bái sháo)*	6g
Calcined Ostreae Concha *(duàn mǔ lì)*	9g
Scrophulariae Radix *(xuán shēn)*	4.5g
Haliotidis Concha *(shí jué míng)*	12g
Tetrapanacis Medulla *(tōng cǎo)*	2.4g

COMMENTARY

ADDITIONAL SIGNS AND SYMPTOMS

- Sensation of heat that is worse in the afternoon (e.g., tidal fevers)
- Heat in the center of the palms and soles
- Night sweats
- Easily fatigued
- Dry mouth and thirst, but unable to drink much
- Dry throat and hoarse voice
- Restless
- Reddish skin
- Lower back pain
- Upper back pain (where the pain feels like a nail going through the chest to the back, that is worse when one inhales)
- Diminished hearing
- Steaming bone syndrome
- Nausea[14]

IF SEVERE, THERE WILL BE DEFICIENCY FIRE THAT ACCOSTS UPWARD:

- Red facial complexion

---

13. The original text prescribed newly-collected Rehmanniae Radix recens *(xiān dì huáng)* 9g.

14. Nausea in this pattern is usually a sign that there is deficiency fire mixed with damp-turbidity.

- Red, burning, or dry eyes
- Sore throat
- Tooth pain
- Insomnia (worse with fatigue)
- Headache
- Tinnitus
- Vertigo
- Lower limbs can be paradoxically cold
- Symptoms are usually worse in the evening and better after 1-3 a.m.
- The pulse is thin and rapid
- The tongue is dry and dark red with a very thin and cracked body. There are often red bumps or nodules on the root of the tongue.

Besides the above important pulse and tongue presentations, a burning or painful sensation at KI-1 *(yǒng quán)* is a key symptom that almost always indicates a pattern of yin deficiency fire.

DISCUSSION

PATTERN: This is a pattern of deficiency fire floating upward, due to yin and blood deficiency, which is located in the Liver and Kidneys.

TREATMENT PRINCIPLE: Tonify the yin and guide deficiency fire downward.

MEDICINAL ANALYSIS

The first set of herbs enriches and nourishes the lower base:

- Rehmanniae Radix *(shēng dì huáng)* and Paeoniae Radix alba *(bái sháo)* enrich the Liver and Kidneys and nourish the blood and Liver and Kidney yin. They also clear deficient heat and cool the blood.
- Scrophulariae Radix *(xuán shēn)* is salty, cold, and enriches the Kidney yin in order to help anchor the fire.

The second set of herbs anchors the ascending deficiency fire:

- Haliotidis Concha *(shí jué míng)* and calcined Ostreae Concha *(duàn mǔ lì)* are heavy substances that direct downward. If there is more yang/fire rising symptomatology, one can use unprepared Ostreae Concha *(mǔ lì)*. If there is more sweating, use calcined Ostreae Concha *(duàn mǔ lì)*.
- Testudinis Plastrum *(guī bǎn)* is salty, balanced, and heavy. It enriches the yin, replenishes the essence, and fortifies water in order to direct fire downward.
- Tetrapanacis Medulla *(tōng cǎo)* is a guiding herb that drains the fire down and out through the urine. This medicinal is light and mild compared to the harsh Alismatis Rhizoma *(zé xiè)* in Six-Ingredient Pill with Rehmannia *(liù wèi dì huáng wán)*. One needs only a small dose for this function.

Dr. Qin's formula is based on Three-Shell Decoction to Restore the Pulse *(sān jiǎ fù mài tāng)*.

Three-Shell Decoction to Restore the Pulse *(sān jiǎ fù mài tāng)*
SOURCE: *Systematic Differentiation of Warm Pathogen Diseases* (1798)

Glycyrrhizae Radix preparata *(zhì gān cǎo)*. 18g
Rehmanniae Radix *(shēng dì huáng)* 18g
Paeoniae Radix alba *(bái sháo)* l8g
Ophiopogonis Radix *(mài mén dōng)* 15g
Cannabis Semen *(huǒ má rén)*. 9g
Asini Corii Colla *(ē jiāo)*. 9g
Ostreae Concha *(mǔ lì)* 15g
Trionycis Carapax *(biē jiǎ)* 24g
Testudinis Plastrum *(guī bǎn)* 30g

---

MODIFICATIONS OF DR. QIN'S FORMULA

Severe yin deficiency heat (e.g., steaming bone syndrome,
heat at night, night sweats, five palm heat):
  Vinegar-fried Trionycis Carapax *(cù chǎo biē jiǎ)*. 12g

Severe steaming bone syndrome:
  Cynanchi atrati Radix *(bái wēi)*. 6g
  Lycii Cortex *(dì gǔ pí)* 6g

Tinnitus:
  Salt-fried Anemarrhenae Rhizoma *(yán chǎo zhī mǔ)* 6g
  Salt-fried Phellodendri Cortex *(yán chǎo huáng bǎi)* 4.5g
  Magnetitum *(cí shí)* 12g

Emotional lability (e.g., pessimistic, depressed, frantic, irritable, and upset):
  Margaritiferae Concha usta *(zhēn zhū mǔ)* 9g
  Fossilia Dentis Mastodi *(lóng chǐ)*. 9g

Sometimes feels hot and sometimes feels cold:
  Two-Solstice Pill *(èr zhì wán)*:
    Ligustri lucidi Fructus *(nǚ zhēn zǐ)*. 6g
    Ecliptae Herba *(mò hàn lián)* 4.5g

For more yin deficiency (dry mouth, no tongue coating):
  Grand Communication Pill *(jiāo tài wán)*:
    Cinnamomi Cortex *(ròu guì)*. 2g
    Coptidis Rhizoma *(huáng lián)*. 4g

  ▶ Grind into powder and add after decoction. Balances the yin and
  yang (slight yellow coating, red tongue tip, palpitations, insomnia).

Severe rising of deficiency fire:
  Cinnamomi Cortex *(ròu guì)*. 2g

Shào yáng disease (e.g., alternating fever and chills, vertigo, or pressure on the chest):

Stellariae Radix *(yín chái hú)* 4.5g

Picrorhizae Rhizoma *(hú huáng lián)* 4.5g
  (with bitter taste)

Sweating:

Tritici Fructus levis *(fú xiǎo mài)* 6g

Oryzae glutinosae Radix *(nuò dào gēn xū)* 6g

Persicae Fructus Immaturus *(bì táo gān)*[15] 6g

> ▶ These are symptomatic and are good for day or night sweats from yin deficiency. If sweating is not stopped, one cannot rebuild the yin. However, if night sweats is the chief complaint, one should consider using Tangkuei and Six-Yellow Decoction *(dāng guī liù huáng tāng)*[16] together with the above three herbs.

Palpitations:

Corni Fructus *(shān zhū yú)* 6g

Schisandrae Fructus *(wǔ wèi zǐ)* 4.5g

Insomnia:

Ziziphi spinosae Semen *(suān zǎo rén)* 9g

Polygoni multiflori Caulis *(yè jiāo téng)* 6g

QUESTION

1. Is tinnitus always related to Kidney and Liver deficiency?

No. There are many reasons why tinnitus occurs. Below are the three major types and distinguishing features:

Liver and Kidney essence deficiency (a chronic high-pitched sound of short duration)

Heat-dampness or phlegm-fire in the Liver and Gallbladder channels (low pitched, like an airplane, that usually lasts for only 1-2 days). There may also be a sensation of one's head feeling large. This type usually comes about from eating inappropriate food or beverages, or hot weather.

Qi and blood deficiency. Chronic and constant low pitch that worsens with fatigue. Nearby sounds sound like they are further away. In addition, there will be a deep and weak pulse and a pale tongue.

A further diagnostic clue is that one can press on the ear: if the tinnitus is eliminated, it is mostly of an excessive nature, if not, it is usually one of deficiency.

---

15. Dried immature peach

16. Angelicae sinensis Radix *(dāng guī)*, Rehmanniae Radix *(shēng dì huáng)*, Rehmanniae Radix preparata *(shú dì huáng)*, Coptidis Rhizoma *(huáng lián)*, Scutellariae Radix *(huáng qín)*, Phellodendri Cortex *(huáng bǎi)*, and Astragali Radix *(huáng qí)*.

12

Epidemic Disease 疫 *(yi)*

CAUSE OF DISEASE

This comes about from infection by perverse qi with damp-heat in the Intestines and Stomach that is constrained and steams.

All of these conditions are contagious and can occur in any season; however, they are more prevalent in summer and autumn.

SIGNS AND SYMPTOMS OF PATTERNS

Latent: Slight chills on the back, lightheadedness and a distended sensation in the forehead, focal distention and fullness in the chest and diaphragm, and achy and numb fingers

Erupting outward: Muddled consciousness, feverishness, sweating from the head, swollen throat, and macular eruptions

Sinking inward (possibly associated with thin mucus and food stagnation): Focal distention and fullness, indefinable epigastric discomfort, blood loss, spontaneous diarrhea, and vomiting roundworms

Underlying desiccated yin fluids combined with stagnation: Delirious speech and mania, black tongue coating, and constipation.

Underlying exhausted yin: Red and hot head and face, feet and knees are icy cold, and fever at night

TREATMENT METHOD

Cold: Clear away filth and transform turbidity.

Heat: Clear the epidemic pathogen and flush away its byproducts.

This is usually an acute type of disease that spreads very quickly. It encompasses diseases such as influenza, scarlet fever, and mumps. Epidemic diseases are very different from common colds or other minor upper respiratory infections. For example, epidemic diseases do not distinguish between young and old and are very acute and severe. They also directly strike the interior, whereas in a common cold the pathogen usually first strikes the exterior and only later is transmitted to the interior. Thus epidemics cannot be resolved by merely promoting sweating; one must vent and discharge the pathogens while separately reducing the pathogens in the exterior and interior.

1. Clear Away Filth and Transform Turbidity (辟秽化浊 *pì huì huà zhuó*)

[PRESENTATION] All cold epidemics such as miasmas from mountain forests and mists

Angelicae dahuricae Radix *(bái zhǐ)*	2.4g
Magnoliae officinalis Cortex *(hòu pò)*	2.4g
Notopterygii Rhizoma seu Radix *(qiāng huó)*	2.4g
Tsaoko Fructus *(cǎo guǒ)*	4.5g
Pogostemonis/Agastaches Herba *(huò xiāng)*	4.5g
Arecae Semen *(bīng láng)*	4.5g
Citri reticulatae viride Pericarpium *(qīng pí)*	4.5g

COMMENTARY

ADDITIONAL SIGNS AND SYMPTOMS

- Chills (predominant) and mild fever
- Strong chills with a mild sense of feverishness, even if the actual body temperature is quite high
- Shortness of breath
- Irritability and restlessness
- Stifling sensation and fullness in the chest and diaphragm
- Nausea or vomiting
- Lack of appetite
- Bloating and gas
- Diarrhea or stools that are loose, sticky, and difficult to fully void
- Headache
- Dizziness
- Puffiness or swelling throughout body and a sensation of heaviness
- Greyish dark face

- Tingling and numbness in various parts of the body
- Achy, heavy joints
- Scanty urine
- The pulse is very deep, wiry, and soggy, and possibly rapid
- The tongue has a swollen, dark pale body with a greasy, sticky, thick, white, grey, or black coating

DISCUSSION

This is also called mountain forest toxic qi and is not that common in clinical practice. It usually occurs in a humid environment and is caused by the inhalation of a pathogen through the nose or mouth, which then directly attacks the middle burner. It results in a pattern of cold-damp stagnation, where dampness is more predominant than cold. Even though the pathogen is primarily in the middle burner, a key component to this treatment principle is the inclusion of medicinals that expel the pathogen outward, because the pathogen originally came from the exterior.

This is a serious condition that may be caused by a parasite or virus, and may have biomedical correlations in such things as Lyme disease or the flu.

MEDICINAL ANALYSIS

SUMMARY

- The nature of all of these medicinals is warm and aromatic such that they vent and discharge the pathogen from the middle, separately reducing the pathogens in the exterior and interior, with an emphasis on the Spleen and Stomach. The warmth causes the cold-damp-turbid pathogen to be evicted.

INDIVIDUAL CHARACTERISTICS

- Notopterygii Rhizoma seu Radix *(qiāng huó)* is acrid and warm; externally it eliminates wind-cold-damp pathogens from the exterior.

- Angelicae dahuricae Radix *(bái zhǐ)*, Pogostemonis/Agastaches Herba *(huò xiāng)*, Tsaoko Fructus *(cǎo guǒ)*, and Magnoliae officinalis Cortex *(hòu pò)* are aromatic, transform dampness, awaken the Spleen, and separately resolve the exterior and interior.

- Citri reticulatae viride Pericarpium *(qīng pí)* regulates the qi and builds up and improves the Spleen and Stomach's transportation function. Arecae Semen *(bīng láng)* regulates the qi, clears away the epidemic, promotes the movement of water, and unblocks and vents the Triple Burner.

- One will usually take this formula for 1-2 weeks. At this point, symptoms should improve (e.g., improved appetite, pulse not as deep, less fatigue, and less chills) and one can switch to a different formula such as:

    —Patchouli/Agastache, Magnolia Bark, Pinellia, and Poria Decoction *(huò pò xià líng tāng)*[1]

---

1. Pogostemonis/Agastaches Herba *(huò xiāng)*, Pinelliae Rhizoma preparatum *(zhì bàn xià)*, Poria rubra *(chì fú líng)*, Armeniacae Semen *(xìng rén)*, Coicis Semen *(yì yǐ rén)*, Amomi Fructus rotundus *(bái dòu kòu)*, Polyporus *(zhū líng)*, Sojae Semen preparatum *(dàn dòu chǐ)*, Alismatis Rhizoma *(zé xiè)*, and Magnoliae officinalis Cortex *(hòu pò)*.

—Patchouli/Agastache Powder to Rectify the Qi *(huò xiāng zhèng qì sǎn)*

Dr. Qin's formula is based on Patchouli/Agastache Powder to Rectify the Qi *(huò xiāng zhèng qì sǎn)* and Reach the Source Drink *(dá yuán yǐn)*.

Patchouli/Agastache Powder to Rectify the Qi *(huò xiāng zhèng qì sǎn)*

SOURCE: *Formulary of the Pharmacy Service for Benefiting the People in the Taiping Era* (1107)

Pogostemonis/Agastaches Herba *(huò xiāng)* 12g
Magnoliae officinalis Cortex *(hòu pò)* 9g
Citri reticulatae Pericarpium *(chén pí)*. 9g
Perillae Folium *(zǐ sū yè)*. 6g
Angelicae dahuricae Radix *(bái zhǐ)* 6g
Pinelliae Rhizoma preparatum *(zhì bàn xià)* 9g
Arecae Pericarpium *(dà fù pí)*. 9g
Atractylodis macrocephalae Rhizoma *(bái zhú)*. 12g
Poria *(fú líng)*. 9g
Platycodi Radix *(jié gěng)* 9g
Glycyrrhizae Radix preparata *(zhì gān cǎo)*. 3g

---

Reach the Source Drink *(dá yuán yǐn)*

SOURCE: *Discussion of Warm Epidemics* (1642)

Tsaoko Fructus *(cǎo guǒ)* 1.5g
Magnoliae officinalis Cortex *(hòu pò)* 3g
Arecae Semen *(bīng láng)*. 6g
Scutellariae Radix *(huáng qín)*. 3g
Anemarrhenae Rhizoma *(zhī mǔ)*. 3g
Paeoniae Radix alba *(bái sháo)* 3g
Glycyrrhizae Radix *(gān cǎo)*. 1.5g

MODIFICATIONS OF DR. QIN'S FORMULA

Poor appetite:

Amomi Fructus *(shā rén)* 4.5g

Amomi Fructus rotundus *(bái dòu kòu)*. 4.5g

Nausea:

Pinelliae Rhizoma preparatum *(zhì bàn xià)*. 6g

Bambusae Caulis in taeniam *(zhú rú)* 4.5g

Diarrhea:

Baked Chebulae Fructus *(wēi hē zǐ)*. 6g

Arecae Pericarpium *(dà fù pí)*. 6g

QUESTIONS

1. *There seems to be quite a few signs and symptoms of dampness. Would one want to add herbs that promote urination to this formula?*

    Even though there may be symptoms like scanty urination, a warming strategy is sufficient to promote urination. There is no need to directly do this with dampness-draining medicinals.

2. Clear Warm Epidemic Disease and Flush Away its Byproducts
(清瘟荡涤 *qīng wēn dàng dí*)

[PRESENTATION] For all warm epidemic diseases when the exterior and interior are completely filled with heat

Gypsum fibrosum *(shí gāo)*	12g
Coptidis Rhizoma *(huáng lián)*	12g
Rehmanniae Radix *(shēng dì huáng)*	9g
Scutellariae Radix *(huáng qín)*	4.5g
Bubali Cornu *(shuǐ niú jiǎo)*[2]	30g
Isatidis/Baphicacanthis Radix *(bǎn lán gēn)*	9g
Lophatheri Herba *(dàn zhú yè)*[3]	4.5g

COMMENTARY

ADDITIONAL SIGNS AND SYMPTOMS

- High fever and strong chills; or if latent, there may be just slight chills on the back
- Bad breath
- Sore throat
- Red face
- Severe headache or distention in the head
- Irritability
- If severe, mania or a maculopapular rash
- The pulse is floating and rapid, with the right pulse stronger than the left
- The tongue has a red body with a white, greasy coating or a yellow, thick coating in later stages. If severe, it will be parched black with prickles.

DISCUSSION

This is a fire-toxin pattern with heat in both the interior and exterior. It usually corresponds to the early stages of severe viral infections such as influenza, mumps, and measles. Although this condition can happen to anyone, children are more susceptible.

Although this pattern does not have a large percentage of dampness or turbidity, epidemic patterns often have a component of foul turbidity and thus one commonly sees manifestations of a lurking damp-heat constraint pattern. When present, the location and degree must be considered, and the formula modified accordingly. If there is extreme damp turbidity—for example, nausea and vomiting, jaundice, stifling sensation in the chest, a pulse felt in the middle depth that is not deep or hidden—one must vent outward and open the membrane source[i] and unblock the interstices and muscle layer of the *shào yáng* with a formula like Reach the Source Drink *(dá yuán yǐn)*.[4]

---

2. The original text prescribed Rhinocerotis Cornu *(xī jiǎo)* 0.6g.

3. The original text prescribed Lophatheri Herba recens *(xiān zhú yè)* 4.5g.

4. See method no. 1 for ingredients.

There are many possible transmutations and presentations for epidemic patterns. One must therefore be flexible in their approach. For example, if there is more exterior than interior involvement, one should emphasize a more acrid, aromatic venting strategy with a formula like Drink to Clear Heat and Resolve Toxicity *(qīng rè jiě dú yǐn)*.[5] With more interior involvement, one should emphasize resolving toxicity and directing the fire downward with a formula like Clear Epidemics and Overcome Toxicity Drink *(qīng wēn bài dú yǐn)*, as in this method. If there is equal involvement of the interior and exterior, consider Double Releasing Powder *(shuāng jiě sǎn)*.[6]

Epidemic conditions are not easy to resolve because if they are not treated correctly, they are especially prone to developing lurking pathogens. For example, a fever may resolve or dramatically diminish after promoting a sweat only to return two or three days later. One may harmonize the interior through purging only to have the condition return again. In such cases there is a lurking pathogen in the interior that has not been fully expelled. Thus one must diligently continue treatment, paying close attention to the transmutations that occur until the condition is cured.

TREATMENT PRINCIPLE: Clear, thrust out, open the orifices, transform maculae, and cool the blood.

MEDICINAL ANALYSIS

- Isatidis/Baphicacanthis Radix *(bǎn lán gēn)* is bitter, cold, clears epidemics, resolves toxicity, and clears and benefits the throat.

- Gypsum fibrosum *(shí gāo)* is sweet and cool and directly enters the Lungs and Stomach to reduce the excess heat, yet it is also able to strongly clear and expel heat and fire from the Triple Burner, and the upper, middle, and lower burners. This should be pre-cooked for 45 minutes.

- Lophatheri Herba *(dàn zhú yè)* is sweet, cold, and light. It enters the Heart, clears heat, eliminates irritability, vents dampness, and expels fire toxin through urination. It also guides the other herbs into the deep collaterals.

- Scutellariae Radix *(huáng qín)* and Coptidis Rhizoma *(huáng lián)* are bitter and cold. They drain the Heart and Lung fire in the upper burner and dry dampness

- Bubali Cornu *(shuǐ niú jiǎo)* is salty and cold, enters the nutritive and blood levels, and is good at clearing fire-heat from the Heart, Liver, and Stomach channels. It can quickly vent and discharge the pathogen, and does not have the side effect of potentially trapping the pathogen, as do many other cold medicinals. It performs the important function of

---

5. Notopterygii Rhizoma seu Radix *(qiāng huó)*, Paeoniae Radix alba *(bái sháo)*, Ginseng Radix *(rén shēn)*, Gypsum fibrosum *(shí gāo)*, Scutellariae Radix *(huáng qín)*, Anemarrhenae Rhizoma *(zhī mǔ)*, Cimicifugae Rhizoma *(shēng má)*, Puerariae Radix *(gé gēn)*, Glycyrrhizae Radix *(gān câo)*, Coptidis Rhizoma *(huáng lián)*, and Rehmanniae Radix *(shēng dì huáng)*.

6. Schizonepetae Herba *(jīng jiè)*, Saposhnikoviae Radix *(fáng fēng)*, Gardeniae Fructus *(zhī zǐ)*, Scutellariae Radix *(huáng qín)*, Angelicae sinensis Radix *(dāng guī)*, Paeoniae Radix alba *(bái sháo)*, Platycodi Radix *(jié gêng)*, Glycyrrhizae Radix *(gān câo)*, Ephedrae Herba *(má huáng)*, Chuanxiong Rhizoma *(chuān xiōng)*, Forsythiae Fructus *(lián qiáo)*, Gypsum fibrosum *(shí gāo)*, Talcum *(huá shí)*, and Atractylodis macrocephalae Rhizoma *(bái zhú)*.

venting pathogenic heat from the collaterals of the Pericardium and heat toxin from the nutritive level and is especially effective if there is mania or the eruption of papules.

- Rehmanniae Radix *(shēng dì huáng)* is especially good at cooling the blood, clearing heat, protecting the yin, nourishing the fluids, and does not cling to the pathogen.

- One should see a result after about 2-3 bags of herbs.

Dr. Qin's formula is based on Clear Epidemics and Overcome Toxicity Drink *(qīng wēn bài dú yǐn)*

Clear Epidemics and Overcome Toxicity Drink *(qīng wēn bài dú yǐn)*

SOURCE: *Achievements Regarding Epidemic Rashes* (1794)

Gypsum fibrosum *(shí gāo)* 24-36g
Rehmanniae Radix *(shēng dì huáng)* 6-12g
Coptidis Rhizoma *(huáng lián)* 3-4.5g
[Bubali Cornu *(shuǐ niú jiǎo)* . . . . 30-120g][7]
Gardeniae Fructus *(zhī zǐ)* 3-18g
Platycodi Radix *(jié gěng)* 1.5-12g
Scutellariae Radix *(huáng qín)* 1.5-12g
Anemarrhenae Rhizoma *(zhī mǔ)* 3-18g
Paeoniae Radix rubra *(chì sháo)* 3-18g
Scrophulariae Radix *(xuán shēn)* 3-18g
Forsythiae Fructus *(lián qiáo)* 3-18g
Lophatheri Herba *(dàn zhú yè)* 1.5-12g
Glycyrrhizae Radix *(gān cǎo)* 1.5-12g
Moutan Cortex *(mǔ dān pí)* 3-18g

---

MODIFICATIONS OF DR. QIN'S FORMULA

High fever:

Lonicerae Flos *(jīn yín huā)* 9g

Dry-fried Gardeniae Fructus *(chǎo zhī zǐ)* 6g

Strong thirst with a very red and dry tongue:

Trichosanthis Radix *(tiān huā fěn)* 9g

Scrophulariae Radix *(xuán shēn)* 6g

Phragmitis Rhizoma *(lú gēn)* 9g

Cough:

Arctii Fructus *(niú bàng zǐ)* 6g

Peucedani Radix *(qián hú)* 4.5g

Cough with blood with a sore throat:

Indigo naturalis *(qīng dài)* 2g

Meretricis/Cyclinae Concha *(gé qiào)* 9g

Callicarpae formosanae Folium *(zǐ zhū)* 6g

---

7. The original text prescribes Rhinocerotis Cornu *(xī jiǎo)*.

271

Sore throat with loss of voice:

Sophorae tonkinensis Radix *(shān dòu gēn)* 6g

Bombyx batryticatus *(bái jiāng cán)* 6g

Cicadae Periostracum *(chán tuì)* 3g

Severe swollen throat (e.g., there is pus and an inability to swallow):

Lasiosphaera/Calvatia *(mǎ bó)* 3g

Belamcandae Rhizoma *(shè gān)* 6g

Scarlet fever with a severe sore throat and copious amounts of pus:

Chrysanthemi indici Flos *(yě jú huā)* 6g

Violae Herba *(zǐ huā dì dīng)* 9g

Taraxaci Herba *(pú gōng yīng)* 6g

Intense headache:

Viticis Fructus *(màn jīng zǐ)* 6g

Prunellae Spica *(xià kū cǎo)* 9g

Celosiae Semen *(qīng xiāng zǐ)* 6g

One may consider using the prepared medicine, Pien Tze Huang[8] at 0.3g twice a day or 0.6g for adults. This is a good remedy for early-stage epidemics as well as a preventative. It is worth keeping in the refrigerator, which will keep it fresh for up to three years.

This pattern can easily lead to loss of consciousness or coma. If one sees a severe condition with a high fever, one can use Calm the Palace Pill with Cattle Gallstone *(ān gōng niú huáng wán)*.

QUESTIONS

1. *Why does Dr. Qin use Isatidis/Baphicacanthis Radix (bǎn lán gēn) instead of something like Lonicerae Flos (jīn yín huā) or Isatidis Folium (dà qīng yè)?*

    Lonicerae Flos *(jīn yín huā)* and Isatidis Folium *(dà qīng yè)* are too superficial for this problem. Isatidis/Baphicacanthis Radix *(bǎn lán gēn)* is not only stronger in clearing toxins, but also able to enter the deep collaterals and organs, whereas Isatidis Folium *(dà qīng yè)* only enters the collaterals, not the organs. This pattern has an organ component (e.g., constipation, urinary blockage, or loss of consciousness).

---

8. Pien Tze Huang (片仔癀 *piàn zî huáng*) is a prepared medicine that contains Bovis Calculus *(niú huáng)*, Moschus *(shè xiāng)*, Notoginseng Radix *(sān qī)*, and snake gall *(shé dân)*. It is manufactured by Zhangzhou Pien Tze Huang Pharmaceutical Company.

13

Treatment Guidelines for

Parasites 虫 *(chóng)*

CAUSE OF DISEASE

Erratic eating habits, qi deficiency, and damp-heat in the middle burner and Stomach cavity with loss of the Spleen's transportation function

"Erratic eating habits" refers to eating too much or too little or eating at irregular times. The loss of the Spleen's transformation function, which in turn can lead to dampness (and possibly heat), produces an environment that allows the parasites to thrive. However, these types of parasitic infections are not very common in the West.

It should be noted that although many young Chinese medicine doctors prefer to solely use Western medicine for the treatment of parasites, many venerated senior physicians still advocate using Chinese herbal medicine. This is because Chinese medicine believes that, for example, children with parasites usually have some Spleen and Stomach deficiency with damp turbidity collecting in the interior. This important etiological factor can be successfully treated with Chinese medicine by using strategies to build up the Spleen and transform dampness. Combined with methods to directly eliminate the parasites, the problem can be cured.

DISEASE MANIFESTATIONS

Indefinable epigastric discomfort, abdominal pain, vomiting of frothy mucus, sallow-yellow complexion, dark color around the orbits and below the nose, a craving to eat uncooked rice, paper, dirt, and charcoal; depression, being downcast with a desire to sleep, and also slight fever and mild chills

Other common symptoms include a large intake of food with a good appetite while still remaining very thin or having an inflated and bulging abdomen with a thin face and limbs, hunger immediately after eating, abdominal pain (especially around the umbilicus), frequent diarrhea, alternating constipation and loose stools, bloating, night sweats on the chest, sparse body and head hair, anal itching that is difficult to endure, the passing of actual parasites through the stool, pale dark face with light patches (worm blotches), nighttime teeth grinding, visible facial blood vessels, multiple small blisters or pimples on the upper and lower lip (most useful when diagnosing children), a blue hue in the sclera or blue nodules at the ends of blood vessels in the sclera. *Note:* The more blue nodules or pimples under the lips, the more parasites there are.

DISEASE LOCATION

- If in the Liver, there will be fear and red or black spots or lines in the eye.

- If in the Heart, there will be irritability in the chest and restlessness.

- If in the Spleen, there will be feverishness with overwork and swelling and increased tension in the limbs.

- If in the Lungs, there will be coughing and wheezing.

This does not refer to parasites actually inhabiting the above organs. Rather, it references the organ that is pathologically affected by the presence of parasites.

TREATMENT METHODS

1. Reduce accumulations and kill parasites
2. Acrid, sour, and bitter descending method

In addition, one should also strengthen the transportation function of the Spleen.

1. Reduce Accumulations and Kill the Parasites (消积杀虫 *xiāo jī shā chóng*)

[PRESENTATION] Worm accumulations that obstruct the middle; enlarged and painful abdomen and childhood nutritional impairment disease

Dry-fried Atractylodis macrocephalae Rhizoma *(chǎo bái zhú)* 4.5g
Quisqualis Fructus *(shǐ jūn zǐ)* 4.5g
Aurantii Fructus immaturus *(zhǐ shí)* 4.5g
Omphalia *(léi wán)* 4.5g
Crataegi Fructus *(shān zhā)* 9g
Carpesi abrotanoidis Fructus *(hè shī)* 4.5g
Chrysomyiae Larva *(wǔ gǔ chóng)* 4.5g

COMMENTARY

ADDITIONAL SIGNS AND SYMPTOMS

- Thin body
- Grinding one's teeth at night
- Red and white points on the inside surface of the lip
- Sallow-yellow complexion
- Reduced appetite (or possibly a predilection to eating strange foods)
- Pruritic rashes around the anus
- Visible parasites in the stools

This method is useful for treating many types of parasites, but especially roundworms. It is often used for infants or children. Strengthening the Spleen is an important component of this treatment method.

MEDICINAL ANALYSIS

- Aurantii Fructus immaturus *(zhǐ shí)* directs qi downward, transforms stagnation, disperses focal distention, and eliminates fullness.
- Dry-fried Atractylodis macrocephalae Rhizoma *(chǎo bái zhú)* builds up the Spleen and dispels dampness in order to reinforce the transporting function.
- Crataegi Fructus *(shān zhā)* disperses all types of food and drink accumulation and stagnation and is especially good at eliminating stagnation due to meat and greasy foods. The Crataegi Fructus *(shān zhā)* available in the West is usually already processed. However, if available, the unprocessed is preferred because it has some antiparasite ability.
- Quisqualis Fructus *(shǐ jūn zǐ)*, Omphalia *(léi wán)*, and Carpesi abrotanoidis Fructus *(hè shī)* kill and expel parasites and eliminate childhood nutritional impairment. Quisqualis Fructus *(shǐ jūn zǐ)* is a gentle, sweet, and warm medicinal that strengthens the Spleen. It is best crushed after removing the seeds from the shells.
- Chrysomyiae Larva *(wǔ gǔ chóng)* is salty and cold and enters the Spleen and Stomach channels. It tonifies the Spleen (protecting it) as well as reducing and guiding out all types of stagnation, thereby aiding in the removal of parasites. It is especially good for children with food stagnation. If it is unavailable, one can substitute Aspongopus *(jiǔ xiāng chóng)*, dry-fried Atractylodis macrocephalae Rhizoma *(chǎo bái zhú)*, dry-fried Setariae (Oryzae) Fructus germinatus *(chǎo gǔ yá)*, or dry-fried Hordei Fructus germinatus *(chǎo mài yá)*.
- One may add dry-fried Arecae Semen *(chǎo bīng láng)* to help kill the parasites, promote the circulation of the Spleen, and help in the removal of toxins.

ANTI-PARASITE SUBSTITUTIONS:

If some of the ingredients above are unavailable, consider these other medicinals that can kill parasites:

Ulmi macrocarpae Fructus preparatus *(wú yí)* 4.5g

Meliae Cortex *(kǔ liàn gēn pí)* 4.5g

Alumen dehydratum *(kū fán)* 6g

Sophorae flavescentis Radix *(kǔ shēn)* 6g

Cucurbitae moschatae Semen *(nán guā zǐ)* 6-9g

steamed Rhei Radix et Rhizoma *(shú dà huáng)* 4-6g

Aloe *(lú huì)* 0.5-1g

Dr. Qin's formula is based on Dissolve Parasites Pill *(huà chóng wán)*.

Dissolve Parasites Pill *(huà chóng wán)*

SOURCE: *Formulary of the Bureau of Medicines of the Taiping Era* (1078)

Carpesi abrotanoidis Fructus *(hè shī)* 1500g
Arecae Semen *(bīng láng)* 1500g
Meliae Cortex *(kǔ liàn gēn pí)* 1500g
Minium *(qiān dān)* 1500g
Alumen *(míng fán)* 375g

MODIFICATIONS OF DR. QIN'S FORMULA

Constipation:

Steamed Rhei Radix et Rhizoma *(shú dà huáng)* 4.5g

Parasites from eating sushi, which often lodge in the
Liver, roundworms, or tapeworms:

Aloe *(lú huì)* 1g

Caryophylli Flos *(dīng xiāng)* 2g

> ▶ Grind these two ingredients into a powder and take either dissolved
> into the decoction or chased with a strained decoction.

One may consider the following to help guide pathogens down and out:

Charred Rhei Radix et Rhizoma *(dà huáng tàn)* 4-6g

Arecae Pericarpium *(dà fù pí)* 6-9g

Pharbitidis Semen *(qiān niú zǐ)* 6-9g

Raphani Semen *(lái fú zǐ)* 6-9g

---

2. Acrid, Sour, Bitter, and Descending Method (辛酸苦降 *xīn suān kǔ jiàng*)

[PRESENTATION] Parasite accumulation; roundworm inversion and vomiting roundworms

Mume Fructus *(wū méi)* 2.4g
Bland Zingiberis Rhizoma *(dàn gān jiāng)* 1.5g
Asari Radix et Rhizoma *(xì xīn)* 2.4g
Dry-fried Zanthoxyli Pericarpium *(chǎo huā jiāo)* 2.4g
Cinnamomi Cortex *(ròu guì)* 0.6g
Dry-fried Coptidis Rhizoma *(chǎo huáng lián)* 1.5g
Massa medicata fermentata *(shén qū)* 9g

COMMENTARY

ADDITIONAL SIGNS AND SYMPTOMS

- Irritability and stifling sensation in the chest and abdomen
- Acid reflux, nausea, or vomiting
- Abdominal pain or discomfort
- Qi gushing up into the chest
- Alternating constipation and loose stools
- Irregular appetite
- Symptoms are intermittent
- Cramping in the gallbladder area
- Food sensitivity, such as discomfort or bloating after eating a small amount of food
- Western medical correlate may be something like chronic gastritis or gastric hypoacidity
- The tongue is pale, moist, and swollen body with teeth marks
- The pulse is weak and especially submerged in the right middle position

MEDICINAL ANALYSIS

SUMMARY

- A useful explanation of the formula's action can be understood through the flavors. The acrid flavor halts the worms. The sour contracts the worms, subduing them and further inhibiting them from moving. Finally, the bitter flavor quiets them (resulting in no activity) and sends them down and out of the Gallbladder. Thus we have acrid, sour, and bitter flavors used together to form the basis of what is called a subduing method. This is also the foundation of Mume Pill *(wū méi wán)*.

- Although the sweet flavor entices the worms to eat or drink the herbs, too much will agitate them. Furthermore, when the worms are too cold, they become agitated. Therefore, to keep them quiet, a small amount of sweet-flavored herbs—Cinnamomi Cortex *(ròu guì)*, Zingiberis Rhizoma *(gān jiāng)*, and Zanthoxyli Pericarpium *(huā jiāo)*—are used to warm the organs inside.

INDIVIDUAL CHARACTERISTICS

- Mume Fructus *(wū méi)* is sour and enters the Liver. As the chief, it causes the other medicinals to focus on this one channel. It quiets roundworms and stops pain.

- Dry-fried Zanthoxyli Pericarpium *(chǎo huā jiāo)*, Asari Radix et Rhizoma *(xì xīn)*, Zingiberis Rhizoma *(gān jiāng)*, and Cinnamomi Cortex *(ròu guì)* are acrid and warm. They drive out roundworms, warm the yin organs, and warm and unblock the blood vessels.

- Cinnamomi Cortex *(ròu guì)* is sweet and aids in relaxing the digestive system.

- Asari Radix et Rhizoma *(xì xīn)* scatters cold.

- Dry-fried Coptidis Rhizoma *(chǎo huáng lián)* is bitter, enabling it to purge the round-worms, and cold, enabling it to clear fire and Stomach heat. The dry-frying makes Coptidis Rhizoma *(huáng lián)* easier on the digestive system, preventing damage to the Spleen and Stomach's yang qi.

- Massa medicata fermentata *(shén qū)* is an assistant that disperses food, builds up the Spleen, and protects the Stomach.

Dr. Qin's formula is based on Mume Pill *(wū méi wán)*.

Mume Pill *(wū méi wán)*

SOURCE: *Discussion of Cold Damage* (c. 220)

Mume Fructus *(wū méi)*.	24-30g
Zanthoxyli Pericarpium *(huā jiāo)*	1.5-3g
Asari Radix et Rhizoma *(xì xīn)*	1.5-3g
Coptidis Rhizoma *(huáng lián)*.	6-9g
Phellodendri Cortex *(huáng bǎi)*	6-9g
Zingiberis Rhizoma *(gān jiāng)*.	6-9g
Aconiti Radix lateralis preparata *(zhì fù zǐ)*	3-6g
Cinnamomi Ramulus *(guì zhī)*.	3-6g
Ginseng Radix *(rén shēn)*	6-9g
Angelicae sinensis Radix *(dāng guī)*.	3-9g

MODIFICATIONS OF DR. QIN'S FORMULA

Abdominal pain:

Aucklandiae Radix *(mù xiāng)*. 4-6g

Bloating and gas:

Arecae Pericarpium *(dà fù pí)*. 6-9g

Dry-fried Arecae Semen *(chǎo bīng láng)*. 6-9g

Hemorrhoids:

Sophorae Flos immaturus *(huái mǐ)* 4-6g

Sanguisorbae Radix *(dì yú)*. 4-6g

Dark urine with slight burning:

Dry-fried Phellodendri Cortex *(chǎo huáng bǎi)* 4-6g

Lower abdominal bloating:

Allii macrostemi Bulbus *(xiè bái)*. 4-6g

If the patient has more severe Spleen and Stomach deficiency, one can incorporate a "regulate the middle and calm the worms method" using Calm Roundworm Decoction *(ān huí tāng)*.[1] Chronic parasitic infections can also lead to anemia; thus sometimes one must first strengthen the patient before killing the parasites. Afterwards, one must resume further nourishing.

---

1. Codonopsis Radix *(dǎng shēn)*, Atractylodis macrocephalae Rhizoma *(bái zhú)*, Poria *(fú líng)*, Zingiberis Rhizoma preparata *(páo jiāng)*, Zanthoxyli Pericarpium *(huā jiāo)*, and Mume Fructus *(wū méi)*.

Appendix I

How to Use this Book

Phase I: If you are new to this book or to writing individualized formulas

In the clinic, this book can easily be used as a manual to look up formulas to carry out a treatment method for a given pattern. One should first try to narrow down the main pathological feature (e.g., phlegm, deficiency, dryness, etc.) that would correspond to one of the thirteen chapters. At the beginning of each chapter are many clues to help with this process of differentiation. Then, one should select the treatment method that best addresses the patient's core presentation (underlying pathodynamic) by reviewing the chief manifestations and accompanying signs and symptoms under each section of the chapter.

It should be noted that whereas the chief manifestation will typically be present, more atypical symptoms are discussed elsewhere in the chapter. In some cases we have pointed out the specific pathodynamic for these occurrences, however most of the time it is up to the reader to do further study to "make sense" of these.

The point is that one can start to hone in on a single pattern by understanding that specific symptoms do not always correspond to certain patterns or pathologies. For example, we can see that weak legs or cold on the upper back can come about from phlegm, weak knees from sunken qi, blurred vision or profuse uterine bleeding from sadness, and extreme sadness from extreme floating qi. These may not be typical or at the front of one's mind; yet not only do they help one choose the correct pathology and treatment method, but perhaps just as importantly, they prevent us from including unnecessary secondary methods, for example, the desire to enrich the yin and replenish the water (tonifying the Kidneys) just because we see weak knees. One should strive to avoid the "symptom A equals pattern B" type of thinking. For example, nocturia is not necessarily related to Kidney deficiency, nor does fatigue necessarily refer to Spleen qi deficiency.

There is nothing special about this process, as we all learn very quickly in school that night sweats do not necessarily mean there is yin deficiency. However, we should always be on the lookout for ways to further refine our diagnostics skills. Thus Drs. Qin and Wu have done a good job of including some of these more interesting diagnostic clues.

Therefore, when one first uses this book to begin writing individualized prescriptions, it is helpful to focus on the key pathology and try to find a core treatment method to utilize. For example, when a patient presents with uncomplicated phlegm-heat lodged in the Lung, treatment method no. 2 in the chapter on phlegm, clear heat and transform phlegm, should be applied. At this point, Dr. Qin's formula can be used as is or with the modifications that he provides.

In this manner, one can usually design a compact formula ranging from 7 to 10 ingredients. Using such a straightforward approach will not only help refine one's diagnostic skills, it can also aid one in troubleshooting cases that do not respond as well as we had hoped. That is, understanding side effects and why they occur provides invaluable feedback towards a fuller understanding of the patient's true condition. This is much more difficult to decipher when complicated formulas are prescribed.

It is important to remember that a large percentage of patients actually do have a single underlying pattern, and that one can solve the problem without diagnosing four, five, or six patterns. I have seen this over and over in my own clinical practice, and we also see this in case studies by great physicians such as Qin Bo-Wei and Ye Tian-Shi. One does not need to make things more complicated than they are.

Thus a central premise of this method of thinking is that if one can clearly diagnose and understand how accompanying symptoms are related to the fundamental underlying pathodynamic, one can then produce coherent and focused formulas.

After one is comfortable with this process, one can move onto the next phase.

Phase II: Understanding patterns on a continuum

Most of the formulas presented in this book address a continuum of pathology. Thus the next level of usage revolves around eliminating medicinals from the core formula, as well as adding others as needed, while still focusing on the single core treatment method. Decisions on which medicinals to add or subtract are related not only to the presenting signs and symptoms, but also to such factors as etiology. For example, if the patient has a cough due to phlegm-heat in the Lungs with lingering external symptoms, one can still use Dr. Qin's core formula for clearing heat and transforming phlegm (p. 9), but modify it by removing Cynanchi stauntonii Rhizoma *(bái qián)* and Eriobotryae Folium *(pí pá yè)* and increasing the dosage of Chrysanthemi Flos *(jú huā)* and Mori Folium *(sāng yè)*. Another example would be the use of a method such as diffuse the Lungs and disperse wind (p. 145). This is a thermally neutral approach for addressing external pathogens. One will learn how to modify the base formula depending upon on how many additional heat or cold symptoms are present.

Such modifications are not always directly found in the commentary, but require an understanding of the method and how each medicinal in a formula relates to it, as well as to the other herbs. The commentary provides examples for guidance on how to start thinking about this for the individual patient. Once one is comfortable with this process, one can move onto the next phase.

Phase III: Combining methods

Sometimes cases require a combination of methods. For example, if the patient primarily has an externally-contracted wind pathogen with developing phlegm-heat in the Lungs, one would combine the treatment methods of diffusing the Lungs and dispersing wind (method no. 1 in Ch. 6, p. 145) with clearing heat and transforming phlegm (method no. 2 in Ch. 1, p. 9). Optimally, one would pick and choose the most appropriate medicinals from each formula creating a new core formula that corresponds to the individual presentation of the patient.

Although this process is inevitable for certain patients, especially those with more complex cases, one should resist the urge to combine too many methods. One of the core principles of this book is learning how to diagnose clearly. One is encouraged to limit the number of patterns that one is diagnosing and to search for the common underlying thread. Therefore, the vast majority of patients can be accommodated with just one or two methods.

Furthermore, when combining methods/formulas, it is also suggested that one limit the number of herbs in the final formula. Merely combining two core formulas and adding 2 to 4 additional modifications, with a total of 16 to 18 herbs, might not be the most effective approach. Again, one of the important themes in this text is learning how to choose just the most appropriate medicinals. Thus, even if you are combining two methods, one should end up with a formula of just 7 to 12 ingredients.

Final thoughts

Any system or method of thinking risks being reduced to a cookbook, or worse, coalescing into a rigid approach whereby, for example, formula A is always prescribed for pattern B. The material presented here should ultimately represent a fluid process that in many respects is the antithesis of the way that many standard TCM texts are used. I believe this is one of the reasons that Dr. Qin organized this text by treatment methods.

When one understands the core principles, and the medicinals and formulas used to achieve those principles, one can eventually transcend the text. In this way, after thorough study and practice, a practitioner might find herself writing formulas that only vaguely resemble Dr. Qin's core formula, yet are completely consistent with the treatment methods and diagnostic system that is presented here. One should, however, not be too hasty to jump ahead of oneself.

This learning process, and the resulting skills that it teaches, really speaks to the essence of herbal prescribing in Chinese medicine. It is hoped that this text will be used as a road-map for this journey.

<hr />

Appendix II

Herbal Processing (炮制 *páo zhì*)

Below is a list of the common processing methods for some of the herbs found in this text. Although the label that one receives from the distributor may, for example, say *bái biǎn dòu*, the herb may actually have been dry-fried, rendering it dry-fried Lablab Semen album *(chǎo biǎn dòu)*.

This list is far from exhaustive and may become outdated. It is presented here merely to demonstrate the current status of a small selection of herbs, and more importantly, to illustrate the importance of thinking about the issue of herbal processing and asking our distributors the appropriate questions. At the time this book was written there are two books in English that have good information on how to prepare medicinals: *Chinese Herbal Medicine: Materia Medica* (3rd Edition) by Dan Bensky, Steve Clavey, and Erich Stöger, and *Pao Zhi: An Introduction to the Use of Processed Chinese Medicinals* by Philippe Sionneau. In addition, we would like to thank Andy Ellis for graciously helping to clarify some of the items presented below.

Herb name in *pin yin*	Typical form in the West
bái biǎn dòu	Usually dry-fried Lablab Semen album *(chǎo biǎn dòu)*, but may be unprocessed Lablab Semen album *(bái biǎn dòu)*
chǎo yì yǐ rén	Sometimes the consumer will receive the popped instead of the dry-fried version
chén pí	dry-fried Citri reticulatae Pericarpium *(chǎo chén pí)*
dà huáng	May be wine-washed Rhei Radix et Rhizoma *(jiǔ xǐ dà huáng)*
dāng guī	May be wine-washed Angelicae sinensis Radix *(jiǔ xǐ dāng guī)*
gǔ yá	May be unprocessed Setariae (Oryzae) Fructus germinatus *(gǔ yá)* or dry-fried Setariae (Oryzae) Fructus germinatus *(chǎo gǔ yá)*
hǎi zǎo	bland Sargassum *(dàn hǎi zǎo)*
hòu pò	ginger Magnoliae officinalis Cortex *(jiāng hòu pò)* or Magnoliae officinalis Cortex *(hòu pò)*
jī nèi jīn	Usually dry-fried Gigeriae galli Endothelium corneum *(chǎo jī nèi jīn)*
kūn bù	bland Eckloniae Thallus *(dàn kūn bù)*
mài yá	May be unprocessed Hordei Fructus germinatus *(mài yá)* or dry-fried Hordei Fructus germinatus *(chǎo mài yá)*
mù xiāng	Usually unprocessed, but may be baked Aucklandiae Radix *(wēi mù xiāng)*
qīng pí	roasted Citri reticulatae viride Pericarpium *(wēi qīng pí)* or possibly dry-fried Citri reticulatae viride Pericarpium *(chǎo qīng pí)*
sāng bái pí	Usually unprocessed, may be prepared Mori Cortex *(zhì sāng bái pí)*
sāng yè	Mori Folium *(sāng yè)* may be mixed with the "frost mulberry leaves" *(shuāng sāng yè)*, which are those gathered after the first frost
shān zhā	May be dry-fried Crataegi Fructus *(chǎo shān zhā)* or unprocessed Crataegi Fructus *(shān zhā)*,
xiāng fù	processed Cyperi Rhizoma *(zhì xiāng fù)* or vinegar-fried Cyperi Rhizoma *(cù xiāng fù)*
xìng rén	Armeniacae Semen amarum *(kǔ xìng rén)*
yuǎn zhì	Usually unprocessed but can be honey-prepared Polygalae Radix *(mì zhì yuǎn zhì)*
zhì fù zǐ	There are a few different preparations available
zhǐ ké	dry-fried Aurantii Fructus *(chǎo zhǐ ké)*
zhǐ shí	dry-fried Aurantii Fructus immaturus *(chǎo zhǐ shí)*
zhì bàn xià	Usually ginger-fried Pinelliae Rhizoma preparatum *(jiāng bàn xià)*, but may also other versions such as Pinelliae Rhizoma preparatum *(fǎ bàn xià)*

Glossary

A list of terms contained in this book, with the Chinese and pinyin, can be found under the Resources tab at the Eastland Press website:

http://www.eastlandpress.com/resources/

However below are some terms that warrant a definition or further explanation.

Ascending counterflow (上逆 *shàng nì*) refers to cough, wheezing, and possibly dry retching. This is a term found originally in the *Inner Classic* meaning a surging counterflow upwards as a result of a disruption of the qi dynamic.

Bloating includes both distention (胀 *zhàng*) and fullness (满 *mǎn*).

Cavernous diarrhea (洞泄 *dòng xiè*) is diarrhea that occurs after eating and contains undigested food. It is usually watery and is hard to control. The intestines become like a tube or cavern through which the stool just flows out.

Cloudy pulse (模糊脉 *mó hú mài*) is a description that Qin Bo-Wei used for a pulse that feels soft; it is a combination of the soggy and sticky (e.g., difficult to move) pulses. It feels as if the surface of the vessel is covered by a tissue and thus one is unable to feel the surface of the pulse clearly. It also can mean that sometimes the pulse is clear and sometimes it is difficult to find. It is usually caused by a combination of factors that stagnate together, such as qi, dampness, food, and phlegm. By contrast, a soggy pulse usually refers only to dampness. Elsewhere, Eastland Press translates this as an *indistinct pulse*.

Dry pulse (干硬脉 *gān yìng mài*) is a pulse that gives the sensation of touching a stick or wood. It is similar to wiry, but much stiffer. It usually represents a somewhat severe yin / essence deficiency or fluid deficiency, which results in vessels that are dry. This pulse is a true visceral pulse, which, as first defined in chapter 19 of the *Basic Questions,* occur when one of the five yin organ's true qi is defeated and exposed. Pulses such as hollow and leather pulse may also have an element of dryness or hardness and may be referred to as a dry pulse. However most of the time the hollow pulse has moisture indicating that the condition is not as severe; a "dry" pulse indicates a more severe presentation. This pulse quality was first defined by Dr. Wu Bo-Ping.

Edgy pulse (促脉 *cù mài*): *see* definition of jumpy pulse below.

Indefinable epigastric discomfort (嘈杂 *cáo zá*) is a type of pathomanifestation that occurs in the Stomach duct and Heart region. A commonly-used definition is provided in the Ming work, *Correct Transmission of Medicine,* by Yu Tuan: "The sign of indefinable epigastric discomfort is like hunger, but not hunger, and like pain but not pain, accompanied by anguish and vexation with no sense of calm. This may be accompanied by belching, or focal distention and fullness, or nausea, and may gradually lead to stomach pain." The pain is relieved by eating, but will return fairly quickly, usually within 30 minutes. Dr. Wu notes that such patients may also feel constant hunger but are easily bloated after eating. It is often caused by phlegm-fire, Liver and Stomach disharmony, Stomach heat, Stomach heat with underlying Spleen deficiency, or blood deficiency. Dr. Wu says that a Spleen deficiency/ Stomach excess pattern is most common.

Jumpy pulse (动脉 *dòng mài*) is a term that Dr. Wu often uses in describing the pulse. It is one that hits your finger with some force and abruptness. As the name suggests, it has a moving, active quality. It is usually associated with heat, but may be associated with cold. It is usually thin, weak, and occurs at a deeper region of the vessel. It is associated more with deficiency. The edgy pulse (促脉 *cù mài*) is very similar in tactile sensation but is more forceful and usually presents in the more superficial aspects of the vessel. It is associated more with excess. Both pulses reflect some measure of activity in the body and typically stagnation of metabolic waste toxins (e.g., heat, dampness, phlegm, etc.) This usage is different from the conventional moving *(dòng)* or rapid-irregular *(cù)* pulses.

Hard pulse (坚脉 *jiān mài*) is a pulse that feels like one is touching a piece of wood and is the opposite of a soft or supple pulse. In this regard, it is similar to a dry pulse, but not as severe, that is, the surface may feel hard like wood, but inside the vessel there is still some moisture. However, it does still reflect yin and fluid deficiency. The harder it is, the closer it is to a dry pulse and consequently the condition is more difficult to treat. This is not a traditional pulse quality.[1]

Promote movement to resolve dampness (or move dampness) (行湿 *xíng shī*) is the ability to break up the dampness and make it less sticky. This is in contrast to drying dampness and promoting the movement of qi. For example, Citri reticulatae viride Pericarpium *(qīng pí),* Cyperi Rhizoma *(xiāng fù),* and Aurantii Fructus *(zhǐ ké)* are able to move the qi and can

---

1. This definition is a combination of Dr. Wu's direct words and my interpretation based on previous conversations with him. More detail, such as a clear differentiation between a dry and hard pulse, could not be verified due to Dr. Wu's failing health in the final stages of editing this book.

assist in the removal of dampness, but do not directly move dampness. Medicinals such as dry-fried Aurantii Fructus *(chǎo zhǐ ké)* and Amomi Fructus rotundus *(bái dòu kòu)* are able to move the dampness.

Panicky throbbing is severe Heart palpitations that are not related to emotional stimulus.

Phlegm inversion (痰厥 *tán jué)* is an inversion pattern that arises when overabundant phlegm causes a qi block and inversion cold in the limbs. In severe cases there can be fainting.

Phlegm and oral-mucus (痰涎 *tán xián)* refers to phlegm and saliva which is especially thin, white, usually profuse, and ejected from the mouth. The term may also refer to phlegm in general.

Quiet the Lungs is a term that Dr. Wu uses to refer to the absence of pathogenic activity, and thus of pathogens and symptoms, in the Lungs.

Soggy pulse (濡脉 *rú mài)* is a quality that feels like a wet blanket or cloth on the pulse. The pulse does not clearly arrive to touch the fingers, meaning that it does not hit sharply or clearly. It may have a slight bit of difficulty arriving (delayed pulse wave). However, if this difficulty in arriving is severe and there is a sticky quality when it touches one's fingers, this is considered a combination of a soggy and sticky pulse, and is probably more akin to the cloudy pulse described above. It may also feel as if it is sometimes there and sometimes not, meaning that the wave is sometimes strong and sometimes weak. It can also have the qualities of a soft pulse. Qin Bo-Wei often found this quality where there was dampness, but it can also be found in qi and yang deficiency. This pulse can occur at any depth. While it is a traditional pulse type, Drs. Qin and Wu apply it in a particular manner.

Soft pulse (软脉 *ruǎn mài)* is one that has a "soft" or spongy feeling with no energy or strength. This pulse is not sticky or difficult to palpate, like a soggy pulse. It can be found in qi or blood deficient patterns or even in externally-contracted patterns. While this is a traditional pulse type, Drs. Qin and Wu apply it in a particular manner.

Spirit radiance (神明 *shén míng)* has multiple meanings but usually refers to the spirit-mind (神志 *shén zhì)* or consciousness/essence-spirit.

Sticky or stagnant pulse (滞脉 *zhì mài)* is one that does not arrive or depart easily, and when it touches the finger it feels sticky. This is not a traditional pulse quality.

Sticky stools can manifest in different ways: 1) incomplete bowel movements; 2) stool that sticks to the toilet bowl; 3) bowel movements that require multiple wipes. This symptom usually corresponds to dampness in the Intestines.

Notes

CHAPTER 1

i. This can be an acute or chronic presentation. The first section, in reference to a "ghost," is usually acute and often occurs in babies or children. It typically occurs when they are half asleep, during the night or day, and their minds are not clear. It can be triggered by watching bad movies, hearing strange sounds, or enduring a stressful event. The second part is in relation to an "evil spirit," which is usually a chronic presentation and is more serious, and often akin to some mental disease. On some days the mind may be somewhat clear and other days very foggy. The point here, however, is that it is caused by phlegm and not by an "evil spirit." Traditionally, though, there was an evil spirit condition that was much more serious. It was often attributed to parasites or to foxes and not to phlegm, hence the disclaimer "but they are not."

ii. This is not chosen for a descending function, but for its ability to eliminate the stagnation that is causing the problem. It also makes use of five-phase theory: move the qi of the Liver to aid in quieting the Lungs. One would therefore not use **Pinelliae Rhizoma preparatum** *(zhì bàn xià)* or **Aurantii Fructus immaturus** *(zhǐ shí)* in this situation. One could also consider using **Bambusae Caulis in taeniam** *(zhú rú)*.

CHAPTER 2

i. Reduce (消 *xiāo*) is also often translated as eliminate, digest, and diminish.

ii. Chrysomyiae Larva (五谷虫 *wǔ gǔ chóng*, screw-worm) is salty and cold and enters the Spleen and Stomach channels. It tonifies the Spleen (protecting it) as well as reducing and guiding out all types of stagnation.

iii. This symptom represents *yáng míng* heat with stagnation.

iv. These last two ingredients are found in an alternate version of the formulas, from the same source.

v. If unavailable, use Glycyrrhizae Radix *(gān cǎo)*. Glycyrrhizae Radix preparata *(zhì gān cǎo)* is too sticky for this situation.

CHAPTER 3

i. This phrase was coined by Dr. Qin (一气化七 *yī qì huà qī*).

ii. Terminological note: All of these terms are similar and essentially relate to dredging (dispersing) and regulating the qi aspect, following the *Inner Classic's* basic idea of "dredging the qi leads to [good] adjustment (疏气令调 *shū qì lìng tiáo*)." Although many attribute varying degrees of movement to these terms, absolute distinctions are still artificial, and may create more confusion than clarity. This is principally because there are varying usages from author to author and text to text.

Dr. Qin himself, who is known for his precise terminology, will use different terms for a single herb depending on the specific context. For example, strong medicinals such as Citri reticulatae viride Pericarpium *(qīng pí)* and Magnoliae officinalis Cortex *(hòu pò)* are noted for breaking up qi [stagnation] (破气 *pò qì*) but are also said to soothe the qi, dredge the qi, regulate the qi, and promote the movement of qi, depending on the situation as well as the medicinals with which they are paired. See discussion starting at the bottom of p. 66 for more on this topic.

In conclusion, one should be aware that some herbs are gentler in their ability to move, such as Citri sarcodactylis Fructus *(fó shǒu)*, and some are more forceful, such as Citri reticulatae viride Pericarpium *(qīng pí)*. Although authors may have differing opinions, throughout this book, clarification on relative strength according to Drs. Qin and Wu is emphasized. In general, however, this class of medicinals is fragrant, acrid, and drying. The more forceful and moving the medicinal, the more attention one must pay to the possibility of damage to the qi, yin, and blood.

iii. This is an extreme presentation which results from so much ascending that it blocks the qi flow, especially in the head. This is seen in some Alzheimer's, epilepsy, Tourette's syndrome, or bipolar presentations.

CHAPTER 4

i. Less commonly, one may see cold and heat occurring together with blood stasis, especially in painful obstruction. For example, many rheumatoid arthritis patients have blood stasis with Kidney yang deficiency. However, after chronic stagnation, they will develop localized heat in the joints. All factors should be addressed simultaneously. One may choose medicinals like Lonicerae Caulis *(rěn dōng téng)* and Lycii Cortex *(dì gǔ pí)* for the heat, but must avoid prescribing overly cold medicinals. A balanced formula that addresses both is Cinnamon Twig, Peony, and Anemarrhena Decoction *(guì zhī sháo yào zhī mǔ tāng)*. Ingredients include Cinnamomi Ramulus *(guì zhī)*, Ephedrae Herba *(má huáng)*, Aconiti Radix lateralis preparata *(zhì fù zǐ)*, Anemarrhenae Rhizoma *(zhī mǔ)*, Paeoniae Radix *(sháo yào)*, Atractylodis macrocephalae Rhizoma *(bái zhú)*, Saposhnikoviae Radix *(fáng fēng)*, Zingiberis Rhizoma recens *(shēng jiāng)*, and Glycyrrhizae Radix *(gān cǎo)*.

ii. This phlegm is from heat causing the body fluids to congeal. It is not uncommon to have phlegm appear as a secondary pathogen due to heat. It is not from Spleen qi deficiency.

iii. Heat can easily cause blockage of menstruation due to stagnation caused from heat. One may then add medicinals such as Leonuri Herba *(yì mǔ cǎo)* or Paeoniae Radix rubra *(chì sháo)*.

iv. *Note:* One would not see severe cases of mania, disturbed Heart spirit, strong heat signs, severe constipation, black, tarry stools, and deep crimson tongue that can occur in a blood level heat pattern treated by Rhinoceros Horn and Rehmannia Decoction *(xī jiǎo dì huáng tāng)*.

v. Ziziphi spinosae Semen *(suān zǎo rén)*, Polygoni multiflori Caulis *(yè jiāo téng)*, and Poriae Sclerotium pararadicis *(fú shén)* may not work in this situation.

vi. Quartz album *(bái shí yīng)* is white quartz. It is sweet and slightly warm and enters the Lung, Kidney, and Heart channels. It warms and moistens the Lungs, warms the Kidneys, calms the spirit, and promotes urination.

vii. Since Rehmanniae Radix preparata *(shú dì huáng)* is cloying, Asari Radix et Rhizoma *(xì xīn)* is added to help circulate the blood. This combination can circulate the blood and warm the gate of vitality, as well as the *chōng* and *rèn* vessels.

viii. The stool itself should not be dry, but may be thin due to swelling of the intestines. This may also manifest simply as a lack of desire to empty the bowels. One may also consider Trichosanthis Semen *(guā lóu rén)* and Allii macrostemi Bulbus *(xiè bái)* to reduce the swelling and promote the bowels.

ix. This suggests a more qi aspect problem, whereas pain that occurs more in the evening or night suggests a more blood aspect problem.

x. This formula is made of equal amounts of charred preparations of the following medicinals that are ground into a fine powder: Cirsii japonici Herba sive Radix *(dà jì)* , Cirsii Herba *(xiǎo jì)*, Rubiae Radix *(qiàn cǎo gēn)*, Imperatae Rhizoma *(bái máo gēn)*, Trachycarpi Petiolus *(zōng lǘ)*, Platycladi Cacumen *(cè bǎi yè)*, Moutan Cortex *(mǔ dān pí)*, Gardeniae Fructus *(zhī zǐ)*, Rhei Radix et Rhizoma *(dà huáng)*, and Nelumbinis Folium *(hé yè)*. This formula can be prepared in advance and kept in a freezer for 1-2 years. To stop bleeding, use 2 tsp boiled in 1 cup water for 2-5 minutes, taken 2-3x/day. It can also be used prophylactically to prevent heavy menstrual bleeding. Begin 1-2 days before onset of menstrual period. It will not stop the bleeding but will make it less heavy and will not cause stagnation. This is very balanced formula; some of the constituents are warm, some cool, some lifting, some binding, and some moving. This formula is effective for gynecological bleeding, nosebleeds, coughing of blood, and blood in the urine.

CHAPTER 5

i. For bone spurs one can add Spatholobi Caulis *(jī xuè téng)*, Angelicae sinensis radicis Cauda *(dāng guī wěi)*, Liquidambaris Fructus *(lù lù tōng)*, and Trachelospermi Caulis *(luò shí téng)*. If there is more pain, add Corydalis Rhizoma *(yán hú suǒ)*, Olibanum *(rǔ xiāng)*, and Myrrha *(mò yào)*. One should be cautious with Drynariae Rhizoma *(gǔ suì bǔ)*, Cibotii Rhizoma *(gǒu jǐ)*, and Psoraleae Fructus *(bǔ gǔ zhī)* because of their warmth; instead, consider combining with Testudinis Plastrum *(guī bǎn)*, Trionycis Carapax *(biē jiǎ)*, Paeoniae Radix alba *(bái sháo)*, and Anemarrhenae Rhizoma *(zhī mǔ)*.

CHAPTER 6

i. This essentially refers to the brain or mind, and is also known as the clear orifices. Manifestations include conditions such as coma, loss of consciousness, or Alzheimer's. The treatment strategy is to open the orifices.

ii. These two are balanced: one is slightly warm and one is slightly cold. Thus, this strategy is more about moving the qi and blood in the channels and guiding medicinals to muscles, joints, and channels versus directly warming the channels.

CHAPTER 7

i. If there is Kidney yin deficiency, one cannot use strong formulas such as Ephedra Decoction *(má huáng tāng)*, Cinnamon Twig Decoction *(guì zhī tāng)*, or Schizonepeta and Saposhnikovia Powder to Overcome Pathogenic Influences *(jīng fáng bài dú sǎn)*. Instead, one can use the formula called Black Paste *(黑膏 hēi gāo)*, which contains Sojae Semen preparatum *(dàn dòu chǐ)* 20g plus Rehmanniae Radix *(shēng dì huáng)* 20g. To make this formula, steam both medicinals (or double-boil them) until soft, then mash together into a paste. One can then take 1-2 teaspoons twice a day in hot water to prevent colds or actually treat external attacks. For example, use when weak patients have not yet actually caught a cold but feel as if they are about to, with slight aversion to wind, slight sore throat, slight fever, red tongue, and a thin, rapid pulse. This is an approach from the early 20th century physician Ding Gan-Ren, who was one of Dr. Qin's most important teachers.

ii. This is Spleen-earth.

iii. The absence of gas demonstrates the severity. Cold will tighten everything up, not allowing for gas. Once gas forms and is passed, usually the tightness has relaxed, and thus is not as severe a presentation.

iv. One can grind the herbs (1.5g each) into a powder and then add the powder to the strained decoction. Do not use cold, moistening medicinals such as Natrii Sulfas *(máng xiāo)*, Aloe *(lú huì)*, or Sennae Folium *(fān xiè yè)*. Rhei Radix et Rhizoma *(dà huáng)* can also be too cold, but it is also drying. The prepared form, steamed Rhei Radix et Rhizoma *(shú dà huáng)*, is warmer, preventing the possibility of more stagnation *(due to the cold)*. If steamed Rhei Radix et Rhizoma *(shú dà huáng)* is unavailable, one may substitute wine-washed Rhei Radix et Rhizoma *(jiǔ xǐ dà huáng)* or charred Rhei Radix et Rhizoma *(dà huáng tàn)*.

CHAPTER 8

i. This type of talking means a lack of control over the mind and speech. There may be difficulty understanding or no real meaning to the words. They may talk to themselves or others.

ii. As noted, Dr. Qin originally used an herb called *lián qiào ké*, which we understand to be a form of Forsythiae Fructus *(lián qiào)* with the seeds removed. This form is lighter and clears and expels heat from the Pericardium, while the commonly available Forsythiae Fructus *(lián qiào)* is colder and works deeper and clears heat more from the Heart.

iii. The larger dosage of Forsythiae Fructus *(lián qiáo)* (compared to the previous method) enables it to work on a deeper level (i.e., more on the Heart than the Pericardium).

CHAPTER 11

i. The three main patterns for cloudy urination are Kidney deficiency, Small Intestine fire, and damp-heat.

CHAPTER 12

i. The membrane source refers to the upper burner diaphragmatic membrane (the membrane and muscles between the abdominal and thoracic cavities).

Symptom Index

I

V

W

Y

Herb and Formula Index

B

bā dàn xìng rén (Pruni Amygdali Semen), 15, 117, 230

bā jǐ tiān (Morindae officinalis Radix), 114, 174, 196

bā xiān cháng shōu wán (Eight-Immortal Pill for Longevity), 111

bā zhèng sǎn (Eight-Herb Powder for Rectification), 195

bái biǎn dòu (Lablab Semen album), 112, 118, 122, 123, 231, 284, xvii

bǎi bù (Stemonae Radix), 13

bái dòu ké (Amomi Pericrapium rotundum), 201

bái dòu kòu (Amomi Fructus rotundus), 19, 50, 51, 52, 122, 123, 196, 198, 201, 203, 204, 206, 219, 222, 268

bái guǒ (Gingko Semen), 26, 92, 118

bǎi hé (Lilii Bulbus), 28, 63, 119, 231

bái hǔ tāng (White Tiger Decoction), 111

bái huā shé shé cǎo (Hedyotis diffusae Herba), 11, 28

bái jí (Bletillae Rhizoma), 107

bái jiāng cán (Bombyx batryticatus), 34, 157, 159, 259, 272

bài jiàng cǎo (Patriniae Herba), 254

bái jiè zǐ (Sinapis Semen), 24, 33, 34

bái máo gēn (Imperatae Rhizoma), 20, 88, 116, 117, 147, 149, 231, 259, 291

bái qián (Cynanchi stauntonii Rhizoma), 9, 10, 11, 12, 13, 280

bái sháo (Paeoniae Radix alba), 24, 25, 64, 66, 67, 85, 86, 87, 88, 89, 92, 96, 100, 101, 115, 119, 127, 128, 150, 152, 153, 155, 159, 236, 237, 251, 255, 258, 261, 262, 270, 292

bái sháo tàn (charred Paeoniae Radix alba), 83, 87, 89, 170

bái shí yīng (Quartz album), 23, 291

bái tōng tāng (White Penetrating Decoction), 174

bái wēi (Cynanchi atrati Radix), 13, 263

bái xiān pí (Dictamni Cortex), 195

bái zhǐ (Angelicae dahuricae Radix), 7, 148, 153, 167, 186, 198, 266, 267, 268

bái zhú (Atractylodis macrocephalae Rhizoma), 45, 47, 48, 49, 51, 71, 72, 73, 75, 76, 81, 100, 105, 106, 120, 121, 122, 123, 125, 126, 131, 132, 167, 168, 169, 180, 186, 195, 198, 201, 203, 204, 205, 208, 223, 268, 270, 278, 291, xvii

bǎi zǐ rén (Platycladi Semen), 67, 68, 69, 112, 119, 131, 246

bái zǐ yǎng xīn wán (Arborvitae Seed Pill to Nourish the Heart), 69, 112

Bambusae Caulis in taeniam *(zhú rú)*, 3, 42, 59, 161, 186, 268, 290
  ginger-prepared *(jiāng zhú rú)*, 223

Bambusae Concretio silicea *(tiān zhú huáng)*, 28, 30, 161, 231

Bambusae Succus *(zhú lì)*, 29, 161

bǎn lán gēn (Isatidis/Baphicacanthis Radix), 149, 269, 270, 272

bàn xià qū (Pinelliae massa fermentata), 16

bāo fù zǐ (baked Aconiti Radix lateralis), 114, 195

bǎo hé wán (Preserve Harmony Pill), 42, 52

běi shā shēn (Glehniae Radix), 116, 117, 128, 229

Belamcandae Rhizoma *(shè gān)*, 272

Benincasae Exocarpium *(dōng guā pí)*, 194, 200, 207, 208, 209, 213, 217, 218

Benincasae Semen *(dōng guā zǐ)*, 16, 194, 195

bí qí (Eleocharitis Rhizoma), 9, 11, 231, 236

bí qí zhī (Eleocharitis Succus), 231

bì táo gān (Persicae Fructus Immaturus), 264

bì xiè (Dioscoreae hypoglaucae Rhizoma), 209, 210

biǎn xù (Polygoni avicularis Herba), 195, 210

biē jiǎ (Trionycis Carapax), 238, 263, 292

bīng láng (Arecae Semen), 41, 42, 43, 44, 45, 55, 196, 211, 213, 266, 267, 268, 276

Bird's nest *(yàn wō)*, 135

Black Gardeniae Fructus *(hēi zhī zǐ)*, 85, 86, 87, 89

Black Paste Formula *(hēi gāo)*, 292

Black Restore the Spleen Decoction *(hēi guī pí tāng)*, 100

Bletillae Rhizoma *(bái jí)*, 107

bò hé (Menthae haplocalycis Herba), 6, 11, 89, 145, 147, 259

Bombycis Faeces *(cán shā)*, 196

Bombyx batryticatus *(bái jiāng cán)*, 34, 157, 159, 259, 272
  processed *(zhì bái jiāng cán)*, 33

Bovis Calculus *(niú huáng)*, 162, 188, 247, 272

bǔ fèi yǎng yīn (Tonify the Lungs and Nourish the Yin Formula), 116

bǔ gǔ zhī (Psoraleae Fructus), 112, 126, 139, 174, 292

bǔ wèi gù biǎo (Tonify the Protective Level and Secure the Exterior Formula), 124

bǔ yáng huán wǔ tāng (Tonify the Yang to Restore Five-Tenths Decoction), 158

I

N

Q

General Index

In this index, each of Qin Bo-Wei's 56 methods is alphabetized and also highlighted with a ▶.

C

D